Nausea

Nausea: Mechanisms and Management

ROBERT M. STERN, KENNETH L. KOCH,
AND PAUL L.R. ANDREWS

OXFORD
UNIVERSITY PRESS

OXFORD
UNIVERSITY PRESS

Oxford University Press, Inc., publishes works that further
Oxford University's objective of excellence
in research, scholarship, and education.

Oxford   New York
Auckland   Cape Town   Dar es Salaam   Hong Kong   Karachi
Kuala Lumpur   Madrid   Melbourne   Mexico City   Nairobi
New Delhi   Shanghai   Taipei Toronto

With offices in
Argentina   Austria   Brazil   Chile   Czech Republic   France   Greece
Guatemala   Hungary   Italy   Japan   Poland   Portugal   Singapore
South Korea   Switzerland   Thailand   Turkey Ukraine   Vietnam

Published by Oxford University Press, Inc.
198 Madison Avenue, New York, New York 10016
www.oup.com

Library of Congress Cataloging-in-Publication Data

Stern, Robert Morris, 1937
Nausea : mechanisms and management / Robert M. Stern, Kenneth L. Koch, and Paul L. R. Andrews.
p.; cm.
Includes bibliographical references and index.
ISBN 978-0-19-517815-9
  1. Nausea. 2. Nausea—Treatment. I. Koch, Kenneth L. II. Andrews, P. L. R.
(Paul L. R.) III. Title.
[DNLM: 1. Nausea. WI 146 S839n 2011]
RB150.N38S84 2011
616'.047–dc22   2010013557

9 8 7 6 5 4 3 2 1

Printed in USA
on acid-free paper

Preface

Our main purpose in writing this book is to bring together from different disciplines the scattered information about nausea that exist, and to add to this review some of our own research findings and theoretical concepts. We know of no other book devoted exclusively to nausea. There are several books with "nausea" and "vomiting" in the title, but in all cases the contents deal primarily with vomiting.

It is ironic that nausea is such a common experience but very little is known about its mechanisms. One obvious reason for this paucity of information is that nausea is a private sensation, as are all sensations, and, therefore, very difficult to study. A second reason is that it falls between the cracks of health-related disciplines. Until recently, many gastroenterologists did not consider nausea a gastrointestinal (GI) symptom. Many textbooks in gastroenterology do not include "nausea" as an index term, and the American Gastroenterological Association began to include "nausea" as an index term in the program for its annual scientific meeting only in 1991. Psychologists studied the sensation of nausea at the beginning of the twentieth century, but since then there has been little interest in nausea with the notable exceptions of research on conditioned taste aversion, the nausea of anti-cancer chemotherapy, and the nausea experienced during motion or, more recently, simulator and space sickness.

We, a research psychophysiologist (Stern), a gastroenterologist (Koch), and a physiologist (Andrews), have been collaborating on various research and clinical issues related to nausea for over twenty years. Where appropriate, we have outlined in this volume not only what we know about nausea but also what we don't know, with the hope that this work will both fill a knowledge gap and stimulate new investigators to join us in our studies of this complex sensation.

The authors acknowledge the contribution to Chapter 1 concerning the ancient use of the word "nausea" by Wilma Olch Stern, as well as her editing of the manuscript.

R.M.S. has benefitted from discussions with or opportunities to work with G. Stacher, G. Adam, A. Mantides, and H. Leibowitz. Many graduate students have contributed to research described in this volume including S. H. J. Uijtdehaage, S. Hu, M. Vasey, E. Muth, P. Gianaros, M. Levine, and M. Williamson. Their contributions to my nausea research is greatly appreciated.

K.L.K. wishes to acknowledge the many patients who taught him insights into the symptom of nausea and to thank Elissa, Jonathan, Christian, Teddy, and Anne, who always supported their Dad's work, and especially Elizabeth, who positively and steadfastly encouraged his medical writing and career.

P. L. R. A. would like to thank all the colleagues with whom he has collaborated and had stimulating discussions about nausea and vomiting over the years and in particular would like to thank (in alphabetical order) Peter Blower, Chris Davis, Mark Friedman, Theresa Hague, Kent Harding, Jan Hawthorn, Charles Horn, Charles Hoyle, Nigel Lawes, Ron Leslie, Keith Lindley, Norio Matsuki, Gary Morrow, Masahiro Nemoto, Peter Milla, Wes Miner, John Rudd, Nathalie Percie du Sert, Catherine Richards, Gareth Sanger, David Tattersall, John Watson, and Bob Young.

Robert M. Stern, Ph.D.
Distinguished Professor Emeritus of Psychology
The Pennsylvania State University
Moore Building
University Park, PA 16802
rs3@psu.edu

Kenneth L. Koch, M.D.
Professor of Internal Medicine
Chief, Section on Gastroenterology
Wake Forest University Baptist Medical Center
Wake Forest University
Winston-Salem, North Carolina 27157
kkoch@wfubmc.edu

Paul L.R. Andrews, Ph.D.
Professor of Comparative Physiology
Division of BioMedical Sciences
St. George's University of London
Cranmer Terrace
Tooting, London, SW17 ORE
United Kingdom
pandrews@sgul.ac.uk

Contents

Section III: Measurement of Nausea

PART II: Management

PART I: Mechanisms

Section I: Present and Past Concepts of Nausea, Prevalence, and Function

Chapter 1

Nausea: Definitions, History, and Function

Nausea is a sometimes difficult-to-describe sick or queasy sensation, usually perceived as being in the stomach, that is sometimes followed by emesis (vomiting). It is a component of a complex protective mechanism that signals us not to eat, and from which we learn to avoid certain foods. Nausea is conceptualized in this volume within an adaptive-evolutionary framework that, as can be seen in the following quote from Robert Boyle's *A Free Enquiry into the Vulgarly Received Notion of Nature*, is not a new approach to its study: "Tis profitable for man that his stomach should nauseate or reject things that have a loathsome taste or smell" (1996/1686, Sect. V., p. 74). It is generally agreed that the function of nausea is to act as a warning signal to protect the organism from the ingestion of toxins. Nausea contributes to a pattern of behavioral adaptation that increases chances of survival. However, there are instances of nausea in humans, such as the nausea following chemotherapy, anesthesia, and surgery, and of motion sickness, that do not appear to be adaptive; although, as we will discuss later, they can be reconciled within the "toxin-defense" hypothesis.

The experience of nausea is difficult to describe and detect in another person, largely because it is a private sensation. One can not tell by appearance alone what sensations another human being or animal is experiencing. And in the case of humans, it is also not possible to be certain that the "nausea" experienced by one person is the same as that experienced by another.

If one is able to ask subjects about their sensations then, assuming that they are being truthful and can accurately describe their sensations, their appearance becomes largely irrelevant. However, if the observer demands independent evidence before believing what a person is reporting, then what can be studied? In the chapters that follow, it is pointed out that changes in the central nervous system (Chapter 4); autonomic nervous system (Chapter 5); an elevated plasma level of antidiuretic hormone (ADH, vasopressin) (Chapter 6), and changes in the frequency and rhythm of the electrogastrogram (EGG) (Chapter 7) are all associated with the sensation of nausea. Appropriate changes measured in these parameters would increase the probability that an observer could conclude that another individual was indeed experiencing nausea.

In brief, the three methods of determining if a person is experiencing nausea are (1) ask the person, preferably using a validated definition; (2) observe behavior; (3) obtain relevant physiological data. However, all three methods have limitations that are discussed in Chapters 8 and 9.

HISTORICAL UNDERSTANDING OF NAUSEA

The sensation of nausea was known in classical antiquity to be induced by irregular motion, such as experienced on shipboard, hence one of its names in Greek, *nausia* or *nautia* from *naus* (ship), and in Latin, *nausea* or *nausia*. The terms most commonly used in Greek for nausea of other causes were forms of the verb *asao*, from *ase*, surfeit or disgust. Words derived from the verb *emeo*, to vomit, are used specifically for that symptom as distinct from nausea. Other terms were used less commonly, such as *akraipalos*, especially for the nausea caused by too much wine, and *bdelugma*, meaning disgust.

In contrast, earlier Egyptian medical texts show little concern with nausea, perhaps because the primary mode of travel via the Nile caused only a minor sense of movement and provided a constant, strong horizon line. We have some understanding of Egyptian medical knowledge from a number of texts listed by Leake (1952, p. 7) and Nunn (1996, p. 25). The largest is a medical papyrus in the University Library of Leipzig purchased in Luxor by Dr. Georg Ebers, for whom it is named (Ebers, 1875). This work of about 1500 B.C.E. consists in part of a miscellaneous collection of diagnoses and prescriptions that contains remedies and folklore from as many as forty sources, some of which are probably as much as 2,000 years older (Bryan & Smith, 1974, pp. xiii–xv). Ailments causing vomiting are included, and among the prescriptions for numerous diseases of the digestive system is a cure for vomiting. The remedy involved drinking a concoction produced by steeping onions in water for four days followed by the beating of part of the mixture to a froth (Bryan & Smith, 1974, p. 51). A loss of appetite, which might indicate nausea, is described as a weariness of eating, a condition that does not allow (the patient) to eat what is in front of him (Nunn, 1996, p. 90). Treatments for "removing sickness of the stomach," and for "causing the stomach to receive food," are listed in another text, the Hearst Medical Papyrus (HMP) of ca. 1500 B.C.E., in the latter case consisting of a mixture of a carminative, chalk, and honey to be swallowed for four days (HMP IV: 4; Leake, 1952, p. 81). The specific ailment in these cases is unclear. The nausea of pregnancy is not treated among the diseases of women, nor are other causes of nausea, such as infection, tumors, or ailments of the vestibular system.

The most extensive documentary corpus of medical texts from antiquity survives from Mesopotamia, where many were recorded on clay tablets that have been recovered in archaeological contexts. The earliest therapeutic manual was compiled in the Ur III period (2112–2004 B.C.E.) with sources that may extend as early as the mid-fourth millennium B.C.E. (Scurlock & Anderson, 2005). By the Old Babylonian period (1894–1595 B.C.E.) diagnostic and prognostic handbooks were compiled in Akkadian. These medical documents are remarkable for the careful observation of clinical symptoms they recorded that permits a modern understanding of medical conditions at the time. In their compendium of medical diagnostic texts, Scurlock and Anderson (2005, pp. 116–154) organize the material by organ systems, including an extensive array concerned with gastrointestinal anatomy and illness. Nausea is uniformly viewed as a precursor to or as concomitant with vomiting rather than a symptom in its own right, and when mentioned it is described as a condition when the "insides will not accept bread and beer," either from loss of appetite or subsequent vomiting. In contrast to the circumlocution used for nausea, several Akkadian terms are used for different types of vomiting, whether the vomiting of blood (*hahu*), vomiting when the stomach is empty (*gasu*), vomiting stomach contents (*paru*), or vomiting bile (*wa-u*).

The most comprehensive treatment of nausea in ancient medical sources occurs in the corpus of (mainly) later fifth-/early fourth-century B.C.E. texts traditionally ascribed to Hippocrates, a physician from the Greek island of Kos, site of a sanctuary of Asklepios, the god of healing. These writings were compiled in the library of Alexandria, Egypt, perhaps as early as the third century B.C.E. This so-called Hippocratic Corpus of about 70 volumes emphasizes medical prognoses based on careful observation and the care of the patient. Discrimination among different causes and treatments of nausea, as distinct from vomiting, were given terms reflective of their cause. The word used for nausea of general medical cause, *ase* (ασπ, from ασαώ), to feel disgusted or nauseated, occurs in *Epidemics* III, Cases III and XII (W. H. S. Jones, 1923, pp. 222–223 and 236–237 resp.).The more specific *nautia* is usually reserved for the nausea of seasickness; however, it is sometimes used for nausea of other causes. For example, in Hippocrates, *Epidemics* IV.41, the word *nausin* is used for nausea in conjunction with a fever (Smith, 1994, pp. 134–135). As mentioned above, the nausea caused by excessive consumption of wine was also known, and the term *akraipalos* for it was used by several authors (Aristotle, *Problemata* 873b11; Athenaeus, I.32d; and Dioscurides, *Medicus* 1.26). In Hippocrates, *Prorrhetic* I.17, nausea with abdominal pain and a fever sufficient to perspire (*asodeos*) is considered a bad sign (Potter, 1995, pp. 174–175); as is nausea without vomiting (*asodees, asodesin*) (*Prorrhetic* I.76 and I.85; Potter, 1995, pp. 186–187 and 188–189). The nausea that accompanies a fever was also noted in *Epidemics* II.3.1d and, as noted above, in IV.41 (Smith, 1994, pp. 48–49 and 134–135 resp.). In *Prorrhetic* I.157 and I.165, nausea (*asodesi*) was recognized as commonly related to a swelling beside the ear, perhaps caused by either a tumor or mastoid infection (Potter, 1995, pp. 208–209 and 210–211 resp.). In *Epidemics* II.1.9 and V.98, trauma and abdominal wounds were noted as other causes of nausea (Smith, 1994, pp. 28–29 and 214–215 resp.).

The nausea that is common in pregnancy was recognized as a distinct symptom by Greek physicians and scientists. In Hippocrates, *Aphorisms* V.61, nausea (*ase*) is given as an indicator of pregnancy (Jones, 1967, pp. 174–175).

In *Epidemics* II.3.1d, fever combined with nausea is associated with miscarriage (Smith, 1994, pp. 48–49). Aristotle, writing in the third quarter of the fourth century B.C.E., refers in *Historia animalium* IX.584a.8 to the separate ailments of nausea (*nautiai*) and vomiting that affect most women after conception, and in 584a.22 to the worst nausea (*asontai*) that can occur later in pregnancy (both in Balme, 1991, p. 481). Causes of nausea specific to women are also discussed by Soranus, a Greek physician from Ephesus of the second century C.E., who probably studied in Alexandria, Egypt, where anatomical investigation was highly developed. Soranus is best known for his comprehensive gynecological and obstetrical work, the *Gynaikeion Pathon* (*On the Illnesses of Women*) (Burguière, Gourevitch & Malinas, 2003; Temkin, 1956). In Book I, 23, Soranus refers to nausea as related to menstruation and in I.36 as a symptom of overeating that leads to vomiting (Temkin, 1956, pp. 20 and 35 resp.). In Book I, 48, he ascribes other causes of the disorder to actions such as the nausea of early pregnancy related to the eating of soil (pica) and in Book II, 40 the nausea and vomiting in infants if moved after nursing, which is likened to motion sickness (Temkin, 1956, pp. 50 and 113 resp.).

Soranus was one of a large number of physicians, some others of whom wrote medical treatises, who were active at one of the numerous healing sanctuaries in the Mediterranean region and at Alexandria, Egypt, from the third century B.C.E. to the second century C.E. (Buck, 1917, pp. 103 ff.). The task of collating this accumulated knowledge and newer theoretical approaches with the Hippocratic Corpus was taken up by a second-century physician, Galen (Cl. Galenus). His prodigious output, totaling more than 600 treatises of which about a third have survived, reflected his knowledge of anatomy gained through the dissection of apes and pigs, and his study at several major healing centers. Galen's treatment of nausea was cursory. All references to the term *nautia* total less than a half column in the index to his collected works known by the early nineteenth century (Kühn, 1827–1833, vol. 20, p. 423) as opposed to vomiting (*vomitus*), with more than four columns of entries (Kühn, 1827–1833, vol. 20, pp. 669–671). In *On the Natural Faculties* III.xii, Galen ascribes nausea to an irritation of the stomach (Kühn, 1827–1833, vol. 2, p. 185; Brock, 1916, pp. 286–287), and in III.vi refers to nausea being invoked when one is forced to eat when disinclined (Kühn, 1827–1833, vol. 2, p. 159; Brock, 1916, pp. 246–247). Elsewhere Galen notes that nausea precedes vomiting (Kühn, 1827–1833, vol. 7, p. 173), and is a sign of fever (Kühn, 1827–1833, vol. 19, p. 514). He provides two remedies for nausea. The recipe for the first, in *Peri Euporiston* (Common Remedies) Book I, calls for two parts sour tree fruit with seeds removed, one part mint, and one part Attic honey to be mixed well in a pottery flask until thickened. The dose is poured off and taken before eating (Kühn, 1827–1833, vol. 14, p. 369). The second, in *Peri Euporiston* Book II, prescribes a tea made by steeping two or three stems of mint with sweet red tree fruit or, alternatively, elder leaves (*Sambuca nigra*) in water (Kühn, 1827–1833, vol. 14, p. 450).

The medical knowledge of the ancient Mediterranean world as compiled by Galen was one of the major sources for later translations of Greek scientific works into Arabic, first by medieval Islamic scholars in the eighth and ninth centuries, most notably Hunain ibn Ishaq, with the support of the Abbassid caliphs and other patrons in scholarly centers in what is now Iraq (Dols, 1984, pp. 8–9) and in the twelfth century by the scholar known in the West as Maimonides, working by that time in Cairo (Bos, 2004, p. xx). Maimonides's 25 treatises were comprised of approximately 1,500 aphorisms drawn from the works of Galen. By the thirteenth century, these Arabic works were translated into Latin, making them available to scholars in Europe, and also into Hebrew versions that circulated mainly in Spain and France (Bos, 2004, p. xxv). Thus, it was primarily the works of Galen, which contain a fairly limited concern with nausea of various causes, that formed the foundation of European medicine. It was not until the early eighteenth century, in the work of the great Dutch physician, Herman Boerhaave (1668–1738) that the primacy of the Hippocratic Corpus was once again recognized. Thus, not surprisingly, it is seasickness that is first mentioned in definitions of nausea and a more serious investigation of the symptom does not occur until the twentieth century, as the sample of definitions of nausea gathered from many sources, shown in Table 1.1, reveals.

Note that all agree that nausea is an unpleasant sensation sometimes followed by vomiting, but there is little agreement as to where it is perceived as occurring. The debate among scientists as to where nausea originates has gone on for many years. For example, Alvarez, a gastroenterologist, in 1940 said, "it is conceivable that nausea is a sensation produced solely in the brain (p. 147)." In contrast, Boring, a psychologist, suggested in 1942, that nausea may be the perception of gastric pain. However, since the sensation can only be produced in the brain, the debate is more about how the pathways leading to the genesis of the sensation are activated.

NAUSEA COMPARED TO OTHER UNPLEASANT SENSATIONS

It may be helpful to examine sensations similar to nausea, such as pain and fatigue, as a means to glean new insights into its function. Both pain and fatigue are unpleasant, but they also provide a warning to avoid or cease certain behaviors, and are, therefore, protective mechanisms that have an evolutionary basis. Pain is a most unpleasant warning that something is wrong in one's body and one usually curtails other activities and seeks the cause. Fatigue is another unpleasant warning, in this case that one must rest and can not continue with usual physical activity.

Sometimes the cause of these sensations is trivial, other times serious or even life threatening. For example, fatigue could signal not enough sleep, overexertion, or even some form of cancer. Sometimes the cause of these sensations is obvious, other times it is difficult to diagnose. Improper lifting of a heavy box

Table 1.1 Definitions of Nausea

We also say that the living being becomes nauseous; that is, that the stomach starts to be emptied through vomiting.	(Galen, second century; Kühn, Vol. 2, p. 193)
Seasickness	(the original sense, 1569; Onions, 1973, p. 1388)
A strong feeling of disgust or loathing	(1619; Onions, 1973, p. 1388)
A sensation which is felt at the back and lower part of the throat; it is not usually associated with pain . . . . Sensation is accompanied by uneasiness in the pit of the stomach, which is denoted by the term 'sinking sensation'; while the brow-ache which is also not an uncommon accompaniment of these sensations must be produced reflexly, and has not been investigated.	(Payne & Poulton, 1928, p. 157)
A psychic experience of human beings which may or may not be associated with vomiting	(Cummins, 1958, p. 710; Borison & Wang, 1953, p. 194)
Inclination to vomit	(Ostler, 1962, p. 326)
An unpleasant sensation ('feeling sick')	(Lewis, 1970, p. 806)
A feeling of sickness with loathing of food and inclination to vomit	(Onions, 1973, p. 1388)
A profoundly unpleasant subjective experience relating to the epigastric region and heralding the approach of frank vomiting	(Reason & Brand, 1975, p. 39)
Denoting not only a specific (if unlocalizable) sensation, but a state of mind and pattern of behavior—a turning away, from food, from everything, and a turning inwards.	(Sacks, 1981, p. 40)
A feeling of sickness with a loathing for food and an inclination to vomit; it is often associated with hypersalivation.	(Bouchier, 1985, p. 980)
A term that is widely used and describes a sensation everyone has experienced. However, no precise definition can be given	(Hanson & McCallum, 1985, p. 210)
An unpleasant sensation of being about to vomit, sometimes culminating in the act of vomiting. The original meaning was seasickness.	(Walton, Beeson & Bodley Scott, 1986, p. 820)
Subjective sensation of humans that is present in many illnesses and is more common than retching and emesis.	(Feldman, Samson, & O'Dorisio, 1988)
An unpleasant—although not painful—sensation usually referred to the gut, and is associated with the desire to vomit or a conviction that vomiting is imminent.	(Andrews & Hawthorn, 1988, p. 160)
A sensation and, as such, it can only be studied with assurance only in human subjects.	(Stricker et al., 1988, p. 295)
Subjective unpleasant feeling referred generally to the epigastrium and abdomen, which may last from a few minutes to several hours	(Sarna, 1989, p.122)

Table 1.1 (*continued*)

A subjective unpleasant sensation associated with the awareness of the urge to vomit. It is usually felt in the epigastrium, and is accompanied by the loss of gastric tone, duodenal contractions and reflux of intestinal contents into the stomach	(Watcha & White, 1992, p. 162)
Feeling sick to your stomach	(Morrow, 1992, p. 573)
Nausea is a subjective feeling	(Del Favero, Tonato & Roila, 1992, p. 69)
An unpleasant sensation of discomfort referred to the upper gut: it is associated with the awareness of the urge to vomit	(Tonato, Roila & Del Favero, 1993, p. 61)
Nausea is not simply " . . . sickness in the stomach . . . " but rather a non-specific term covering a complex reaction of different physiological and psychological systems to a change in autonomic activity of some nausea-evoking stimulus	(Muth et al., 1996, p. 511)
A feeling of sickness in the stomach, combined with a loathing of food and an inclination to vomit.	(Spiegl, 1996, p. 105)
The wombles, an old English word that means "A rolling or uneasiness in the stomach; a feeling of nausea"	(Spiegl, 1996, p. 167)
A visceral sensation experienced by healthy individuals as well as patients.	(Kiernan et al., 1997, p. 257)
A psychic experience of humans that defies precise definition	(Lee & Feldman, 1993, p. 509)
An unpleasant sensation vaguely located in the upper abdomen and chest which heralds vomiting or fainting but which may also occur without dramatic issue.	(Blakemore & Jennett, 2001, p. 491)
Nausea is entirely subjective and is commonly described as the sensation (or sensations) that immediately precede vomiting. Patients state that they feel as if they are about to vomit, or use such terms as "sick to the stomach" or "queasy."	(Quigley, Hasler & Parkman, 2001, p. 263)
An unpleasant sensation usually referred to the stomach and sometimes followed by vomiting	(Stern, 2002, p. 589)
An unpleasant sensation, vaguely referred to the epigastrium and abdomen, and often culminating in vomiting.	(Dorland, 2003, p. 1223)
The feeling that you might vomit	(MASCC, 2004, p. 1)
Nausea is an unpleasant psychic experience vaguely associated with the epigastrium and duodenum which often culminates just before vomiting	(Himi et al., 2004, p. 46)
A feeling of sickness with an inclination to vomit	(Soanes & Stevenson, 2006)
Nausea is an aversive experience that often accompanies emesis, and is a distinct perception, different from pain and stress	(Horn, 2008, p. 431)
Nausea is an unpleasant wavelike feeling in the back of the throat and/or stomach that may or may not result in vomiting	[National Cancer Institute (NCI), 2009]

could cause pain in the lower back, or the pain could be caused by secondary gain brought about by reinforcement of prior complaints following a back injury. In common with these examples it is apparent that nausea is an unpleasant sensation, the causes of which may be trivial or serious, and obvious or difficult to diagnose. In many cases where the cause is difficult to pinpoint and the condition difficult to treat, there may be a large psychological component, such as the example of a child who reports nausea at breakfast many mornings prior to going to school.

THE NAUSEA-EMESIS RELATIONSHIP

Some describe nausea as the sensation one experiences prior to vomiting. However, the authors of this volume reject that idea and will provide evidence that nausea and vomiting are not on a simple continuum. Nausea is sometimes assumed to be the conscious awareness of unusual activity in the so-called vomiting center in the brain stem, first described in detail by Borison and Wang (1953). However, despite numerous references to a vomiting center in the literature, the existence of such an anatomically well localized structure and its relationship, if any, to nausea remain controversial (Miller, 1993).

Blum, Heinrichs, and Herxheimer (2000) have indicated that most individuals report that nausea is more commonly experienced than vomiting, nausea feels worse, nausea is more disabling, and nausea lasts longer than vomiting. But most published research on the control of nausea and vomiting is actually about vomiting and not nausea, ignoring the more common and more troublesome symptom of nausea.

Nausea is frequently followed by vomiting, and sometimes the symptoms of nausea abate following vomiting. It is this sequence of events that may lead one to the assumption that nausea and vomiting are on a continuum. However, there are situations where nausea is present in varying degrees, but the individual does not vomit. For example, some individuals receiving chemotherapy for cancer and 28% of women in the first trimester of pregnancy experience nausea, but do not vomit (Gadsby, 2000). And there are other situations where individuals vomit with little or no sensations of nausea, e.g., astronauts in space. Oman, Lichtenberg, and Money (1990) provide the following quote from an astronaut on Spacelab I: "I wasn't nauseous, I just had stomach discomfort. It just didn't feel right, and I was doing things to keep my activity down. But I don't think I really slowed down until 2 to 5 min before I vomited. And at that point, you say, 'Oh, I think I better take it easy' and then the next thing you know, you've gone beyond the point of no return" (p. 239).

As is discussed in Chapter 14, ondansetron and other 5-HT$_3$ receptor antagonists are antiemetics that effectively reduce vomiting following chemotherapy, but such agents do little to relieve nausea (e.g., Levitt et al., 1993). Roscoe et al. (2000) studied the effectiveness of 5-HT$_3$ receptor antagonists in preventing the nausea and vomiting of 1,423 cancer patients who received chemotherapy. They found that over time, as a higher percentage of patients received the 5-HT$_3$ agents, reports of emesis decreased but reports of nausea did not.

In studies of a more recently developed drug, the NK$_1$ receptor antagonist aprepitant (Emend), cancer patients receiving chemotherapy reported a significant reduction in emesis but less reduction in nausea (Hesketh et al., 2003a; Poli-Bigelli et al., 2003). In these studies, approximately 50% of the patients who received aprepitant in addition to their other medications reported nausea; and this figure was not significantly different from nausea reports of patients in the control group that did not receive aprepitant.

To summarize, even though the introduction of 5-HT$_3$ and NK$_1$ receptor antagonists has improved the treatment-related side effects in patients receiving anticancer chemotherapy, it is clear that these agents are more effective against vomiting than against nausea. If nausea is viewed as a point on the same continuum as vomiting, then it should, in theory, be easier to reduce nausea than vomiting. But as the studies described above indicate, this is not the case.

THE FUNCTION OF NAUSEA

As stated above, it is generally agreed that nausea acts as a warning signal to protect the organism from the ingestion of toxins. It is a pattern of adaptation that increases chances of survival. Davis et al. (1986) discuss the role of nausea and vomiting in each of three levels of toxin defense. As can be seen in Table 1.2, the first level is nausea and avoidance evoked by smell and taste, a level of defense against toxins highly developed in rodents, who cannot vomit and, therefore, for whom the next two levels are irrelevant. According to Davis et al., the second level refers to "the detection of toxins by receptors in the gut followed by a central reflex producing an appropriate response, nausea, to prevent further consumption, inhibition of gastric motility to confine the toxin to the stomach, and, if necessary, vomiting to purge the system of the already ingested (but not necessarily yet absorbed) toxin" (p. 66). The third level of defense, according to Davis et al., refers to toxin sensors in the area postrema that detect circulating toxins in the blood and provoke vomiting.

Treisman (1977) had previously suggested a fourth level of toxin defense, an early warning system that is extremely sensitive to disturbances in sensory input or motor control. Treisman pointed out that in situations such as motion sickness, nausea and vomiting occur to an apparently inappropriate stimulus—sensory conflict caused by unusual movement—rather than the ingestion of a toxin. He states that such false alarms (e.g., the nausea of motion sickness, anxiety, anticipation of chemotherapy) are to be expected considering the importance of toxin defense to the survival of the organism and the evolutionary novelty of the situations. It can also be argued that the consequence of a "false alarm" to a stimulus that is in reality innocuous is preferable to the consequences of a failure to respond to a "real" stimulus. This argument has been made particularly for pregnancy sickness (Nesse & Williams, 1998).

Table 1.2 The Hierarchical Organization of the Defense Mechanism for Protections of the Organism Against Toxins

Level of defense mechanisms	Location of toxin	Type of sensor and location	Effect	Resultant action
First-level defense	External to gastrointestinal tract	1. Smell and taste 2. Peripheral	(a) Avoidance (b) Nausea	(a) Learned aversion for potential toxins
Second-level defense	Intragastric	1. Gastric chemoreceptors 2. Near the absorptive site	(a) Nausea (b) Gastric motility ↓ (c) Avoidance (d) Vomiting	(a) Learned aversion (b) Confining toxin to one area (c) Ejection of toxin
Third-level defense	Within the vascular system	1. Area postrema (CTZ) 2. Within the CNS	(a) Nausea (b) Gastric motility ↓ (c) Vomiting	(a) Ejection of toxin (b) Confining toxin (c) Learned aversion

Reproduced with permission from Davis et al.,1986.

Reports of nausea are common in patients suffering with anxiety, such as generalized anxiety disorder (Marten et al. 1993). Marten et al. reported that 58% of patients from four clinics diagnosed with generalized anxiety disorder reported nausea as an associated symptom. Research has shown that individuals reporting anxiety have an abnormally low threshold for any type of threat to their well-being (Mathews, 1990). Therefore, extreme anxiety may lower an individual's threshold for the detection of toxins resulting in loss of appetite or nausea. It has been found that high anxiety contributes to greater side effects, more nausea and vomiting, from chemotherapy (Jacobsen et al., 1988) and from the anticipation of chemotherapy (Andrykowski, 1990). See Chapter 3 for a further discussion of the relationship of anxiety to nausea.

As stated above, nausea acts as a warning signal indicating that there may be something wrong with food being approached or eaten. The survival value of avoiding foods that have made one nauseated in the past, conditioned taste aversion (CTA), is obvious (see Chapter 8 for a detailed discussion of CTA and related phenomena). CTA has been demonstrated in animals ranging from the garden slug to humans (Garcia, Quick & White, 1984). As Bernstein has stated, "learned food aversions combine with innate food aversions (unlearned responses to tastes such as sour and bitter that warn of toxins or spoilage) to guard the internal milieu from potentially damaging ingesta (1999, p. 229)."

CTA was clearly demonstrated in the laboratory by Garcia and Koelling (1966). They let rats taste saccharin and then injected them with lithium chloride, which produces visceral malaise ("nausea"). After that experience, the rats would not drink saccharin when offered on a later occasion. Subsequent studies by Garcia and others demonstrated that unlike typical classical conditioning studies, the interval between ingestion of the to-be-conditioned substance and nausea can be very long, and conditioning may require only one trial. Additional findings indicated that there is something unique about the taste–nausea relationship. Garcia and his co-workers found that when taste cues were followed by other types of noxious stimuli such as electric shock, rats did not develop conditioned taste aversion. And visual and auditory stimuli followed by nausea also failed to produce conditioned aversion. Garcia argues that the theoretical significance of this unique readiness to make connections between taste and nausea is a by-product of the evolutionary history of mammals. Natural selection favors organisms that quickly learn what not to eat. But whereas conditioned taste aversion may have evolved as an adaptive warning signal of the danger of ingested toxin, CTA can also lead to the avoidance of foods that are not poisonous and may be nutritious. An example would be a pediatric cancer patient who drank a glass of milk prior to chemotherapy, became severely nauseous following chemotherapy, and subsequently would not drink milk.

In several studies of motion sickness described in Chapter 15, (e.g., Stern et al.,1987a; Koch & Stern, 1994) it was demonstrated that nausea provoked by a rotating optokinetic drum (see Figure 7.1) is accompanied by abnormal dysrhythmic electrical activity in the stomach and little or no contractile activity. See Chapter 7 for a discussion of the relationship of this abnormal gastric activity to nausea. In short, the stomach is functionally shut down and not emptying. This demonstrates that nausea not only acts to prevent the ingestion of toxins or other substances that might make one ill, but nausea is also accompanied by physiological changes in the stomach that delay the passage of possibly toxic food into the intestine and subsequent absorption. This also occurs in rats, which lack a vomiting reflex (Andrews & Horn, 2006). Wolf (1943) made a similar observation after examining gastric activity of human participants who were exposed to a variety of nauseating stimuli. He stated in conclusion, "Nausea occurred only during phases of inhibition of gastric motor activity" (p. 882). Davis et al. (1986) made a similar point in their discussion of their second level of defense against the ingestion of toxins.

This protective action of the stomach when food that is not pleasant is ingested was demonstrated in a modified sham feed study with healthy human participants (Stern et al., 2001a). One group chewed and spit a cooked frankfurter, while the second group chewed and spit a cold sausage made from tofu, an experience that was rated as disgusting by the subjects. The effects of these two eating experiences were measured with the electrogastrogram (EGG).

As can be seen in Figure 1.1, normal 3 cpm gastric activity increased in the group that chewed and spit the frankfurter but decreased in the group that chewed and spit the cold tofu sausage. The decreased 3 cpm response of the tofu group is an example of decreased cephalic-vagal reflex activity that inhibited normal gastric functioning, and protected the organism.

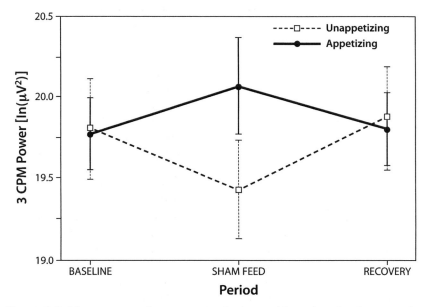

Figure 1.1 Mean power at 3 cpm expressed as natural log values for the group that was sham fed appetizing food and the group that was sham fed unappetizing food for the baseline period, the sham-feed period, and the first 5-min recovery period. The difference in 3 cpm power during sham feeding was significant ($p < 0.05$). Reproduced with permission from Stern et al., 2001a.

Unpublished results from one of our laboratories (RMS) have shown that after an overnight fast, the electrical activity of the stomach is often unstable, showing considerable dysrhythmia, the same pattern seen when subjects report nausea. And subjects often report mixed sensations of hunger–nausea. Note that Boring (1942) reported that, "Nausea can be perceived, and includes gastric pains, which may in exceptional circumstances be confused with hunger." (p. 563). This complex hunger–nausea sensation has been reported by individuals who are breaking a fast of several days (Duncan, 1962). It is interesting that people who are very hungry, who might be expected to approach any and all food with gusto, sometimes act more cautiously and are choosey as to what they will eat. One possible explanation is that under conditions of prolonged food deprivation, one might be inclined to ingest almost anything, including toxins, and so as a protective mechanism during a prolonged fast, one's threshold of acceptable foods shifts, becomes more selective, and favors bland familiar foods. In fact, Jacobs and Sharma (1969) reported that food-deprived rats and dogs discriminated more when fed than freely fed animals.

Related to this phenomenon of a shift in the threshold of acceptable foods is Hook's (1978) and Profet's (1992) theory about the nausea of "morning sickness." Both Hook and Profet propose that the nausea of pregnancy is a mechanism for screening out toxins to protect the embryo. Profet has suggested that during the first trimester of pregnancy there is a recalibration of the chemoreceptor trigger zone in the area postrema (see Chapters 4 and 5 in this volume) and a shift in the mother's threshold for taste and smell; i.e., they become keener. As a result of this threshold shift, previously desired foods with strong taste and/or odors, such as coffee, strong smelling cheese, etc., are nauseating and are thus avoided. See Chapter 12 in this volume for further discussion of the nausea of pregnancy in general and Profet's theory in particular. Although there is not yet agreement as to whether pregnancy sickness serves an adaptive prophylactic function, in most situations nausea provides one with a warning not to eat and/or what not to eat.

In the chapters that follow, what is known about the mechanisms and management of nausea is summarized, but it is often concluded "we don't know enough." One reason for this lack of knowledge stated above is the inherent difficulty in studying private sensations. But another reason for the paucity of information about nausea is the fact that the study of nausea "falls between the cracks" of our traditional disciplines. The authors of this volume—a psychophysiologist, a gastroenterologist, and a physiologist—have combined their knowledge and present in the chapters that follow not only what is known about nausea but also what needs to be learned about the mechanisms involved in nausea before new and more efficacious treatments can be developed.

Chapter 2

Prevalence of Nausea from Various Causes

Thomas (2000), in a chapter entitled the "Economic Impact of Nausea and Vomiting," estimated that nausea and vomiting costs the U.S. economy between 4 and 10 billion dollars per year. And the cost in human suffering is, of course, immeasurable. Rub, Andrews, and Whitehead (1992) inquired about the prevalence of nausea during the past 12 months in 596 otherwise healthy people. Women reported significantly more nausea than men, and overall, 54% of the subjects reported at least one incident of nausea. The authors also reported a decrease in prevalence of nausea with increasing age. More recently, Camilleri et al. (2005) reported the prevalence and socioeconomic impact of upper gastrointestinal (GI) disorders in the United States based on telephone interviews with 21,128 adults. With regard to nausea, they found that 11.9% of females reported experiencing nausea at least once during the previous three months, and 6.8% of males reported nausea during the same period. The relevance of gender, age, and other personal status variables to the experience of nausea will be discussed in Chapter 3, along with the complex interaction of inherent and psychological factors. In this chapter we discuss the prevalence of nausea associated with gastrointestinal diseases and disorders, diabetes, pregnancy, postoperative surgery, chemotherapy treatment for cancer, and provocative motion.

PREVALENCE OF NAUSEA ASSOCIATED WITH GI DISEASES AND DISORDERS

Garthright, Archer, and Kvenberg (1988) estimated that acute GI infections with nausea and vomiting account for medical expenses of $1.25 billion and are associated with $21.8 billion in lost productivity. Blum, Heinrichs, and Herxheimer (2000), in summarizing the results of the 1993 National Health Interview Survey, reported that 43% of respondents were nauseous on more than three occasions during the past six months. Of those reporting nausea, 65% said that at least on some occasions it was due to food poisoning and 58% reported that sometimes a "stomach virus" caused their nausea. Blum et al. also pointed out that people 18–44 years old with annual incomes under $10,000 reported much more frequent nausea and vomiting due to indigestion during the previous year than people over 40 years old and with incomes over $10,000. Frank et al. (2000) reported that the results of the Domestic/ International Gastroenterological Surveillance Study (DIGEST) revealed that 15% of U.S. and Canadian subjects reported experiencing nausea associated with abnormal upper GI functioning during the previous three months.

PREVALENCE OF NAUSEA ASSOCIATED WITH DIABETES

Patients with diabetes mellitus are classified as being in one of the following two groups:

Type 1, insulin-dependent (5–10% of all diabetics) or
Type 2, non-insulin-dependent

In one of the first published studies of the prevalence of nausea and other GI symptoms in both Type 1 and Type 2 diabetics, Enck et al. (1994) compared symptom reports of diabetic patients with those of matched healthy controls. They reported finding no differences in reports of upper GI symptoms between Type 1 diabetics and control subjects; however, Type 2 diabetics reported significantly more nausea than controls (11.8% vs. 2.9%). Schvarcz et al. (1996), on the other hand, reported that long-term Type 1 diabetics reported significantly more nausea during the previous three months than matched healthy controls (22.7% vs. 9.1%). The authors added that they found increased frequency of upper GI symptoms in females and in patients with poor glycemic control.

Maleki et al. (2000) studied reports of GI symptoms in a community-based sample of both Type 1 and Type 2 diabetics and compared their responses to matched healthy controls. Results for reports of nausea showed no difference between either group of diabetic patients and controls. In general, the authors reported finding few differences in reports of GI symptoms between their community-based sample of diabetics and healthy controls. In contrast to these findings, Bytzer et al. (2001) sampled 15,000 adults, 423 with diabetes, and found that all 16 GI symptoms included in the questionnaire were reported more frequently by diabetics compared with controls. The questionnaire also included, for diabetics, items about glycemic control. The authors reported that an increased prevalence rate of GI symptoms for diabetics was associated with self-reports of poor glycemic control. Wilm and Helmert (2006), using the German Federal Health Services survey from 1987, 1991, and 1998, compared responses of over 18,000 adults to questions about diabetes and GI symptoms. Nausea was the only GI symptom to be more prevalent in diabetics than non-diabetics. The authors reported that 12% of diabetics reported nausea vs. 6% of nondiabetics, and female diabetics reported more nausea than male diabetics.

In summary, the results of the above studies of the prevalence of nausea in diabetic individuals are equivocal, but the majority indicates a greater prevalence of nausea in diabetics than healthy controls. Some of the variability in the results may be a function of the different questionnaires used, the lack of data on gastroparesis, autonomic neuropathy, and glycemic control.

PREVALENCE OF NAUSEA ASSOCIATED WITH PREGNANCY

Gadsby, Barnie-Adshead, and Jagger (1993) and Gadsby (1994) reported that in England, 8.5 million working days are lost every year because of the nausea and vomiting of pregnancy (NVP). The authors go on to say that severely affected women miss a mean of 62 hours of work during their pregnancy. For further discussion see Gadsby (2000).

The nausea of pregnancy is usually thought of as two conditions: the very serious condition of hyperemesis gravidarum, and the more common condition referred to as the nausea of pregnancy ("morning sickness").

Hyperemesis gravidarum refers to a condition in which a pregnant woman continues to have severe nausea and vomiting during the second and third trimester. The nausea and vomiting can be so frequent and severe that the nutritional status of the mother and the safety of both the mother and fetus are at risk. Fortunately, most investigators report that the prevalence of hyperemesis gravidarum is less than 1%. See, for example, Fairweather (1968) and Kallen (2000).

Normal nausea of pregnancy is common, usually beginning during the fourth to sixth week of pregnancy and tapering off by the twelfth week. According to Blum, Heinrichs, and Herxheimer (2000), prevalence reports vary from one study to another (from 65 to 75%) because of the usual difficulties of assessing nausea, and cultural differences in reporting nausea and other symptoms of discomfort.

Approximately four million pregnant women in the United States and 350,000 women in Canada experience NVP each year (Emelianova et al., 1999). Nausea of pregnancy affects women in all socioeconomic strata, but different attitudes exist among women in regard to the symptoms. According to Mazzotta et al. (2000), American women more often perceive that drug therapy for NVP poses increased risks for fetal malformations than do Canadian women, for whom the nausea and vomiting symptoms raised concerns for their unborn child. American women with NVP experienced larger weight loss, more hospitalizations, and more time lost from paid employment compared with Canadian women.

In a large prospective multicenter study of pregnant women in the 1960s (Klebanoff et al., 1985), vomiting occurred in 56% of the women (excluding those with hyperemesis gravidarum), was more common in the first pregnancy, in younger women, in women with fewer than 12 years of education, in nonsmokers, and in women weighing 170 lbs. or more. Significantly more nausea and vomiting occurs in the first trimester in women with multiple gestations compared with single gestation pregnancies (87% versus 73%, $p < 0.01$) (Brandes, 1967). Järnfelt-Samsioe, Samsioe, and Velinder (1983) reported that the peak incidence of nausea in their study was in the first trimester (91%), and only 3% reported nausea in the last trimester. They also reported that nausea was reported by 50% of the participants in the morning, whereas the nausea peaked in the evening for 7% of the participants, and 36% experienced nausea constantly.

A more recent prospective study of 160 pregnant women by Lacroix, Eason, and Melzack (2000) recorded details of nausea and vomiting on a daily basis. This study revealed the impressive burden of the NVP symptoms. In this study, 74% of the women reported nausea. "Morning sickness" occurred in only 1.8% of the women, whereas 80% of the women reported that nausea lasted all day. The overall duration of nausea averaged 35 days. Furthermore, only 50% of the women had relief of nausea by the 14th week of gestation. Nausea had disappeared by week 22 in 90% of the women. Nausea was rated with the McGill Nausea Questionnaire (Melzack et al., 1985), a validated questionnaire used in other medical conditions. The mean nausea index for the chemo-therapeutic agent 5-Fluorouracil, was 3.3, whereas the mean nausea index for women during peak nausea at 11 weeks was 1.85. Thus, on average, the nausea experienced by these women with NVP was comparable to that induced by a moderately nauseogenic chemotherapy agent. Lacroix, Eason, and Melzack (2000) also found significant relationships among NVP and low educational level, middle to low income, and part-time work. Thus, socioeconomic factors, as well as the pathophysiological factors described in "The Nausea of Pregnancy" (Chapter 12, in this volume), also influence NVP symptoms.

According to Semmens (1971), NVP is more common in Westernized countries and more prominent in urban populations compared with rural populations. Nausea and vomiting of pregnancy is rare in African, native-American/Eskimo, and some Asian populations except for the industrialized Japanese populations. Thus, nausea and vomiting are not uniformly associated with the condition of pregnancy. Genetic differences, as well as socioeconomic differences, may have a role in the prevalence of nausea and vomiting.

The presence of NVP has been associated with decreased risk of miscarriage, perinatal death, low infant birth rate, and preterm birth. Furthermore, a meta-analysis of 11 studies confirmed the significant association between NVP and decreased risk of miscarriage (Brandes, 1967; Järnfelt-Samsioe, Samsioe & Velinder, 1983; Tierson, Olsen & Hook, 1986; Weigel & Weigel, 1989). These findings plus concerns about drug therapy (described in the treatment section of Chapter 12, in this volume) have tended to reduce efforts to treat NVP. The true burden of nausea and vomiting also is not appreciated in a variety of medical disorders that range from diabetic gastropathy to the suffering endured during nausea and vomiting related to cancer chemotherapy. The same lack of appreciation of the burden of symptoms appears to be true for NVP.

Smith et al. (2000) used the Rhodes index of nausea and vomiting (see Chapter 9, in this volume) and the SF-36 Health Survey in evaluating 593 pregnant women presenting with NVP. Nausea was the most troublesome symptom in terms of duration and intensity for these women. Low SF-36 Health Survey scores for physical functioning and social functioning were found, with major negative effects on working, household duties, and parenting. Ninety-six percent of the women were distressed by their nausea at a mild to moderate level, and 28% had greater distress from the nausea. Retching was reported by 72% of the women from the nausea. Retching was less distressing than nausea; vomiting occurred in 44% of the women and was considered a mild distress. Over half of the women took time off from work: 28% changed their work schedule, 4% left work all together, and 55% had frequent sick days.

Psychosocial morbidity in Canadian patients with NVP was assessed by Mazzotta et al. (2000) in a structured interview. Those women with severe nausea and vomiting had more frequent depression, more often considered termination of pregnancy, reported adverse effects of the illness on their relationships with spouses, and also perceived that their symptoms would adversely effect their baby. These same psychosocial issues were also reported by women with mild nausea and vomiting, indicating that simply categorizing these patients by the number of the episodes of nausea or vomiting per day does not reflect the true suffering and dysfunction associated with NVP.

PREVALENCE OF NAUSEA ASSOCIATED WITH SURGERY AND ANESTHESIA

Postoperative nausea and vomiting (PONV) has a significant impact on the overall functioning of surgical centers (Hirsch, 1994; Westman, 1999). It has been estimated that PONV increases the cost per surgical patient by over $415 (Quigley, Hasler & Parkman, 2001). It is difficult to report with confidence the prevalence of postoperative nausea (PON) because of the many different contributing factors, including type of surgery, anesthesia, antiemetics, prior surgeries, history of motion sickness, and other factors such as gender and age that have been previously mentioned as risk factors for nausea.

The difficulty in quantifying the prevalence of PON can be seen in the results of a study of 104 patients who had laparoscopic foregut procedures (Bradshaw et al., 2002). The results show the importance of time-since-surgery in prevalence of PON. Immediately following surgery, while the patients were still in the postanesthesia care unit (PACU), 30% reported nausea; however, after the patients were moved to the nursing care unit, 60% reported nausea. And the authors reported that 60% of the patients who received antiemetics prior to surgery reported nausea, whereas 64% of the patients who did not receive antiemetics reported nausea. In a more recent retrospective study of 3641 patients who had inpatient surgery with a general anesthetic at Duke University Hospital (Habib et al, 2006a), while still in the PACU 16% reported nausea and 3% vomited. However, after leaving the PACU, 40% reported nausea and/ or vomiting. All subjects had at least two risk factors for PONV and 79% received prophylactic antiemetics.

The effect of the stage of the menstrual cycle on the prevalence of PON in female patients is another factor that has been studied by several investigators. Harmon et al. (2000) studied the effects of menstrual cycle irregularity on PON following laparoscopy. They reported that 20% of women with regular menstrual cycles reported nausea, but 40% of women with irregular menstrual cycles reported nausea. The effect of the actual stage of the menstrual cycle on PONV is controversial. Some investigators think that the stage makes a difference. For example, Beattie et al. (1991) studied 235 women who had tubal ligation and found that reports of PONV were highest on day 5 of the menstrual cycle and lowest on days 18–20. However, Eberhart, Morin, and Georgieff (2000) in a review article, state that the stage of the menstrual cycle has no impact on PON/PONV. Inconsistencies in the results of studies of the effects of the stage of the menstrual cycle on PONV are not surprising when one considers the many additional factors mentioned above that effect nausea and vomiting and may have varied from study to study.

The effects of another variable on PON, orthostatic function, were studied by Pusch et al. (2002). The participants, 200 women who were scheduled for elective gynecological surgery, were given an orthostatic test the day before surgery. Of the women who were classified as having normal orthostatic function, 31% reported PON, whereas 78% of the women who were classified as having orthostatic dysfunction reported PON.

PREVALENCE OF NAUSEA ASSOCIATED WITH CHEMOTHERAPY TREATMENT FOR CANCER

The nausea associated with chemotherapy is usually divided into the following three temporal periods:

a. Acute Nausea—Nausea that occurs during treatment or within 24 hours.
b. Delayed Nausea—Nausea that begins after an 18- to 24-hour period during which the patient is free of nausea.
c. Anticipatory Nausea—Nausea that occurs before or in anticipation of treatment.

Overall Reports of Chemotherapy-Induced Nausea

Several studies of chemotherapy-induced nausea were conducted in the early 1990s. In a review article, Bovbjerg et al. (1990) reported that chemotherapy-induced nausea varied from 25% to 75% of patients, depending on the particular cytotoxic drug and dosage. Note that this review was done in 1990 prior to the introduction of the 5-HT$_3$ receptor antagonists, but as was reported by Roscoe et al. (2000), the prevalence of chemotherapy-induced nausea has not changed. Graves (1992) reported that the nausea of 30% of chemotherapy patients cannot be controlled with any drug. Tonato (1994) reported that nausea cannot be controlled in 30–40% of chemotherapy patients who are treated with cisplatin, one of the most nauseogenic cytotoxic drugs used in chemotherapy. Clark and Gralla (1993) found that 90% of chemotherapy patients who received high dosages of cisplatin experienced nausea. And more recently, Neymark and Crott (2005) summarized the results of three European Organization for Research and Treatment of Cancer trials of cisplatin-based chemotherapy and reported that between 42 and 59% of patients reported at least one episode of nausea.

A study from the University of Rochester Cancer Center, in cooperation with 18 other cancer centers (Hickok et al., 2003), provides considerable data on the prevalence of nausea following chemotherapy in 360 cancer patients. All patients received ondansetron with dexamethasone as antiemetics on the day of treatment and received one of the following cytotoxic drugs: doxorubicin, cisplatin, or carboplatin. The authors reported that 76% of the cancer patients experienced nausea at some time between infusion of the cytotoxic drug and the following five days even though they had all received a 5-HT$_3$ receptor antagonist antiemetic prior to chemotherapy. Nausea was reported by 61% of patients who received carboplatin; 75% of those who received cisplatin; and 86% of patients who received doxorubicin. One-third of the patients reported nausea on at least four consecutive days following their chemotherapy; 22% reported nausea on all five days.

In a two-center study supported by Merck (2003), of 550 cancer patients who were given cisplatin and standard antiemetic therapy, 56% reported nausea from one center and 61% from the second center. When patients were given the NK$_1$ receptor antagonist, aprepitant, in addition to standard antiemetic therapy, overall reports of nausea from patients in the two centers dropped only to 52% and 51%. The decrease in reports of nausea with aprepitant was not statistically significant from the first study but it was from the second because in the second study the control group, against which the aprepitant group was compared, reported a higher level of nausea.

It should be noted that several studies have found that both physicians and nurses tend to underestimate markedly the prevalence of nausea, particularly the delayed nausea that frequently follows chemotherapy. For example, Grunberg et al. (2004) found that more than 75% of 24 physicians and nurses underestimated the prevalence of delayed nausea reported by 298 cancer patients. Liau et al. (2005) compared reports of nausea from 107 chemotherapy patients with the estimates of 37 health care providers. They reported that the nurses and physicians underestimated reports of acute nausea by 16% and delayed nausea by 30%.

Acute and Delayed Nausea

Clark and Gralla (1993), as well as several other investigators, have observed that the 5-HT$_3$ receptor antagonists do not relieve delayed nausea. Hickok et al. (2003) reported that the percentage of acute nausea varied as a function of the cytotoxic drug received during chemotherapy. Of the patients who received doxorubicin, 55% reported nausea on the day of treatment; 43% of patients treated with cisplatin reported acute nausea; and 25% of patients who received carboplatin reported nausea on the day of treatment. The nausea caused by doxorubicin, compared to the other two drugs, was more likely to be moderate or severe. According to the Hickok et al. (2003) study, 73% of their patients reported nausea some time during the delay period, and 36% experienced nausea only during the delay period (they did not experience any acute nausea). The peak severity of nausea that occurred during the delay period tended to be higher than the peak severity that occurred on the day of chemotherapy. Delayed nausea also varied as a function of cytotoxic drug. Of those patients treated with doxorubicin, 83% reported delayed nausea; 75% of patients who received cisplatin reported delayed nausea; and 56% of patients who were treated with carboplatin experienced delayed nausea. As mentioned above, the results from the two centers that were supported by Merck (2003) indicated that with standard antiemetic treatment 52% and 60% of patients reported delayed nausea. With the addition of aprepitant, reports of delayed nausea from the two centers dropped to 49% and 47%.

Anticipatory Nausea

Many cancer patients receiving chemotherapy suffer from anticipatory nausea. That is, these patients experience nausea prior to receiving chemotherapy, often during the hours prior to their next treatment and often at the sight or smell of the clinic or someone associated with the clinic where they previously received treatment that resulted in nausea and/or vomiting. It is thought that anticipatory nausea is a classically conditioned response, and, for most patients, it is not relieved by any known drug or treatment. Approximately 25 to 50% of cancer patients suffering from anticipatory nausea and/or vomiting delay one or more scheduled courses of chemotherapy, or even refuse further treatment (Laszlo, 1983). Watson, McCarron, and Law (1992) studied 95 adult cancer patients being treated with mild to moderately emetic cytotoxic drugs and determined that 23% reported anticipatory nausea. Tye et al. (1997) investigated the prevalence of anticipatory nausea among 59 pediatric cancer patients, all of whom were treated with ondansetron; 59% indicated at least mild anticipatory nausea.

In 1998, Stockhorst, Klosterhalfen, and Steingrüber published a review article summarizing what was known at that time about the prevalence of anticipatory nausea. The reported prevalence of anticipatory nausea ranged from 26 to 57%. The authors point out that there is a high correlation between degree of acute and/or delayed nausea, and anticipatory nausea. That is, the greater the nausea experienced at chemotherapy session X, the greater the probability of anticipatory nausea prior to chemotherapy session X+1. The probability of anticipatory nausea also increases with a decrease in the interval between chemotherapy sessions.

It is difficult to summarize the data relevant to the issue of the prevalence of nausea resulting from chemotherapy because of the variability from study to study. Some possible explanations for the variability reported both within and between studies follow:

a. Different subjects, e.g., age, gender, diagnosis, stage of disease
b. Different cytotoxic drugs and dosages
c. Different antiemetic drugs administered
d. Different number of previous treatments and different intervals since last treatment

e. Different methods for determining frequency, severity, and duration of nausea

PREVALENCE OF NAUSEA ASSOCIATED WITH PROVOCATIVE MOTION

At one time it was thought that susceptibility to motion sickness was limited to the "delicate in health" or those possessing a "neurotic disposition" (Reason & Brand, 1975). In other words, nausea was thought of as a sign of weakness. However we now know that this is not true; rather motion sickness is a normal response of healthy individuals, and nausea is one of the primary symptoms of motion sickness. Quantifying the prevalence of nausea reported during motion sickness in the general population is difficult because the values obtained will depend on the method of assessing symptoms, the sample studied, and the nature of the motion. According to Reason and Brand (1975), "all individuals possessing an intact vestibular apparatus can be made motion sick given the right quality and quantity of provocative stimulation, although there are wide and consistent individual differences in the degree of susceptibility" (p. 29). Furthermore, most studies of the prevalence of motion sickness do not provide separate figures for prevalence of nausea of their subjects. We will assume that in such studies the values given for prevalence of motion sickness are estimates of values for prevalence of nausea while motion sick, but it should be pointed out that some subjects who experience and report motion sickness have symptoms such as dizziness and no nausea.

Reason (1967) reported that 90% of a sample of 300 college students reported a history of motion sickness. Reason and Brand (1975) developed a Motion Sickness Questionnaire (MSQ) that has been used by many investigators to assess individuals' history of motion sickness. The use of this and other questionnaires used to measure nausea is described in Chapter 9 (in this volume). The prevalence of motion sickness in trains has always been low, 0.13% (Kaplan, 1964), but may have changed in modern high-speed trains. Prevalence of seasickness was estimated by Chinn (1951) to be 25–30% during moderate turbulence during the first two or three days on an Atlantic crossing. We would expect the prevalence of seasickness to be lower today thanks to better design of ships and new antinausea drugs and products that were not available 50 years ago. We conclude the same to be true for air travel; the prevalence of airsickness has probably dropped due to better design of planes, their ability to fly higher to avoid turbulence, and the use of medication and products that prevent or reduce nausea. Data from Reason's (1967) questionnaire of British college students revealed that 57% had experienced nausea while riding in cars. A more recent study (Turner & Griffin, 1999) of 3256 bus travelers in England revealed that 28% reported feeling ill on at least one trip and 13% reported nausea.

Three additional areas in which motion sickness is of concern include motion sickness in the military, in microgravity (space sickness), and in virtual environments (cybersickness).

Prevalence of Motion Sickness in the Military

Motion sickness in peacetime is unpleasant but not fatal. Motion sickness that incapacitates military personnel can be fatal. For example, if troops being put ashore in small amphibious craft are suffering from severe motion sickness they might not be able to fire their weapons accurately or evade enemy fire. Studies of amphibious operations following World War II showed that 11% of the U.S. troops in landing craft suffered severe motion sickness during mild swells, and 60% were sick when the sea was rough (Tyler, 1946).

Air sickness continues to be a problem for the military for at least two reasons: military planes must often make maneuvers that provoke motion sickness, and military pilots can not take anti–motion sickness drugs because of the undesirable side effects such as drowsiness. (See Chapter 3 in this volume, "Adaptation," for a discussion of training programs to help pilots who would otherwise be disqualified because of their susceptibility to airsickness.) A design issue that has increased reports of motion sickness in military vehicles is the decrease in available vision outside of the tank, plane, or ship. Newer designs of these vehicles include electronic sensing systems that communicate position to the operator on a computer monitor. But the absence of normal vision of the terrain in front of the tank makes the operator more susceptible to motion sickness. The modern tank operator becomes more like the child in the back seat of a moving car rather than the driver. Lerman et al. (1992) discuss the problem of motion sickness in tank drivers and the even more severe symptoms of motion sickness experienced by individuals using a tank simulator (see the section below on cybersickness). In conclusion, the prevalence of motion sickness increases in any vehicle that creates a sensory mismatch, usually by depriving the operator of visual or other sensory inputs that normally accompany other signals to the brain.

Prevalence of Motion Sickness in Microgravity (Space Sickness)

Astronauts who are susceptible to space motion sickness (SMS) usually begin to experience symptoms within the first hour of orbital flight, and symptoms usually resolve within 48 hours. Restriction of movement decreases SMS. Note that there were no reports of SMS from the Mercury and Gemini missions, both small vehicles that restricted movement. Gorgiladze and Bryanov (1989) reported that up to the date of their study, 48% of the Russian cosmonauts reported SMS. Davis et al. (1988) reported that 35% of the Apollo crew members reported SMS, and 60% of the Skylab astronauts reported experiencing SMS. Davis et al. also reported that for the first 24 space shuttle flights, 67% of the crewmembers reported symptoms of SMS.

Prevalence of Motion Sickness in Virtual Environments (Cybersickness)

Virtual environments (VE) range from IMAX films that entertain to head-coupled PC-based virtual environments that are used to train astronauts.

Use of a VE has the great advantage of creating a particular environment without all of the actual sensory inputs being present; e.g., the training cockpit of a new jet plane that presents visual information on a wide screen or head-mounted glasses but doesn't move. Since VEs by their very nature create sensory mismatch, immersion in such systems provokes in some people symptoms of cybersickness, including nausea.

It is difficult to determine the prevalence of nausea provoked by VEs since it will depend on the nature of the VE and the nature of the participants, but some examples follow. Regan and Price (1994) immersed 146 subjects in a VE for 20 minutes, and 61% reported symptoms including nausea. These symptoms caused 5% of the participants to terminate the session early. In another study, Stanney et al. (2003) exposed subjects to a VE for 15–60 minutes. They reported that 80% experienced symptoms of cybersickness, and 13% had to terminate the session early. Kim et al. (2005) exposed 61 participants to a VE and correlated their degree of cybersickness with several physiological measures. They found that severity of cybersickness correlated positively with tachygastria, eyeblink rate, heart period, and EEG delta waves. In conclusion, designers of VEs must consider the fact that the greater the sensory mismatch created, the greater the probability that some users will experience symptoms of cybersickness including nausea.

CONCLUSIONS

Studies of the prevalence of nausea probably understate the severity of the problem. Blum (2000) noted the tendency of sufferers not to report nausea. The absence of a clinically observable event in the case of nausea also leads to its underreporting. Apfel (2010) has referred to the prevalence of nausea in postoperative patients after release from the ambulatory surgical centers now commonly used in medical practice. For cancer patients, 5-HT_3 receptor antagonists, while reducing the incidence of vomiting, often delay the onset of nausea until the patient has left the health care facility (see Chapter 14, in this volume). The lack of consistency in the measurement of nausea, as described in Chapter 9 (in this volume), also brings into question the results of studies of the prevalence of nausea described above.

Chapter 3

Nausea as a Protective Control Mechanism with a Dynamic Threshold

As was mentioned in Chapter 1, nausea is a symptom of a complex protective control mechanism with multiple detectors that inhibits food intake in certain situations, such as when the available food is perceived as disgusting, or when the available food has been previously associated with nausea and/or vomiting(conditioned taste aversion). Nausea also inhibits food intake when the stomach and the related control mechanisms are not functioning normally because of factors such as the ingestion of a toxin, some form of pathology, or stress and/or anxiety.

THE CONCEPT OF A DYNAMIC NAUSEA THRESHOLD

It is proposed that each individual has a dynamic threshold for the complex control mechanism—nausea—that may change from moment to moment. As is depicted in Figure 3.1, the threshold depends on the interaction of certain inherent, or relatively fixed, characteristics of an individual, e.g., age, gender, and genetic factors, and more changeable psychological states such as anxiety, expectation, anticipation, and adaptation that probably accounts for much of the inter- and intraindividual variation in the response to nauseogenic stimuli. It is hypothesized that the threshold level affects the individual's cognitive appraisal of both the nauseogenic stimulus and his/her bodily changes in response to the nauseogenic stimulus. The appraisal is thought to affect both selective attention, as well as one's evaluation of threat and coping ability, and it is this changing appraisal that modulates the response to the chemotherapy drug, spoiled food, motion, etc.

What follows is a description of some of the factors that have been studied, but the list is neither exhaustive nor are the factors included here thought to be independent.

Inherent Factors

There are at least three inherent factors that have been found to affect the nausea threshold of healthy individuals: age, gender, and genetic factors, and they frequently interact.

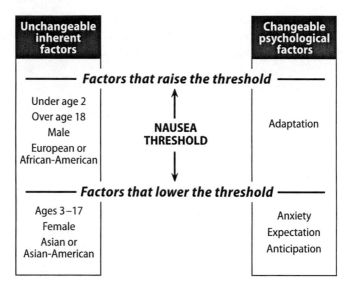

Figure 3.1 Inherent and changeable psychological factors that are thought to interact to induce a nausea threshold. Reproduced with permission from Stern and Koch, 2006.

Age

In an unpublished study from one of our laboratories (RMS) of the reaction of infants (6–20 months old) to exposure to a rotating drum, no reactions suggesting motion sickness were noted. The absence of motion sickness in infants can be attributed to their lack of the development of congruent sensory signals to their brains. That is, sensory mismatch, the cause of much motion sickness, may not occur in infants because they lack the repeated experience of certain sensory signals, primarily visual and vestibular, usually occurring together. Reason and Brand (1975) reported that infants below the age of two are generally immune to motion sickness, susceptibility is greatest between two and twelve, and motion sickness is rare beyond the age of 50. Rub, Andrews, and Whitehead (1992), in a study of the prevalence of nausea and vomiting during a 6-month period, reported that both decreased with age. Researchers studying the nausea of chemotherapy (e.g., Morrow, 1989) have indicated that older patients report less nausea than younger patients. Kenny (1994), in a review of risk factors for postoperative nausea and vomiting, reported that children were twice as susceptible as adults. And Cohen et al. (1994) reported that a questionnaire given to 16,000 postoperative patients revealed that younger patients and females reported more nausea and vomiting than older patients and males. However, these studies did not report differences in nausea as a function of type of surgery or anesthetic.

Gender

Numerous reports in the motion sickness literature indicate that women report more symptoms than men (e.g., Reason & Brand, 1975); however, they might not experience greater physiological changes. Bos et al. (2007) recently reported the results of a questionnaire of seasickness symptoms given to 2840 passengers on several ships. According to the authors, female symptom ratings were 1.5 times as great as men's and peaked at age 11. However, male symptom ratings peaked at age 21, indicating an interaction between age and gender. Symptom ratings decreased with older ages and the gender difference was not seen. Jokerst et al. (1999a) used an optokinetic drum and collected both subjective reports and EGG data from the stomach and concluded that, indeed, women reported more symptoms than men, but they did not show greater disturbances in gastric activity. The chemotherapy literature also indicates that women report more nausea than men receiving the same drugs. In a study of the side effects of opioids, Cepeda et al. (2003) reported that women had significantly more nausea and vomiting than men. And Koivuranta et al. (1997), in a study of 1107 inpatients, reported significantly more postoperative nausea in women than men, as did Watcha and White (1992).

Genetic Factors

There are many studies in the motion sickness literature describing group differences in susceptibility to nausea and other symptoms that are attributed to genetic factors. (See Chapter 15, in this volume). For example, in the first of three studies, Stern et al. (1993) reported that 15 Chinese subjects experienced significantly more symptoms of motion sickness than 15 European American or 15 African American subjects. Furthermore, the Chinese subjects showed significantly greater abnormal gastric activity during drum rotation than the other two groups. Since the Chinese subjects in this study had recently come to the United States, it was possible that nonbiological factors such as child-rearing practices or diet may account for the difference in susceptibility. To rule out this possibility, in a second study, Muth et al. (1994) tested Asian Americans, U.S.-born children of Asian parents, and obtained similar results. In the third of this series of studies, Stern et al. (1996) again showed hyper-susceptibility to motion sickness provoked by a rotating optokinetic drum among Asian subjects.

Klosterhalfen et al. (2005a) compared nausea and other symptoms of motion sickness in European and Chinese subjects who were exposed to a rotating chair while they moved their head. Rotation time tolerated by the European subjects was significantly greater than that for the Chinese subjects. Klosterhalfen et al. (2006) again compared nausea and other symptoms of motion sickness in European and Chinese subjects but in this study used a rotating optokinetic drum rather than a rotating chair. They again reported finding significantly greater rotation tolerance for the European subjects.

Jordan et al. (1995) compared the incidence of hyperemesis gravidarum between Pacific Islanders and non–Pacific Islanders living in Wellington, New Zealand, during a 5-year period and concluded that the incidence was significantly greater among Pacific Island women, especially Samoans. Cepeda et al. (2003), in a study of the side effects of opioids mentioned above, reported that white subjects had more nausea and vomiting than black subjects.

Tremblay et al. (2003) examined the role of genetic factors in susceptibility to the nausea and vomiting that frequently accompanies chemotherapy. They reported that variations in the 5-HT$_3$B receptor gene are related to the effectiveness of antiemetic treatment (see Chapter 14, in this volume).

Psychological Factors

A hypothesis as to why the same nauseogenic stimulus may cause different responses in the same individual on different days is based on the assumption that changeable psychological factors interact with inherent factors to modulate the response. For example, if a person were particularly anxious on the third day of a series of six days of chemotherapy treatment, he/she might be expected to have a very low nausea threshold and, therefore, appraise the chemotherapy procedure and/or his/her bodily reactions to it as a greater threat than usual and experience more nausea and vomiting than usual.

There is considerable overlap among the following psychological factors, and, indeed, what one psychologist refers to as "anticipation," for example, another investigator may label as "expectation."

Anxiety

Reports of nausea are common in patients with various anxiety conditions such as generalized anxiety disorder, according to Marten et al. (1993). Research has shown that anxious individuals are hyperalert to any type of threat, and therefore extreme anxiety would be expected to lower their threshold for the detection of toxins, among other things, resulting in loss of appetite and/or nausea. Haug, Mykletun, and Dahl (2002) conducted a community survey of factors that effect nausea and reported that anxiety disorders were the strongest risk factor for nausea. In addition, it has been found that high anxiety contributes to greater side effects, including more nausea and vomiting, from chemotherapy (Jacobsen et al., 1988) and from the anticipation of chemotherapy (Andrykowski, 1990). In the hypothetical example given above, the person who was very anxious on the third day of his/her chemotherapy may have appraised the procedure as more threatening on that particular day and paid more attention to the procedure and to his/her bodily responses to the chemotherapy drug, in essence, getting caught up in a positive feedback loop that resulted in severe nausea and vomiting.

Expectation

Several studies have found that expectations about nausea prior to initial chemotherapy treatment can lower that individual's nausea threshold and in so doing affect appraisal of the procedure and one's bodily responses (e.g., Haut et al., 1991). This would be predicted by response expectancy theories such as that proposed by Kirsch (1999). Specifically, Kirsch states that if an individual is presented with information that indicates that sickness may result due to exposure to some new stimulus (such as information from clinic staff about potential chemotherapy side effects before the first treatment) and the stimulus exposure itself supports that prediction, then the (nausea) response to the stimulus is likely to be augmented more so than if either the response expectation or the stimulus were not present together. The results of a study by Levine, Stern, and Koch (2006) demonstrate the importance of the strength of the expectation and the strength of the nauseogenic stimulus in determining the results. Prior to being exposed to a rotating optokinetic drum, three groups of subjects were given placebos. One group was told that the pills would reduce nausea, a second group was told that the pills would increase nausea, and a third group was told that the pills were a placebo. The first group reported the same degree of nausea as the placebo-control group. The surprise finding was that the group that was told that the pills would increase their nausea reported significantly less nausea than the other two groups and significantly less of the abnormal gastric activity that usually accompanies nausea. A tentative explanation is that these subjects had a strong negative expectation that was not supported by the actual stimulus; and when their bodily reaction was not very great, the contrast caused an increase in their nausea threshold, an appraisal of the stimulus as not very noxious, and reports of little nausea.

Gianaros et al. (2001) reported that the greater the amount of abnormal gastric activity immediately prior to chemotherapy, the greater the probability that the patient experienced nausea during and/or following the chemotherapy. One interpretation of this finding is that prior to treatment, those subjects who had an expectation of experiencing nausea during chemotherapy had a lowered threshold for nausea. This may have contributed to the abnormal pretreatment gastric activity, to which they paid attention and appraised as evidence of the seriousness of the threat and/or their inability to cope. And this may have led to the development of nausea during their subsequent chemotherapy. This would be another example of nausea resulting from a positive feedback loop. It should be noted that if health care providers are not required to tell patients what side effects they may experience from chemotherapy, they may experience a much lower incidence of nausea than if they are told, according to anecdotal reports in Greek chemotherapy patients compared to U.S. estimates following the same chemotherapy protocols (personal communication; Chief, Oncology Department, Athens Naval Hospital, 1996).

Anticipation

According to Morrow (1993), approximately 25% of cancer patients report nausea in anticipation of chemotherapy following treatment sessions during which they experienced nausea. Anticipatory nausea is thought to be a learned response; it is seldom reported by patients who do not experience nausea during previous treatments. Data tend to support a classical conditioning model with the chemotherapy nurse or the sight or smell of the clinic acting as the conditioned stimulus, the chemotherapy drugs acting as the unconditioned stimulus, and nausea and vomiting being the unconditioned response. Morrow points out that anxiety may play a pivotal role in raising the probability of anticipatory effects prior to subsequent treatment. The precise role of anxiety in increasing anticipatory nausea is not understood at this time, but there are several possible avenues including increasing posttreatment nausea and vomiting (which has been shown to increase subsequent anticipatory nausea), and/or increasing the classical conditioning process by alerting or sensitizing the patient.

Adaptation

Adaptation has been defined by Parker and Parker (1990) "as a semi-permanent change of perception or motor response that serves to reduce or eliminate a perceived discrepancy between or within sensory modalities or the errors in motor acts induced by this discrepancy" (p. 249). Nausea and other symptoms of space motion sickness can be conceptualized as side effects of adaptation to weightlessness as the astronauts adjust to the discrepancy between normal visual function and altered vestibular function, among other sensory conflicts.

Hu et al. (1991) and others have studied the effects of exposing healthy volunteers to sensory conflict in the laboratory several times and observing a decrease in symptoms such as nausea as indications of adaptation. The stimulus situation used was a rotating optokinetic drum, which creates normal vestibular signals in the subject but abnormal and conflicting visual signals. Visually, the participant has the illusion that he/she is rotating and the drum is still. An initial attempt by one of the authors (RMS) to adapt subjects to vection-induced nausea in a rotating optokinetic drum by bringing them back for a second session one week later was a failure. However, comments from two astronauts concerning their pre–space flight training in the KC-135 aircraft, which they refer to as the Vomit Comet, were most helpful. The astronauts indicated that almost everyone gets nauseated and/or vomits the first time they ride in the roller-coaster-like training plane that gives them their first experience of weightlessness; and if they don't get to ride in it again for several days, it is like starting all over and they get sick again. Stern et al. (1989) redesigned their adaptation study in the rotating drum and instead of a 7-day intersession interval, used a 48-hour interval. With the shorter intersession interval, most subjects showed a significant reduction in abnormal gastric electrical activity and symptoms of motion sickness, and by the third session the subjects were practically asymptomatic. Hu and Stern (1999) demonstrated that adaptation to the sensory conflict of a rotating optokinetic drum was completely retained by most subjects for one month and partially retained for one year. And Williamson, Higgins, and Stern (2003) have shown that adaptation to a rotating drum transfers from the laboratory to car sickness. For additional information about the retention and transfer of adaptation to stimulus rearrangements see Parker and Parker (1990).

One of the first attempts to adapt aviators to motion sickness using a ground-based procedure was reported by Popov (1943). He theorized that adapting individuals to strong vestibular signals, such as experienced by regular use of a trampoline and gymnastic exercises, would reduce airsickness.

The U.S. Air Force (Levy, Jones & Carlson, 1981) and the U.S. Navy working together with the United Kingdom Admiralty Research Establishment (Dobie & May, 1994) have developed programs to help pilots in training who would otherwise be disqualified because of their susceptibility to airsickness. One program includes a biofeedback procedure, and the other treatment involves cognitive-behavioral management of motion sickness. Both programs result, when successful, in the individual's gradually adapting to stimuli that had previously made him/her airsick. For a more complete discussion of adaptation to airsickness see Stott (1990).

In conclusion, nausea is a symptom, an unpleasant sensation of a protective mechanism elicited by the interaction of inherent factors and changeable psychological states. Individual differences in the experience of nausea are a function of one's nausea threshold at a certain point in time. Psychological factors such as anxiety, expectation, and anticipation are thought to lower the threshold, and adaptation raises it. It is hypothesized that the threshold changes affect cognitive appraisal of the nauseogenic stimulus and/or the bodily changes that follow exposure to the nauseogenic stimulus; and it is the appraisal that modulates the response to the nauseogenic stimulus. A difficult problem facing health care providers/researchers is how to reduce selectively this very effective protective mechanism, nausea, when it is not needed.

Section II: Physiology of Nausea

Chapter 4

The Central Nervous System and Nausea

The brain can be conceived as being a functionally specialized piece of gut tissue that evolved at the consuming end of the gut as a tool for recognizing food.
—(Max, 1992, p. 18)

INTRODUCTION

"What is the neuroanatomical substrate subserving the subjective sensation of nausea?" This question was posed in a summary of the discussions of a meeting in 1986 on Nausea and Vomiting Mechanisms and Treatment. The authors commented, "there was very little discussion during the meeting about the cause(s) of nausea and even less about its control (Davis et al., 1986)." Unfortunately we still do not have the answer to this question and this hampers the development of treatments that are as effective against nausea as against vomiting; for this reason nausea is often referred to as the "neglected symptom" (Foubert & Vaessen, 2005).

In humans, nausea must, at some point, be an expression of the activation of structures within the brain leading to the genesis of a sensation with qualities different and hence distinguishable from other sensations. The inputs to the brain by which nausea (and vomiting) can be induced are well characterized, but little is known about the way in which the information is processed within the brain leading to the genesis of the sensation itself. There is a paucity of brain imaging studies in humans experiencing nausea, so to obtain an insight into how and where the sensation may be generated we will draw on studies from animals and humans of processing of visceral and vestibular information and studies of neural pathways of conditioned taste aversion in animals, which, arguably, has features in common with nausea (see Chapter 8, in this volume). Comparative studies have identified common features of the pathways processing fundamental sensations such as pain, hunger, and satiety; and if, as we believe, nausea is in the same category, then there should be some common features in processing between species in which we can demonstrate nausea or have a high degree of suspicion that it or some closely analogous sensation is present. However, we must be mindful of substantial differences in cerebral cortical anatomy between primates, cetaceans, and other mammals (Craig, 2009a; 2009b; Dunbar & Shultz, 2007; Marino, 2007;

Craig, 2002; Butler & Hodos, 1996). Knowledge of the brain pathways involved in the genesis of nausea is a critical prerequisite to identification of the neurotransmitters and receptors in the pathway as targets for drugs to alleviate nausea. However, anatomical and physiological studies of the way in which afferent information from the viscera is "processed" centrally have come primarily from studies in the rat (lacking an ability to vomit), cat, dog, and to a lesser extent the ferret and nonhuman primates.

In addition to the conscious sensation aspect of nausea there are also a number of physiological changes mediated by the autonomic nervous system (see Chapter 5, in this volume). Some of these changes can be viewed either as accompanying nausea or as prodromata to vomiting. The central neural control of these changes will be discussed, as, perhaps with the exception of the secretion of vasopressin (see Chapter 6, in this volume) and the changes in the EGG (see Chapter 7, in this volume), although they are not considered to be directly involved in the genesis of the conscious sensation, they may be useful surrogate markers for the presence of nausea in experimental human studies and perhaps some animals. In addition these autonomic responses reflect central nervous system activity and hence provide a window through which the brain can be studied indirectly. The final sections of this chapter discuss some approaches to further study of the central nervous system pathways involved in nausea and evolutionary aspects.

CONVERGENCE AND DIVERGENCE OF PATHWAYS IN THE BRAINSTEM

Convergence in the Nucleus Tractus Solitarius

The three "classical" inputs by which nausea and vomiting can be induced, namely the vestibular system via the vestibular nuclei (Chapter 15, in this volume), the area postrema (Chapter 6, in this volume), and the abdominal and cardiac vagal afferents (Chapter 5, in this volume), all converge in the nucleus tractus solitarius (NTS) in the brainstem. (Note that Saper, 2002, correctly points out that NTS is the abbreviation for *nucleus tracti solitarii*; however, in this book we will use the commonly used but imprecisely translated version "nucleus tractus solitarius.") As the brainstem is the location of the coordinating mechanism for vomiting, it seems probable that vomiting induced by cerebral cortical inputs (e.g., anterior cingulate cortex area 25 and rostral 24; for references see Devinsky, Morrell, & Vogt, 1995) also involves projections to the brainstem. The limbic system (including the cingulate cortex) is known to have a major influence on autonomic nervous system function via inputs to the NTS. The NTS is also the primary projection site for gustatory and other information from the oropharynx (glossopharyngeal, facial, and vagus nerves), although these afferents terminate in the more rostral parts compared to the abdominal vagal afferents, which terminate more caudally in the medial NTS (Loewy, 1990; Berthoud & Neuhuber, 2000). Outputs from the area postrema terminate in the dorsomedial NTS (i.e., the same site as the abdominal vagal afferents) (Figure 4.1). Tract tracing studies in the cat show that the medial and inferior vestibular nuclei project to the middle and lateral regions of the NTS, but electrophysiological studies identified NTS neurons with a convergent vestibular and abdominal vagal afferent input (Yates et al., 1994).

Processing in the Nucleus Tractus Solitarius

The NTS should not be viewed as a "simple brainstem relay nucleus," as a few key facts will serve to illustrate: it is estimated to have over a million synapses in the rat (Andresen & Kunze, 1994); it monitors the major physiological systems (e.g., cardiovascular, respiratory, and gastrointestinal) and has outputs that can eventually influence all major brain regions; and it is neuro-chemically diverse, with well over 40 neuroactive substances and receptors shown to be present (Miller & Leslie, 1994). Although it may be described as an integrative nucleus for visceral information, it is clear that the relevant infor-mation encoded in the original input signals (e.g., from the gut) is conserved and directed to ensure the correct motor or sensory response whether it be gastric relaxation and a sensation of comfortable fullness or nausea and vomit-ing. Relatively little is known of the way in which an input signal, such as that originating from an abdominal vagal afferent, is "processed" during its journey through the NTS to the point where it impinges on a neuron with an output outside the NTS, and even less is known about the neurophysiology of the rela-tionships between the area postrema and the NTS. However, in both cases responses are rapid; abdominal vagal afferent stimulation in the conscious ferret evokes licking and emesis within 10–15 seconds of the onset of high fre-quency stimulation, and a range of intragastric stimuli (e.g., copper sulphate and hypertonic solutions) evoke emesis in ~10 minutes (Andrews et al., 1990b). In humans subcutaneous apomorphine can induce nausea within a minute and vomiting in three minutes (see Figure 4.2; Cannon et al., 1983), a latency for emesis comparable to that in the ferret (Andrews et al., 1990b).

Studies in the dog, investigating the gastrointestinal motility changes prior to and during emesis, revealed that for exemplar agents acting via the abdominal vagal afferents (intragastric copper sulphate) and the area postrema (apomorphine), the dose required to evoke the motility changes was lower than that for induction of vomiting (Lang & Marvig, 1989). These observations provide additional support that the motor response required is encoded in the original signal originating from the vagal afferents and area postrema projected to the NTS.

Information processing in the NTS is not fixed, as its own synapses show plasticity (Chen & Bonham, 2005) and the NTS receives descending modula-tory inputs from more rostral brain structures such as the vestibular nuclei, hypothalamus, and limbic system (see below). There is some evidence that the blood-brain barrier may be "leaky" in the NTS itself (Gross et al., 1990), but irrespective of this the projection of NTS dendrites into the area postrema

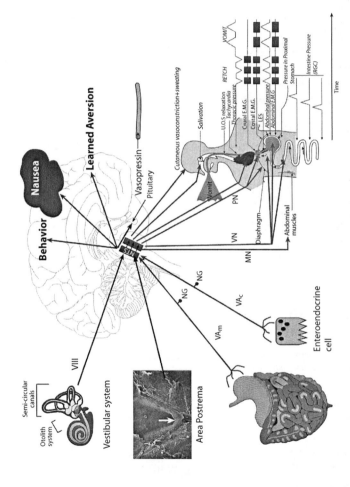

Figure 4.1 A diagrammatic summary of the main afferent pathways capable of inducing nausea and vomiting converging on the nucleus tractus solitarius (NTS): Vestibular system (semicircular canals and otoliths via cranial nerve VIII and the vestibular nucleus); area postrema and the abdominal vagal afferents (VA_M-vagal afferent mechanoreceptors, VA_C-vagal afferent mucosal chemoreceptors, NG-nodose ganglion). The NTS sends outputs to the major motor nuclei (located in the more ventral parts of the brainstem; motor nuclei such as the ventral respiratory group (VRG), Bötzinger neurons, presympathetic neurons) responsible for the mechanical events of retching and vomiting [e.g., VN-abdominal vagus nerve from dorsal motor vagal nucleus mediating lower esophageal sphincter (LES) relaxation, gastric relaxation and giant retrograde contraction of the small intestine; P-phrenic nerve with nuclei in C_3–C_5 driven from VRG; MN-spinal motor neurons], the prodromata of vomiting often associated with nausea (mediated by sympathetic and parasympathetic nerves) and the rostral projections (predominantly via the parabrachial nucleus [PBN]) leading to vasopressin secretion (hypothalamus–posterior pituitary) and the more complex responses requiring cerebral cortical involvement including the genesis of the sensation of nausea itself. UOS-upper esophageal sphincter; EMG-electromyogram. See text for details.

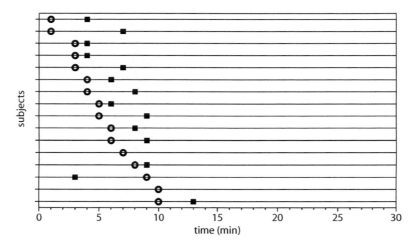

Figure 4.2 Time to the onset of nausea (circles) or vomiting (squares) in 15 healthy volunteers who received apomorphine (0.03 mg/kg sc.). The study by Cannon et al., 1983 also included three subjects who did not respond to apomorphine and are not shown in this figure. Note the rapid onset of the responses and that nausea usually precedes vomiting by a few minutes. In one subject vomiting preceded nausea and in two subjects only nausea was evoked by apomorphine. Replotted from data in Fig. 26.2, Lee & Feldman, 1983.

(Morest, 1960) as well as the inputs from the area postrema itself make it likely that its function may also be modulated by systemic factors (e.g., hormones from the gut). The extent of the connectivity between the area postrema and the nuclei in the dorsal brainstem should not be underestimated, as the area postrema also sends outputs to the dorsal motor vagal nucleus, the dorsal nucleus of the spinal trigeminal tract, and the lateral parabrachial nucleus (Shapiro & Miselis, 1985). Lawes (1991) has proposed that the area postrema is a component of a system of interconnected paraventricular nuclei located within two principal synapses of the area postrema and which are broadly involved in protecting the organism from noxious stimuli, particularly those related to ingestion. This anatomically defined system of interconnected nuclei extends from the forebrain to the hindbrain and includes nuclei in the brain stem (e.g., NTS, DMVN) involved in the autonomic and somatic motor components of vomiting, hypothalamic nuclei (e.g., supraoptic and paraventricular) involved in the endocrine response to nauseogenic and emetic stimuli, and the central nucleus of the amygdala implicated in conditioned taste aversion.

There is a wealth of evidence that transmission through the NTS is subject to substantial modulation by systemic agents including gut hormones, descending neural inputs, primary afferent inputs, and transmitters released within the NTS itself (Chen & Bonham, 2005; Travagli et al., 2006). In view of this it is therefore reasonable to postulate that the NTS (or the parabrachial nucleus, see below) may "gate" the onward transmission of information, and it is this that determines whether nausea will be induced. It is interesting to note that Borison and Wang (1953) commented on the possibility that "nausea represents the conscious awareness of certain subcortical autonomic processes." Limited evidence for the presence of intrinsic pathways capable of modulating the processing of emetic inputs comes from observations of either the induction or enhancement of emetic responses by antagonists of particular receptors and also by the antiemetic effects of some receptor agonists. For example, in animal models the opioid receptor antagonist naloxone can induce emesis as well as potentiate the emetic responses to apomorphine, cisplatin, and intragastric copper sulphate (Rudd & Naylor, 1995; Rudd et al., 1999) and reduce the threshold for the dose of an agent required to induce emesis (Lang & Marvig, 1989). Feeding in the Siberian tiger (*Pantheria tigris altaica*) is reduced by naloxone, and emesis ensues when novel food is paired with naloxone (Billington et al., 1985). In humans naloxone has been shown to enhance the emetic response in patients undergoing chemotherapy and the apomorphine-induced nausea score in volunteers (Kobrinsky, 1988; Kobrinsky et al., 1988) as well as reduce the latency to induce the symptoms of motion sickness (Allen et al., 1986). These observations are consistent with the relatively broad spectrum, antiemetic effects of selective opioid receptor agonists (Rudd & Naylor, 1995; Rudd et al., 1999). Similarly, there is evidence that cannabinoid$_1$ (CB$_1$) receptor agonists have antiemetic effects and that CB$_1$ receptor antagonists can induce emesis (Darmani, 2001) and enhance emetic responses in animal models (Van Sickle et al., 2001; 2003), although there are some potential issues concerning the pharmacological properties of one of the agents used. A low incidence of nausea has been reported as the main adverse event in one study of the appetite-suppressing effect of a CB$_1$ receptor antagonist (Rimonabant) in obese patients (Pi-Sunyer et al., 2006). Other agonists shown to have antiemetic effects act at the 5-HT$_{1A}$, GABA$_B$, and ghrelin receptors (see Sanger & Andrews, 2006 for references). The site(s) at which these various agents are acting to modulate the emetic pathways has not been identified but has been argued to be the NTS because of the location of receptors/transmitters and also of evidence from general electrophysiological studies of the NTS. These limited studies establish that in principle the emetic pathways are subject to modulation and provide a theoretical basis for proposing that the rostral projection of information from the NTS may be subject to "gating" and this could be a determinant of the occurrence of nausea (cf., descending modulation of pain pathways).

Divergence and NTS Outputs

If the NTS is the major nucleus where the emetic inputs converge, then it follows that the outputs from the NTS must be responsible—either directly or indirectly—for the induction of both nausea and vomiting. A question that arises from this is, "where do the pathways responsible for nausea and vomiting diverge?" The answer to this question has a practical implication, as the divergence point would theoretically be the last point at which a single drug could be targeted to affect both nausea *and* vomiting.

Based on the observation that the entire neural circuitry required for coordinating the autonomic and somatic motor outputs required for prodromata, retching, and vomiting are located in the brainstem, whereas for induction of nausea and the associated release of vasopressin (AVP) into the blood a rostral projection of signals to "higher" regions of the brain is required, the divergence is most likely to occur in the NTS itself, although the parabrachial nucleus should not be excluded. It should be noted that this view is most easily supported in relation to nausea and vomiting induced by vagal afferent and area postrema activation. As for nausea induced by cerebral inputs, olfactory stimuli, and the vestibular system a case can be made that the brainstem may not be involved in the genesis of the sensation, although it is needed for prodromata because of the requirement to connect with the autonomic efferents arising from the brain stem and spinal cord. However, for vomiting induced by the same inputs the brainstem is essential. Even in the case of inputs to the area postrema, its direct connections to the lateral parabrachial nucleus (Shapiro & Miselis, 1985) could be involved in the rostral projection of signals relating to nausea as opposed to vomiting, which would be via the NTS projection.

The next sections examine in more detail how the outputs from the NTS could lead to either nausea or vomiting. The NTS sends projections to 25 other brain nuclei or regions (for reviews and references for the summary below, see Loewy, 1990b; Leslie, Reynolds & Lawes, 1992; Saper, 2002), but the extensive influence of the NTS outputs can be grouped as follows:

- Autonomic motor nuclei in the brainstem (dorsal motor vagal nucleus-DMVN, nucleus ambiguus-NA) and spinal cord (intermediolateral horn-ILH), cranial nerve nuclei (V, VII, IX), and the nucleus ambiguus innervating the pharyngeal striated muscle. It is these outputs that are primarily responsible for the autonomic and somatic motor events of vomiting and its prodromata, including events more associated with nausea, such as cold sweating. These outputs are discussed primarily in the section on the brain-stem pathway involved in vomiting.
- Rostral nuclei involved in the processing of visceral and gustatory information such as the lateral parabrachial nucleus (Saper, 2002) and the A1 catecholaminergic cell groups (Harris & Loewy, 1990). The parabrachial nucleus is the major nucleus at which the primary outputs from the NTS terminate and as a consequence is also the main relay for the projection of information received by the NTS to "higher" nuclei.
- Forebrain structures involved in endocrine functions including the multiple hypothalamic subnuclei such as the paraventricular nucleus involved in vasopressin secretion (Harris & Loewy, 1990) and limbic

system nuclei including the central nucleus of the amygdala involved in behavioral responses (Cechetto & Saper, 1990).
- Cortical structures presumed to be involved in "interoception" (e.g., anterior insula) (Loewy, 1990b).

Central Pathways for Vomiting

The pathways for coordinating the motor outputs responsible for retching and vomiting as well as the autonomic changes that precede and accompany these events are all in the brain stem. Thus retching and vomiting as well as prodromata such as swallowing, licking, and salivation can be elicited in decerebrate animals such as the dog, cat, ferret, and *Suncus* (see Figure 4.3). Chronically decerebrate rats will exhibit the same orofacial behavioral rejection

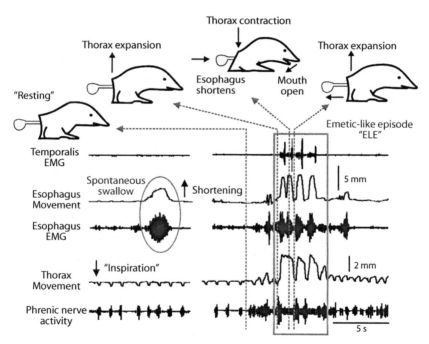

Figure 4.3 Swallowing and "emesis" in an arterially perfused decerebrate preparation of *Suncus murinus* (house musk shrew). Records show the overall posture of the animal (upper row), efferent activity in the phrenic nerve, electrical activity recorded from temporalis and esophageal muscle, and thoracic movement. The left-hand panel shows activity during a spontaneous swallow (note that the activity is confined to the esophagus) and the right-hand panel shows an "emetic-like episode" evoked by the VR1 receptor agonist resiniferatoxin (40 nM) added to the perfusate. Note the activity in the temporalis muscle associated with mouth opening, the rhythmic contraction and expansion of the thorax, and change in phrenic nerve activity, both of which begin before esophageal shortening is recorded. Redrawn with permission from data in Smith, Paton, and Andrews, 2002.

sequences in responses to oral application of quinine as do intact rats (see Grill, 1985 for review), although decerebrate rats do not demonstrate "bait shyness" (Grill & Norgren, 1978a; 1978b). The brain stem contains the pathways required for this gustatory rejection response (Travers & Travers, 2005), as is the case for vomiting (in emetic species), but both nausea and conditioned taste aversion require the presence of more rostral brain structures. Anencephalic newborn humans also show orofacial rejection responses to unpleasant substances placed on the tongue as is also the case for healthy newborns (Steiner, 1973).

The brain-stem pathways coordinating the diverse motor output pathways involved in retching and vomiting have mainly been studied in decerebrate paralyzed dogs, cats, and ferrets (Fukuda et al., 2003; Onishi et al., 2007; Grelot & Miller, 1997) with the pathways being similar among these species. Isolated studies in patients with discrete lesions involving the dorsal vagal complex, e.g., metastatic malignant melanoma (Baker & Bernat, 1985), astrocytoma (Wood et al., 1985), and CNS lupus (Sawai et al., 2006), where nausea and vomiting are prominent symptoms, indicates that the same dorsal brain-stem pathways are involved in humans. However, it is not known whether the neurotransmitters/cotransmitters and receptor types and their distribution are the same in the animal species as in humans at each site in the pathway. Such differences could contribute to some of the difficulties in translation of results from animal to human studies investigating antiemetics or identification of substances with emetic liability (Holmes et al., 2009, and Chapter 8, in this volume).

The NTS is at a focal point receiving direct inputs from the main pathways capable of induction of vomiting, namely, the abdominal and cardiac vagal afferents, the area postrema, and the vestibular nuclei as well as indirect inputs from "higher" brain regions (see below). The NTS can access all the relevant motor nuclei responsible for the mechanical events of retching and vomiting as well as the prodromal and accompanying signs mediated largely by the autonomic nervous system (see Chapter 5, in this volume). The major brain-stem nuclei/regions and their outflows together with the major motor events are summarized as follows:

- *Dorsal motor vagal nucleus* (DMVN). The DMVN provides the main vagal outflow (Loewy, 1990a) to the lower esophagus (longitudinal shortening), lower esophageal sphincter (relaxes), proximal stomach (relaxes), and the small intestine (retrograde giant contraction). There is also some evidence from the ferret that the DMVN may also be involved in the inhibition of the crural diaphragm (Niedringhaus et al., 2008a; 2008b).
- *Superior and inferior salivatory nuclei.* These nuclei located in the ventrolateral medulla dorsal to the facial nucleus are the source of the facial (VII) and glossopharyngeal (IX) outflows driving salivation (Loewy, 1990a). Sympathetic efferents originating in the spinal cord are also involved, driven from the brain stem.

- *Nucleus ambiguus.* This also provides a vagal outflow and sends projections to the striated muscle of the pharynx (upper esophageal sphincter inhibition), larynx and the esophagus (longitudinal shortening), and the heart (tachycardia by reduced vagal drive) (Loewy, 1990a).
- *Rostral ventrolateral medulla.* This is the site of origin of the presympathetic neurons projecting to the spinal cord to synapse with the preganglionic sympathetic outflows originating in the intermediolateral cell column supplying the heart (tachycardia), the arterioles (vasoconstriction), sweat glands (sudomotor responses), and adrenal medulla (adrenaline secretion) (Loewy, 1990b).
- *Retrofacial nucleus and the ventral respiratory group.* These are the major sites regulating the spinal outputs to the diaphragm (phrenic nerve) and abdominal muscles (abdominal motor neurons) that provide the major force for the oral expulsion of the contents of the stomach (vomiting). Fukuda et al. (2003) have provided evidence from studies in dogs and ferrets (Onishi et al., 2007) for a central pattern generator (CPG) in the region of the retrofacial nucleus. It is proposed that when the CPG receives an appropriate emetic input from the NTS via a 'prodromal sign center' located in the reticular area dorsally adjacent to the semicompact part of the nucleus ambiguus, it coordinates the outputs from the premotor nuclei (Bötzinger complex, pre-Bötzinger complex, ventral respiratory group) supplying the phrenic nerve nucleus (spinal cord C3, 4, 5) and the abdominal motor neurons. In addition to these well-known outflows, neurons in the ventral respiratory group project to the sacral spinal cord, where they are proposed to be involved in pudendal motorneuron-mediated tightening of the urethral and anal sphincters during vomiting (Miller et al., 1995).

The coordination of the entire motor act of retching and vomiting is impressive, with gastric relaxation preceding the occurrence of the retrograde giant contraction, which in turn must reach the stomach before retching can commence (see Chapter 5, in this volume). The primary differences between retching and vomiting apart from the expulsion of the gastric contents are the intensity of diaphragm and abdominal muscle activation and the inhibition of the contraction of the crural fibers of the diaphragm (contributing to the esophageal antireflux barrier) to facilitate expulsion during the vomit (see Figure 4.1). The coordination is particularly impressive when the speed with which these events take place is considered, especially in small mammals such as the house musk shrew with a retching frequency of ~ 4 Hz (Andrews et al., 1996). Preliminary studies in the ferret indicate that the gastric volume is inversely related to the number of retches that precede a vomit, but further studies are required (Andrews et al., 1990a). Additional studies are needed to understand fully the coordinating mechanism and especially the neurotransmitters involved in the outputs from the NTS and in the CPG itself, as these sites would be logical targets for pharmacological intervention with the expectation of efficacy against vomiting induced by activation of diverse inputs.

The brain-stem pathways enabling vomiting are highly conserved. In mammals the act of vomiting involves coordination between motor activity in the gastrointestinal tract and the respiratory system, with the diaphragm providing the major propulsive force. This interaction is facilitated by the proximity and connectivity in the brainstem of the relevant nuclei. Such an interaction between the respiratory and gastrointestinal systems is also required for the act of vomiting in "lower" vertebrates such as fish and amphibians (see Chapter 8, in this volume), but in these cases the gastrointestinal tract plays more of an active role in the expulsion of gut contents.

CENTRAL PATHWAYS FOR NAUSEA

This section reviews the projections from the NTS to the "higher" regions of the brain in an attempt to identify where the sensation of nausea may be generated. The approach used is to compare knowledge of anatomical pathways with information from animal studies investigating patterns of Fos expression in response to emetic and other stimuli. The brain pathways involved in conditioned taste aversion in the rat have been relatively well studied, and in view of the parallels between this phenomenon and nausea (see Chapter 8, in this volume) these studies provide useful additional information. We will initially focus on the outputs from the NTS, but will return to the issue of whether these are the only routes by which nausea can be induced. For simplicity we will review three aspects separately: (1) Endocrine and other effects mediated via the hypothalamic nuclei; (2) Lessons from conditioned taste aversion; and (3) Higher projections of visceral afferent information.

Endocrine and Other Effects Mediated Via the Hypothalamic Nuclei

As is discussed in Chapter 6 (in this volume), a rise in plasma vasopressin (AVP) has been shown to be produced by a range of emetic stimuli acting via the vagal afferents, the area postrema, and the vestibular system. The origin of the vasopressin is the posterior pituitary via activation of the hypothalamic paraventricular and supraoptic nuclei. Electrical stimulation of the abdominal vagal afferents and apomorphine stimulates the secretion of plasma vasopressin in anesthetized ferrets (Hawthorn et al., 1988) (see Figure 6.6, p. 132); thus, consciousness is not a requirement for this response, at least via the vagus and the area postrema. In the ferret, utilizing CCK and lithium chloride, stimuli argued to evoke behavioral signs of nausea, Billig, Yates, and Rinaman (2001) reported an increase in Fos expression in the neurons in the dorsal vagal complex (including the AP, NTS, and DMVN) with a population of the Fos positive neurons also being positive for tyrosine hydroxylase (catecholaminergic) or glucagon-like peptide-1 (GLP-1). Increased Fos labeling was also demonstrated in the paraventricular nucleus (PVN-medial parvocellular, lateral and medial magnocellular [sends axons to the posterior pituitary], and posterior) with a high proportion of the Fos positive neurons shown to be either AVP or oxytocin positive. The supraoptic nucleus (SON) also showed an increase in Fos positive neurons, and again these were shown to be either vasopressin (AVP) or oxytocin (OT) positive. In the rat, lithium chloride has been shown to increase the number of Fos positive neurons in the NTS (Olson et al., 1993) as well as in the SON and PVN, with many other cells being either oxytocin or vasopressin positive (Olszewski et al., 2000). The increase in plasma oxytocin concentration induced by intraperitoneal lithium chloride in the rat is not affected by area postrema ablation (Curtis et al., 1994), supporting an involvement of the abdominal visceral afferents in this response. The anorectic response to lithium chloride was still present in the area pos-trema–ablated animals, but the conditioned taste aversion response was abolished (Curtis et al., 1994). Gastric distension in the rat has also been shown to increase the number of Fos positive neurons in the AP, NTS, SON, and PVN, with the number of Fos positive neurons in all regions markedly reduced by vagotomy, perivagal capsaicin, or systemic (but not intracere-broventricular, i.c.v.) granisetron (a 5-HT$_3$ receptor antagonist; Mazda et al., 2004). Fluorogold labeling was used to demonstrate that Fos expressing neurons in the NTS projected to the PVN. A "minimally injurious" concentration of hydrochloric acid in the stomach increased Fos expression in the NTS, SON, and PVN (Michl et al., 2001) and intragastric administration of the "bitter" T2R taste receptor agonist denatonium to rats increased Fos expression in the visceral region of the NTS and the hypothalamic paraventricular nucleus (Hao, Sternini, & Raybould, 2008). A small increase in Fos expression was reported in the parvocellular and magnocellular regions of the PVN but not in the SON of rats treated six hours earlier with a relatively high dose of cisplatin (Horn, Ciucci & Chaudhury, 2007). It should be noted that this study also found evidence for large decreases in Fos activation at lower doses and at different time points following the same stimulus so some caution needs to be exerted in extrapolating from one stimulus to another.

In this context the main projection route from the NTS to the hypothalamus is by projections from the lateral parabrachial nucleus which receives the major output from the visceroceptive portion of the NTS (Saper, 2002). This route is of particular interest because one of the two output pathways from the area postrema is to the lateral parabrachial nucleus, the other is to the NTS (Miller & Leslie, 1994). The ferret study of lithium chloride and CCK by Billig, Yates, and Rinaman (2001) reported Fos expression in the parabrachial nucleus as did a rat study using lithium chloride (St Andre, Albanos & Reilly, 2007), the intragastric denatonium study in the rat described above (Hao, Sternini & Raybould, 2008), and a study of cisplatin in *Suncus* (De Jonghe & Horn, 2009). Overall the parabrachial nucleus located in the pons is regarded as the "second" major brain-stem relay nucleus, with the NTS being the first.

The above studies are consistent with the hypothesis that stimuli acting either via the abdominal vagus or the area postrema to induce "nausea" or conditioned taste aversion activate the hypothalamic SON/PVN via projections from the NTS and parabrachial nucleus. It must be noted that increased Fos expression in the SON/PVN is not specific for emetic stimuli but that such changes also occur in response to pain, immobilization stress, and—less surprisingly—osmotic challenge (Pacak & Palkovits, 2001).

In addition to the brain stem and hypothalamic structures shown to be activated by stimuli inducing "nausea" or CTA, Fos expression studies have shown increased labeling in the central nucleus of the amygdala and the bed nucleus of stria terminalis (BNST) (Olson et al., 1993; Billig, Yates & Rinaman, 2001; Horn, Ciucci & Chaudhury, 2007; St Andre, Albanos & Reilly, 2007; De Jonghe & Horn, 2009). The Fos response to cisplatin measured in the rat six hours after administration was reduced by abdominal vagotomy in the caudal and middle NTS and the central nucleus of the amygdala but not in the rostral NTS, the area postrema, or the SON/PVN (Horn, 2009).

Although the focus of the above discussion was primarily to review evidence for a brain stem-to-hypothalamic pathway involved in the elevated plasma AVP seen in emetic species and OT in the rat in response to emetic/CTA-inducing stimuli, it is important to appreciate that not all neurons in the SON and PVN project to the posterior pituitary and are involved in regulation of the plasma levels of OT and AVP. For example parvicellular PVN neurons produce corticotrophin-releasing hormone (CRH), which via the hypophyseal portal system regulates ACTH secretion (Nussey & Whitehead, 2001) and parvicellular PVN neurons influence the autonomic outflows via descending projections to the brain stem (e.g., NTS, DMVN, NA, parabrachial nucleus, locus coeruleus) and the spinal cord (van der Kooy et al., 1984; Willet et al., 1987; Loewy, 1990). The PVN together with the lateral hypothalamus is also involved in control of food intake. The parvicellular PVN also sends ascending projections to the amygdala (Loewy, 1990), providing a substrate for an involvement in aversive responses.

The hypothalamus in general and the PVN in particular are in a pivotal position to regulate the key physiological changes observed in a subject experiencing nausea: reduction/cessation of food intake (Berthoud, 2008); elevation of plasma AVP (OT in rat) and ACTH (see Chapter 6, in this volume); and modulation of autonomic outflow, especially that to the sympathetic system (ILH of spinal cord: adrenaline secretion, vasoconstriction, see Chapter 5, in this volume). Thus while some of the events such as salivation, gastric relaxation, and retrograde giant contraction of the small intestine (see Chapter 5, in this volume) can be mediated purely by brain-stem pathways, the endocrine and anorectic effects reflect an involvement of the hypothalamus.

Lessons from Conditioned Taste Aversion

Conditioned taste aversion (CTA) is argued to be a model for the study of nausea in rodent species lacking the vomiting reflex (see Chapter 8, in this volume, for detailed discussion). In an experimental setting, the formation of CTA usually requires a temporal linkage of information regarding the taste of a substance (conditioned stimulus) with a perception of visceral malaise ("nausea"—unconditioned response) caused by an illness-inducing substance (unconditioned stimulus). This linkage leads the animal to avoid the conditioned stimulus if exposed in the future, and if tested it should show aversive (rejection) behaviors if it is placed in the mouth. In the rat, according to Parker (2006), while conditioned taste avoidance can be induced by "*almost any substance that changes a rat's physiological state*," the aversive response is only induced by substances with the potential to induce emesis in responsive species . These learned avoidance and aversive responses when related to food would have survival value in the wild and in this context requires activation of the gustatory pathway and visceral malaise ("nausea") pathways and a convergence of the information at some point for the linkage to be made. There are striking parallels between the pathways involved in processing the two sets of information (Saper, 2002). Gustatory afferents from the tongue and oral cavity project predominantly to the more rostral parts of the NTS via the chorda tympani (VII), lingual (glossopharyngeal, IX), and superior laryngeal (vagal, X) nerves (Loewy, 1990). From the NTS the major projection is to the medial parabrachial nucleus, also known as the "pontine taste area." From here the major projection is to the medial part of the ventroposterior parvicellular nucleus of the thalamus (VPpc, also known as the ventroposterior medial parvicellular nucleus, VPMpc) with less substantial projections to the lateral and paraventricular hypothalamus, bed nucleus of stria terminalis, substantia innominata, and the central nucleus of the amygdala. The primary output from the VPMpc is to the dysgranular insular cortex and in the rat is the location of the primary gustatory cortex (Saper, 2002), but in gyrencephalic animals it is located in the ventral part of the parietal lobe along the banks of the lateral sulcus (Brodmann's area 43). The parabrachial nucleus also sends a direct projection (i.e., not via the thalamus) to the cortex; but, in contrast to those projecting via the indirect route, they terminate in the agranular (not dysgranular) and lateral prefrontal cortex (Saper, 2002). Saper (2002) argues that as these neurons do not respond to specific visceral stimuli, this pathway may be more involved in behavioral responses to food rather than visceral sensation.

There are reciprocal connections between all the key nuclei such that the insular cortex sends outputs (direct and indirect) to subcortical (e.g., central nucleus of the amygdala, lateral hypothalamus, parabrachial nucleus, NTS) structures enabling modulation of ascending information and also autonomic outflows (Loewy, 1990; Cechetto & Saper, 1990).

Lesioning studies in the rat have shown that neither the basolateral amygdala nor the central nucleus of the amygdala is required for the induction of conditioned disgust/aversive reactions (to lithium chloride); the taste avoidance response induced by lithium was reduced by lesions of the basolateral amygdala but not the central nucleus of the amygdala (Rana & Parker, 2008). In addition, rats with lesion of the gustatory (insular) cortex could learn to avoid drinking fluids previously paired with lithium but did not show aversive/disgust reactions to the fluids when placed in the mouth (Kiefer & Orr, 1992). This finding is similar to the results of another study which reported in addition that the increase in Fos expression in the intermediate region of the NTS that accompanies the formation of CTA was reduced (Schafe & Bernstein, 1998). It is worth noting that the intermediate region of the NTS has been proposed to be involved in the hedonic (aversion and reward) aspects of taste, whereas the rostral part deals with the sensory aspects (Sewards, 2004). Furthermore it is argued that this separation is reflected in the entire pathway through the parabrachial nucleus, thalamus, and gustatory cortex. Overall, it appears that while learned avoidance responses involve subcortical structures (e.g., basolateral amygdala), for learned aversive/disgust responses cortical structures are required.

The above description of pathways relevant to CTA is based primarily on the rat, and it must be noted that in primates a secondary cortical taste area is located in the orbitofrontal cortex, which is also the location of the secondary olfactory cortex (see below; Rolls, 2004). This region, in addition to having neurons responding to the classical taste stimuli (bitter, salt, sweet, sour), also has neurons responding to the taste of glutamate (produces the umami taste in humans), texture, and astringency of food. The latter may be of particular relevance as astringent and bitter tastes in primates evoke a gustofacial rejection reflex that is considered to be an adaptive response to avoiding foods with low nutritional value or that are toxic (Hladik & Chivers, 1994). It is argued that the "reward value" of taste is represented in the orbitofrontal cortex of primates, and furthermore this region receives convergent olfactory and visual inputs. Lesion of this area also alters food preferences (Rolls, 2004).

Returning to the detailed information available from the rat, there are striking parallels between the processing of gustatory information and that arising from the visceral afferent inputs to the NTS and the AP. The major route for projection of visceral afferent information to the cerebral cortex is as follows: visceral afferents terminate in the NTS, projections to the parabrachial nucleus, then to the ventroposterior thalamus (VPpc), and finally to the dysgranular and granular parts of the anterior insular cortex ("primary interoceptive /visceral cortex"). In rats, malaise induced by acute lithium chloride administration was associated with an increased Fos expression in the insular cortex, and inactivation of this region reduced the signs of malaise induced by the lithium (Contreras, Ceric & Torrealba, 2007). Nausea and vomiting can be relatively common side effects of lithium therapy in humans (Yung, 1984). Other central projections shared by the two pathways include the lateral and PVN hypothalamus, bed nucleus of stria terminalis, and the central nucleus of the amygdala. The granular part of the insular cortex also has major projections to broadly the same subcortical structures as the dysgranular ("gustatory") region including the amygdala (basolateral), except that the "gustatory" insular cortex projects to the "gustatory" (rostral) region of the NTS, whereas the "visceral" insular cortex projects to the "visceral" (more caudal) region of the NTS (Loewy, 1990b).

From the above outline it is clear that there are multiple opportunities for the convergence between gustatory and visceral information (i.e., the CS and the US) required for the formation of CTA. Apart from the close proximity of the termination of gustatory and abdominal visceral (vagal afferent) information in the insula (i.e., dysgranular and granular), neurons responding to both inputs have been reported in this region (Saper, 2002). In addition, descending pathways from the insula are available for the animal to mount the appropriate behavioral, autonomic, and endocrine responses.

Studies of glucagon-like peptide-1 (GLP-1) provide further insights into the pathways involved in the formation of CTA and the reduction in food intake associated with visceral illness which in some settings may itself be an indicator of nausea (see Chapter 8, this volume). Injection of GLP-1 into the hypothalamic PVN reduced food intake in the rat, but this was not the case when it was injected directly into the central nucleus of the amygdala (Kinzig, D'Alessio & Seeley, 2002; McMahon & Wellman, 1997). Conversely GLP-1 administration into the hypothalamus did not induce CTA, whereas it was possible to induce CTA by GLP-1 injection into the amygdala when it was paired with a flavor. Furthermore, a GLP-1 antagonist injected into the amygdala reduced the CTA induced by lithium chloride (Kinzig, D'Alessio & Seeley, 2002). The latter has also been demonstrated with injection of a glutamate receptor antagonist (MK-801) into the amygdala (Tucci, Rada & Hernandez, 1998) and depletion of noradrenaline in the basolateral amygdala (Borsini & Rolls, 1984). The GLP-1 study provides evidence for a separation of the sites involved in visceral illness (central nucleus of the amygdala) and anorexia (hypothalamus and brain stem). Furthermore, the studies are consistent with earlier electrolytic lesion studies which showed that bilateral lesion of the amygdala in the rat prevented the acquisition of CTA as well as the expression of the associated fos-like immunoreactivity in the intermediate NTS (Schafe & Bernstein, 1998). Reversible blockade of the amygdala by local injection of tetrodotoxin provides further evidence that the amygdala is required for the acquisition rather than expression of CTA (Roldan & Bures, 1994).

In summary, lesions to either the insular cortex or the amygdala can prevent the acquisition of CTA (rat). The most likely pathway is that different regions of the insular cortex receive information on both the taste of a substance and on any gut inputs indicating "visceral malaise" that occurs contemporaneously, with this information being passed to the amygdala, which, via its outputs to the hypothalamus, the brain stem, and the cortex (e.g., cingulate cortex) mediates the endocrine, autonomic responses, and behavioral responses to illness.

The nature of the conscious perception of visceral events will be discussed in the concluding part of this chapter, but two related aspects will be highlighted here. First, it is not necessary for the animal (rat) to be conscious when the illness-inducing agent is administered for an aversion to be acquired (Garcia, Hankins & Rusiniak, 1974). This observation may also be used to argue that even awake animals (as exemplified by the rat) do not need to be consciously aware of the visceral malaise for either the formation of the aversion or for the genesis of the associated endocrine, autonomic, and behavioral responses. Second, in species where conditioned taste aversion paradigms have been used for predation control such as in coyotes, we need to consider what occurs when the animal encounters the prey to which it has been averted. Coyotes fed meals of lamb (flesh, skin, and wool) laced with lithium chloride eventually "ran away from the lambs and retched" (Garcia, Hankins & Rusiniak, 1974). Was this response an "automatic" one triggered by the smell/taste of lamb, or did the smell/taste of lamb trigger the conscious recall of a memory of an unpleasant experience?

Higher Projections of Visceral Afferent Information

The level of the brain at which the afferent signals evoke a conscious sensation recognizable as nausea is not known, but it is likely to be at sites in the telencephalon, although diencephalic structures such as the thalamus cannot be excluded. This section will review pathways by which visceral afferent information and information from other structures involved in nausea and vomiting, such as the vestibular and olfactory systems, can also access these structures. This analysis is intended to illustrate the available substrates based on knowledge of pathways (mainly animals) and limited imaging studies in humans. Studies of pain pathways in humans have also drawn attention to the importance of descending modulation (via the periaqueductal gray), anticipation of, and attention to, aversive stimuli (Van Oudenhove, Coen & Aziz, 2007). It is likely that similar factors are also involved in the "nausea pathway(s)."

Studies primarily in the rat, cat, and more recently monkey show that the major projection route for visceral afferent information from the brain stem (NTS, PBN) is to the insular cortex (granular region) either directly or indirectly via routes including the hypothalamus or the ventroposterior parvicellular thalamic nucleus (VPpc). Electrophysiological studies have also shown a vagal afferent projection to the primary somatosensory cortex (S1) in the rat, but in the cat a projection was demonstrated to cortical area 3a but not 3b, which is equivalent to S1 (Ito & Craig, 2003). Ito and Craig (2003) propose that 3a, the cingulate cortex, and the insular cortex comprise a "visceral afferent cortical network" with the data from the cat being supported by brain imaging studies in humans (see below). The insular cortex also receives inputs from the basolateral amygdaloid nucleus and the infralimbic cortex (Cechetto & Saper, 1990). The insula sends outputs to the amygdala, hypothalamus, PAG, and brainstem and via these connections is able to initiate and modulate autonomic outflows.

An extensive study of electrical stimulation of the forebrain in macaque monkeys identified a number of sites from which vomiting could be induced (Robinson & Mishkin, 1968). The authors comment that the onset of vomiting was "heralded by the animal becoming quiet, pale, and sweaty" and "animals who did vomit usually presented a prodromal phase of pallor, increased salivation, quietness, and *the appearance of nausea*" (our italics). The regions from which vomiting was most reliably induced were the amygdala, the nucleus ventralis anterior of the thalamus, anterior perforated area, and the hippocampus. Although this study does not provide evidence that stimulation of these structures can induce the sensation of nausea, it does show that vomiting and some of the autonomic prodromata can be evoked from "higher" regions of the brain from structures implicated in the processing of visceral afferent information. Arguably the observed quiescence is an indication that the animals became aware of an altered internal state.

Brain imaging studies in humans that have involved painful and nonpainful stimulation of the gastrointestinal tract (usually esophagus and rectum/anal canal) provide some insights into the pathways which may be involved in humans although such studies have not had nausea as a primary focus (Aziz et al., 2000; Kern & Shaker 2002; Derbyshire, 2003; Elke et al., 2003; Stephan et al., 2005; Dunckley et al., 2005; Lawal et al., 2005; Vandenbergh et al., 2005; Coen et al., 2007; Ladabaum, Roberts & McGonigle, 2007). Overall, these studies have shown an involvement in humans of the same major nuclei, such as the parabrachial nucleus, hypothalamus, thalamus, cingulate cortex, and insular cortex, as have been implicated in visceral afferent processing in animals. In humans the thalamic projections are to the cortical "visceral sensory/ pain neuromatrix" (Van Oudenhove, Coen & Aziz, 2007). This terminology encompasses several cortical structures activated by visceral afferents: SI/SII somatosensory cortices, cingulate cortex ("limbic motor cortex"), insular cortex ("limbic sensory cortex"), prefrontal cortex (orbitofrontal cortex, dorsolateral prefrontal cortex). These regions are variously responsible for processing the sensory, cognitive, and emotional components of the response to painful visceral stimulation (Coen et al., 2007). Attention has focused on the insula, which is not a pain specific region, although the anterior region has been implicated in the emotional response to visceral pain (Coen et al., 2007). It has been termed the "interoceptive cortex" and, as was described above, has been identified in animal tract tracing studies as the major cortical site to which visceral afferent (including vagal) information projects. In humans the insular cortex has been shown to be activated by esophageal and gastric distension including at noxious levels (Aziz et al., 2000; Elke et al., 2003; Stephan et al., 2005; Vandenbergh et al., 2005; Ladabaum, Roberts & McGonigle, 2007).

The majority of brain imaging studies have investigated either esophageal or rectal distension and while these have identified regions involved in signaling both noxious and nonnoxious sensations, there are relatively few studies involving stimulation of structures commonly associated with the induction of nausea such as the stomach. Progressive distension of the distal stomach in healthy volunteers evokes a gradation of sensations including bloating, pain, and nausea (Ladabaum et al., 1998; also see Chapter 5, in this volume). A related PET study identified an increase in activity in the caudate nucleus, anterior cingulate cortex, thalamus, and insula, but it was not possible to relate the activation of a particular structure to a specific sensation because there was strong correlation among the symptoms (Ladabaum et al., 2001). A further study by Ladabaum, Roberts, and McGonigle (2007), using fMRI, investigated the effect of noxious fundic distension and identified activation of the insular cortex, anterior and posterior cingulate cortex, right frontal lobe, and the inferior parietal lobes of the brain. The results of this study are broadly similar to other studies investigating the brain activity induced by fundic distension with the major difference being in whether the primary somatosensory cortex (S1) was one of the structures activated (Vandenbergh et al., 2005) or not (Lu et al., 2004; Ladabaum, Roberts & McGonigle, 2007).

In the section above on CTA pathways it was noted that the orbitofrontal cortex was a second gustatory cortical area and also received olfactory information. To this can be added information from the viscera including that arising from proximal gastric distension (Vandenbergh et al., 2005), supporting its role as an area integrating different modalities of sensory information including those relating to food intake. It is interesting to note that Vandenbergh et al. (2005) reported that they found "no evidence for a functional neuroanatomic divergence in the processing of noxious and innocuous gastric stimuli." Finally, the dorsolateral prefrontal cortex is implicated in attention to visceral sensations.

The introduction of electrical stimulation of the vagus nerve as a treatment for epilepsy and depression resistant to conventional therapy has given rise to imaging studies attempting to understand the mechanisms. A study using fMRI showed that transcutaneous stimulation of the left cervical vagus increased activity in the left locus coeruleus, thalamus (L>R), left prefrontal cortex, bilaterally in the postcentral gyrus, left posterior cingulate gyrus, and the left insula (Dietrich et al., 2008). The results are similar to an earlier study using implanted electrodes, which showed most intense activation in the insular cortex and the thalamus (Narayanan et al., 2002). The auricular branch (Alderman's nerve) of the vagus nerve has also been the subject of an fMRI study using transcutaneous stimulation (Kraus et al., 2007) with increased activity evoked in the insula, precentral gyrus, and thalamus. Although we have highlighted the brain regions activated by vagal stimulation, the studies also report regions deactivated by stimulation and these include the amygdala, hippocampus, parahippocampal gyrus, superior temporal gyrus (Kraus et al., 2007), posterior cingulate gyrus, nucleus accumbens, and cerebellum (Henry et al., 1998; Dietrich et al., 2008). Overall, these human vagal stimulation studies confirm the brain regions implicated in the processing of visceral afferent information in both humans and laboratory animals described above, and provide additional support for the view that conclusions about the processing of visceral afferent information drawn from animals have broad applicability to humans. But caution needs to be exercised because of differences between the pathways of humans and of nonhuman primates and other mammals (e.g., rat) particularly in the forebrain. In relation to animal models of pain, Craig (2009a) makes the point that poststroke central pain can not be modeled in rats because they lack the pathway (lamina I–medial dorsal thalamus–anterior cingulate cortex) implicated but which is present in primates. However, he also notes that in contrast to humans even monkeys do not appear to have the pathway required for the re-representation of the lamina I information in the anterior insular cortex, and concludes provocatively that, "the available evidence indicates that neither rodents nor monkeys can experience feelings in the same way that humans do."

In the section above we have taken a limited view of the genesis of the sensation of nausea as arising by activation of the area postrema and the abdominal vagal afferents via their projections to the NTS, parabrachial nucleus, and subsequent rostral projection of information mainly via the thalamus to the insular cortex. However Craig (2002; 2003; 2009b) argues that a wider view should be taken regarding interoception and its relationship to the question, "How do you feel?" It is proposed that visceral sensation and pain are both components of a common interoceptive system that monitors the physiological condition of the body and are both involved in homeostasis (Craig, 2002; 2003; 2009b). Furthermore it is proposed that these sensations are intimately involved in consciousness and the sense of self. Both gut pain and nausea are examples of a deviation from an internal sense of a state of normality or even well-being requiring the organism to be alerted to the changed state, classify it broadly as pleasant or unpleasant, and take appropriate action (e.g., behavioral, autonomic, endocrine) to attempt to return the body to a normal state with different "levels" of the brain being responsible for particular aspects. For example, the brain stem mediates the reflex responses of salivation, proximal stomach relaxation (see Chapter 5, in this volume), and vomiting; the hypothalamus secretion of vasopressin and ACTH; the insula and somatosensory cortex and the orbitofrontal cortex conscious awareness and associative (nausea with food) aspects respectively; and the insula, together with the cingulate cortex the more complex autonomic "emotional" responses via the descending pathways to the hypothalamus, brain stem, and spinal cord.

The pathways involved in this more general view of interoception have been the subject of detailed reviews by Craig (2002; 2003; 2009b) and will only be summarized here together with some aspects that are of particular relevance to nausea. Figure 4.4 illustrates the pathway by which information from the visceral afferents could reach the cortex. The key elements are that the small diameter (Aδ and C-fibers) afferent fibers project from the viscera indirectly (via lamina I) in sympathetic (e.g., greater splanchnic) and directly in parasympathetic (e.g., vagus) nerve trunks to the NTS and the parabrachial nucleus in the brainstem. These two nuclei in turn project to the basal region of ventromedial nucleus of the thalamus (VMb, also known as parvicellular ventroposterior medial nucleus, VMpc). Another thalamic nucleus, the posterior region of the ventromedial nucleus (VMpo) receives a direct input from lamina 1 (i.e., not via the NTS or PBN) and furthermore this nucleus does not receive an input from the "parasympathetic" afferents. The output from the thalamic nuclei (VMb and VMpo) is to the mid and posterior regions of the dorsal insular cortex (ibid). The visceral afferent inputs, including those from the gut,

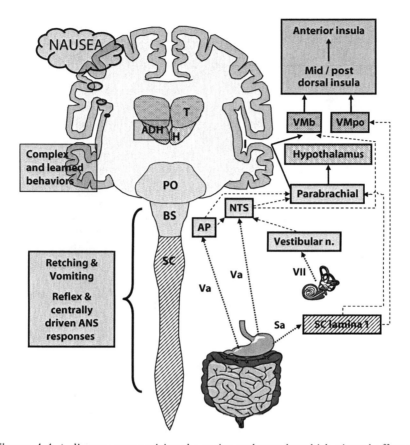

Figure 4.4 A diagram summarizing the major pathways by which visceral afferent information is proposed to reach the cerebral cortex (particularly the insular region) and may lead to the induction of the sensation of nausea. The pathways shown combine those described by Craig (2002) for a primate with pathways involved in the processing of abdominal vagal afferent information and projections of the area postrema and vestibular system (see Loewy, 1990, Yates, Miller & Lucot, 1998 and Saper, 2002) thus providing a pathway by which nausea could be induced by their activation. The diagram highlights the hierarchical processing of the information by matching shading of brain structures on the CNS outline with specific structures indicated in the "pathway boxes" on the right side of the figure. Primary afferent pathways are indicated with a dotted line (….), second order projections with a dashed line (----) and higher order projections with a solid (_____) line. The boxes on the left side indicate the functional consequences of the pathway activation at the various CNS levels. Abbreviations: ANS-Autonomic Nervous System; AP-Area Postrema; BS-Brain Stem; H-Hypothalamus (particularly Posterior hypothalamus, supraoptic and paraventricular nuclei); I-Insular region of the Cerebral Cortex; NTS-Nucleus Tractus Solitarius; PO -Pons; Sa -Greater Splanchnic Nerve Afferent Fibres; SC-Spinal Cord; T-Thalamus ; Va-Abdominal Vagal Afferent Nerves; Vestibular n.-Vestibular Nerve Nucleus; VIII-Vestibular Nerve; VMb-The basal region of the ventromedial thalamic nucleus; VMpo-The posterior region of the ventromedial nucleus of the thalamus.

received by this "interoceptive cortex" provide circumstantial evidence that it is involved in the genesis of the sensation of nausea especially when induced by stimuli acting in the gut, although other emetic pathways could input to the insula via their projections to the NTS and PBN. In humans the information reaching the mid/posterior dorsal insula is then "re-represented" in the anterior insula with the information from the "parasympathetic" afferents in the left anterior insula and that from the "sympathetic" afferents in the right anterior insula (Craig, 2002). Imaging studies of the left and right insula in subjects experiencing nausea induced by stimuli acting in the upper gut should be able to identify the relative contributions of the vagal (parasympathetic) and splanchnic (sympathetic) afferents in the genesis of the sensation. In humans further projection of information from the anterior insula to the orbitofrontal cortex occurs where the hedonic valence (pleasant/unpleasant, approach/avoid) is assigned.

Craig (2002; 2003; 2009b) makes a number of important points regarding the differences in the pathway between non primates and primates and between human and non-human primates that have implications for the study of nausea in animal models (see Chapter 8). For example several components of the pathway are either absent in non primates (e.g., NTS input to VMb, lamina I to VMpo) or primitive in nonprimates (VMpo). And in addition, there appear to be differences between humans and nonhuman primates in the lateralization of interoceptive information in the right anterior insula, which appear to be related to the sense of self.

The above studies raise a number of important questions about the sensations experienced by animals and the extent to which it is possible to study such sensations in animals with substantial differences in the development of specific brain pathways and nuclei. Studies of pathways responsible for the genesis of the sensation of nausea in humans are not only essential for development of treatments for use in humans but are also needed to assess the appropriateness of animal models and related welfare issues.

The above studies have focused on the central projection of visceral afferent information, but nausea and vomiting can also arise from olfactory and vestibular inputs so it is appropriate to conclude this section on central projections with a discussion of how information from both systems reaches the cortex.

Olfactory Pathways

The conscious perception of olfactory stimuli is by a pathway from the olfactory bulb via the olfactory tubercule and the medial dorsal nucleus of the thalamus to the orbitofrontal cortex (neocortex); but, uniquely for a sensory system, another pathway from the olfactory bulb projects directly to the olfactory cortex (located in a phylogenetically ancient region of the cortex) from which there are widespread projections to areas of the brain involved in motivation, memory, and emotion (Butler & Hodos, 1996; Felten & Józefowicz, 2003). It has been commented that, "there are so many structures that receive olfactory connections that listing those parts of the brain to which olfactory projections do not have access might be easier" (Bear, Connors & Paradiso, 1996). This extensive influence reflects the diverse roles of olfaction and receptors in the olfactory epithelium in the identification of food, assessment of its quality (is it putrid?) and its enjoyment (e.g., the aroma of fresh baked bread, white truffles, or wine), aversive responses, hunting prey by scent trails, respiration (apnea, sniffing, sneezing), mood (e.g., alerting and relaxing aromas), maternal bonding, mating, navigation, and behavioral responses to conspecifics (e.g., scent marking in dogs) and other species (e.g., skunks). In addition to the olfactory nerve, the nasal epithelium is also supplied by the trigeminal nerve, which gives rise to sensation of irritation that can contribute to the overall olfactory sensation. Stimuli with an action on both the trigeminal and olfactory nerves are termed "bimodal"; whereas those with an action on only the olfactory nerve are termed "pure olfactants," with both pleasant and unpleasant smelling substances being capable of inducing irritation (Zelano et al., 2007).

Nausea can be evoked by unpleasant odors (e.g., the "rotten egg" smell of hydrogen sulfide), but it is difficult to separate induction by a direct pathway (cf., area postrema, vagal afferents) as opposed to induction via a learned association. The latter has been documented as an element involved in the anticipatory nausea and vomiting associated with anticancer chemotherapy, where the smell of the hospital can evoke a recollection of the nausea and vomiting experienced when chemotherapy was given in the same setting (Morrow et al., 2002b; see also Chapter 14, in this volume). Brain imaging studies investigated the patterns of activity in response to both real and imagined pleasant (strawberry) and unpleasant (rotten eggs) odors and demonstrated that in both cases activity was higher in response to the unpleasant odor in the left frontal piriform cortex (primary olfactory cortex) and the left insula, although activity was also increased in the orbitofrontal cortex (Bensafi, Sobel & Khan, 2007). Although innate rejection responses to bitter-tasting substances have been demonstrated in neonates (Steiner, 1973), we are not aware of similar studies using olfactory stimuli; however, it appears likely that such responses exist as it is known that reaction time to unpleasant olfactory stimuli is faster than to pleasant ones (Jacob et al., 2003).

The survival advantage of a link between the odor of foods and any subsequent illness is clear, but there appears to be little research on this topic. A study by Yeshrun et al. (2009), attempting to explain why childhood olfactory memories can be so intense, tested whether the memory of the linkage between an odor (pleasant or unpleasant) and an object encountered at the same time was "stronger" when that odor was encountered for the very first time. Using behavioral tests and hippocampal imaging they showed that this was the case. Exposure during childhood to a food ("object") with an unpleasant odor which was ingested and subsequently induced illness (nausea and vomiting) would potentially have life-long survival value, especially as it is argued that the emetic reflex is more easily induced in children than adults, although direct experimental evidence is lacking. However there are examples of food in many cultures which although having smells suggestive of the odor of vomit (e.g. rancid, acidic, fermented) are nevertheless eaten, indicating that it is possible to overcome the revulsion to certain odors probably by observation of the behavior of conspecifics (usually parents). For example the Durian fruit (*Durio zibethinus*) when ripe is said to have an odor like stale vomit (Davidson, 1999), and airlines in Southeast Asia are reported to refuse to allow it in the cabin because of the unpleasant penetrating smell. Davidson (1999) also recounts being told by a Swedish naval office that tins of the salted fermented surströmming herring were opened on deck because of the smell. Adult human vomit has a characteristic persistent unpleasant odor which humans seek to avoid. A drawing by P. Boone from 1651 entitled, "Allegories of the senses; the sense of smell (reaction to vomiting)," shows two men holding their nose while viewing a third projectile vomiting (Wellcome Images L0019338; images.wellcome.ac.uk). An ability to detect and avoid a place where a human has vomited (if they were not observed doing so) has survival value, as vomit is a route by which infectious pathogens such as *Helicobacter pylori* and Norovirus can be transferred (Marks et al., 2000). Caul (1994) estimated that vomiting can release >30 million virus particles, whereas only 10–100 particles may be required for an infectious dose.

Vestibular Pathways

The vestibular system is essential for the genesis of motion sickness (Yates, Miller & Lucot, 1998). In the section above on the brain stem, the projections from the vestibular system to the vestibular nuclei and dorsal vagal complex were outlined, providing the substrate by which vestibular stimulation could induce vomiting and the accompanying autonomic changes. The vestibular system also sends direct projections to the cerebellum, which is involved in somatomotor control, to the spinal cord for postural adjustments to head and neck muscles and limb extensor muscles, and to the extraocular muscles to coordinate the movements of the eyes with those of the head (Felten & Józefowicz, 2003). The descending vestibular pathways to the dorsal vagal complex also provide a pathway by which nausea could be induced by activation of pathways ascending from the brain stem (Yates, Miller & Lucot, 1998). Nausea could also be induced by ascending pathways from the vestibular nuclei to the thalamus (posterolateral thalamus), lateral postcentral gyrus, insular cortex, and temporoparietal cortex. Several fMRI studies in humans have investigated the brain regions activated by galvanic (e.g., Bense et al., 2001; Stephan et al., 2005) or caloric (e.g., Fasold et al., 2002) vestibular stimulation, but these have not been intended to induce nausea, although stimulus parameters used did evoke feelings of motion or nystagmus in the subjects. Galvanic stimulation, which activates the vestibular afferents arising from both the semicircular canals and the otoliths, evokes activity in diverse nuclei including: anterior and posterior insula and retroinsular regions, inferior/middle frontal gyrus, superior temporal gyrus, temporoparietal cortex, precentral gyrus, basal ganglia, thalamus, anterior cingulate gyrus, parahippocampal gyrus and hippocampus, supplementary motor area, and the cerebellum (crus I, vermal lobule IV) (Bense et al., 2001; Stephan et al., 2005). Of particular relevance to nausea is the activation of the anterior cingulate gyrus and the anterior region of the insula, both areas linked to the processing of visceral information and autonomic responses to visceral stimulation (see above).

Motion (both real and illusory) provides a stimulus that is relatively easy to control and amenable to pharmacological intervention. A study using a revolving chair investigated the effects of placebo, dimenhydrate (an antihistamine), and ginger root capsules on the reported gastrointestinal sensations using a psychophysical approach (Mowrey & Clayson, 1982). This study is of interest because it reveals the time course of the change in the intensity of the gastrointestinal sensations, and power function analysis showed "knees" in the plots (see Figure 4.5). They propose that this marks the transition from activation of sensory pathways involved in nausea to those involved in vomiting or its prodromata. It would be interesting to combine such a study with the real time measurement of autonomic nervous system function discussed in Chapter 5 (in this volume). The effects of the two interventions were most marked on the first ("nausea") components, with ginger capsules being more effective than dimenhydrate or placebo.

Miller et al. (1996) used magnetoencephalography to investigate cerebral cortical regions in subjects experiencing nausea induced by head movement during yaw-axis rotation. A region 2–3 cm in diameter in the inferior frontal gyrus was activated by this stimulus, but not by speech, finger movement, or exaggerated breathing (see Figure 4.6). It was noted that the number of dipoles (an index of neuronal activation) was related to the intensity of nausea. It is worth noting that the inferior frontal gyrus was also shown in fMRI studies to be activated by galvanic vestibular stimulation (Bense et al., 2001; Stephan et al., 2005) and caloric vestibular stimulation (e.g., Fasold et al., 2002). The same subjects were studied during nausea induced by ingestion of syrup of ipecac. This revealed that the same cortical region was active as during motion-induced nausea, and furthermore that the 5-HT$_3$ receptor antagonist ondansetron reduced both the intensity of ipecac-induced nausea and the number of dipoles. The Miller et al. (1996) study appears to be unique; similar studies need to be undertaken using more modern methods of brain imaging (see below).

The diverse studies reviewed above from both humans and animals demonstrate that there are anatomical pathways by which signals from the pathways known to be capable of inducing nausea (and vomiting) can access the highest level of the brain where it is assumed that they enter consciousness. This provides a theoretical framework for the genesis of the sensation, but does not tell us how it is encoded or even where it is experienced: is there a "nausea sensory cortex" and is the association of the sensation with the upper abdomen due to signals from the gut or a phenomenon analogous to referred pain? There are a large number of outstanding issues and these are addressed in various ways in the subsequent sections.

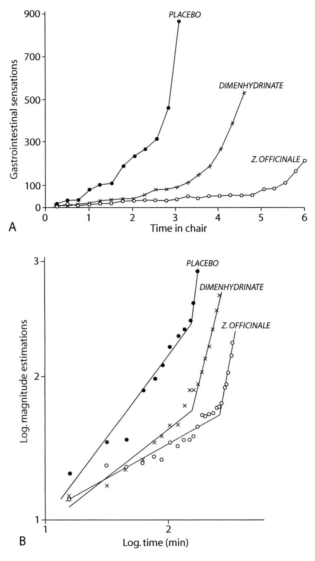

Figure 4.5 Upper Panel A. The effect of three treatments on the magnitude of gastro-intestinal symptoms induced by rotation in healthy volunteers. Data are plotted as geo-metric means of estimations of the sensation magnitude. *Z. officinalis* was given as two gelatin capsules of powdered ginger rhizome; gelatin capsules containing chickweed herb were used as placebo; and Dramamine (dimenhydrinate) was given at a dose of 100 mg. The mean times for which the subjects could tolerate the chair were signifi-cantly different between each group. Lower Panel B. A logarithmic plot of the data in the upper panel. Note the "knees" in the plots, which can be indicative of a change in the sensory mechanisms. This may mark the transition from the sensory experience of nausea to the more imminent onset of vomiting (if the stimulus continued). Reproduced with permission from Mowrey and Clayson, 1982.

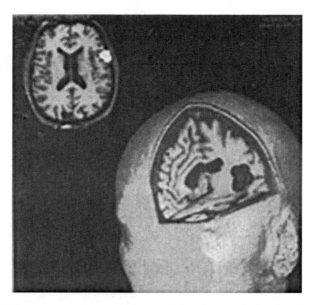

Figure 4.6 The pattern of current dipoles indicative of neuronal activation in the inferior frontal gyrus in a subject made nauseous by oral ingestion of ipecac syrup (5 ml). This study used magnetic source imaging on one side of the head only. Reproduced with permission from Miller et al., 1996.

NAUSEA, THE BRAIN, AND CONSCIOUSNESS: SOME EVOLUTIONARY CONSIDERATIONS

The protective function of vomiting in removing food containing toxins from the body is clear. In some species (e.g., dogfish, saltwater crocodile, owl) it is also used to remove indigestible residues from the stomach (Andrews, Sims & Young, 1998; Andrews et al., 2000; Darolova, 1991), while in others it is used in defense (e.g., petrel; Matthews, 1949) and in the modified form of regurgitation to feed the young (e.g., African wild dog; Van Lawick-Goodall & Van Lawick-Goodall, 1970). Evidence that the act of vomiting itself is aversive is lacking, and there are anecdotal reports of positive sensations following vomiting. What then are the advantages of having the conscious sensation of nausea so intimately linked to vomiting? This touches on the evolution of consciousness and the nature of consciousness in nonhuman animals as the question arises whether animals other than humans experience a similar sensation.

Studies in anencephalic humans and decerebrate animals (rat) have shown reflex rejection (tongue protrusion, increased salivation) of bitter-tasting substances when placed in the mouth (Steiner, 1973; Grill, 1985), a response that must be innate and presumably linked to the survival value of recognition of the relationship between naturally occurring bitter-tasting substances (particularly alkaloids in plants) and toxicity (Glendinning, 2007). However, in the examples given there is no evidence of a conscious perception of the bitter taste so the response to be elicited must be encoded in the original afferent signal from the taste buds. Humans can learn to override innate rejection mechanisms to ingest substances such as coffee, dark chocolate, chilli, and bitter aperitives that innately would be rejected (Logue, 1991).

In decerebrate and anesthetized animals it is possible to induce retching and vomiting preceded by increased salivation, licking, and swallowing in response to emetic agents present in the stomach or abdominal vagal afferent stimulation (Andrews & Wood, 1988; Andrews et al., 1990b). Thus in mammals and arguably vertebrates in general the gustatory and gastrointestinal rejection reflexes would enable an animal to survive encounters with potentially toxic foods. In the rat (and probably all rodents) where the vomiting reflex is lacking, it has been argued that neophobia, nibbling type ingestion patterns, as well as taste related reflexes and learned behavior provide the major lines of defense (Davis et al., 1986; Andrews & Horn, 2006), but rats may also have enhanced detoxification mechanisms (e.g., cytochrome P450 subfamilies, proteases; Gibbs et al., 2004). Rejection of toxic foods has also been reported in animals such as the sea slug, sea anemone, and sea squirt (see Chapter 8, in this volume) with "simple" nervous systems fundamentally different in organization from those in vertebrates and where there is no evidence for "higher" levels of cognition. Aversions may not need particularly complex nervous systems as, for example, in the nematode *C. elegans* olfactory aversion has been demonstrated as a mechanism by which the organism avoids ingestion of potentially lethal pathogenic bacteria (Zhang, Lu & Bargmann, 2005) with the behavior mediated by a 5-HT-gated ion channel (MOD-1). Studies of *Drosophila melanogaster* larvae have revealed an endogenous mechanism regulating the ingestion or rejection of noxious food (Wu, Zhao & Shen, 2005). The larvae are voracious feeders and when food is available will reject food adulterated with quinine; however, when food-deprived they will feed on the food containing quinine. This behavior is mediated by the neuropeptide F receptor (NPFR1, which is related to the mammalian NPY receptor family) since overexpression of NPFR1 in the central nervous system was able to induce feeding on the contaminated food. The NFPR1 signaling itself is modulated by an insulin-like signaling pathway (Wu, Zhao & Shen, 2005). Although this is not an example of a learned behavioral response, it provides a further example of a "simple" system capable of making choices about ingestion or rejection of food and initiating an appropriate behavioral sequence of either remaining at the food source or continuing to forage for unadulterated food. Conditioned aversive responses to toxic food have been reported in fish (Gerhart, 1991), where the cerebral hemispheres are rudimentary (see Chapter 8, in this volume).

The above brief review shows that both rejection of ingested contaminated food and avoidance of potentially toxic food can both be accomplished by animals with "simple" nervous systems but lacking higher cognitive capacity. In the light of this we need to consider the evolutionary advantage of having a specific conscious sensation of nausea as a component of the body's defensive system against ingested toxins and, as humans are the only species in which we can be certain that nausea exists, we will view this from a human perspective and use it as a basis to comment about other species where possible. In attempting to consider nausea in humans in an evolutionary context, we must recall that our ancestral environment presented different challenges from our current one especially in modern developed societies.

Learned Aversions

In humans, nausea can certainly give rise to learned (Pavlovian) aversions, but, as noted above in rats, the animal does not need to be conscious at the time of the visceral illness for a learned aversion to form. The presence of a specific nonpainful conscious sensation indicative of visceral illness allows humans to set the occurrence of the sensation in the context of concurrent events (e.g., sea travel) or events that have occurred recently (e.g., ingestion of a meal many hours earlier, a cycle of chemotherapy). The ability to make a conscious link between the sensation of nausea and the recollection of recent events may make a more robust linkage between the two, and in addition the entire context within which these events happened can be recalled (e.g., type of food, location, season of the year, restaurant in which a meal was eaten). This may confer a survival advantage in food selection especially for a species with an omnivorous diet. It would be interesting to know at what age humans first become consciously aware of the sensation of nausea especially as anecdotally food aversions formed early in life sustain throughout life. The study by Bernstein (1978) of learned taste aversions in children receiving chemotherapy included a 2-year-old child, but as individual data were not reported we do not know if they developed an aversion. An additional question is, "How many times a year nausea and vomiting are triggered in response to contaminated food?" A survey of almost 600 participants ranging in age from 18 to 91 years revealed an incidence of vomiting attributed to food poisoning of 9.5% (Rub, Andrews & Whitehead, 1992).

Altered Internal State

Nausea and visceral pain are two distinct sensations that provide an awareness of an altered internal state. It is interesting to consider why there should be two separate sensations rather than just one that indicates a negative deviation from normal. Clearly they must be conveying different information advantageous for survival. Studies of individuals with congenital absence of somatic pain sensations provide clear evidence for the survival advantage of such pain signaling as these individuals suffer frequent injuries as children (McMurray, 1950). Pain is usually evoked in the gut by distension (e.g., pyloric obstruction), contraction (e.g., colonic spasm, reflex response to mucosal irritation, or luminal distension), inflammation (e.g., *Helicobacter pylori* gastritis, reflux esophagitis), and ischemia (may be secondary to muscle spasm, ischemic mesenteric syndrome). There do not seem to be similar studies of individuals lacking visceral pain sensitivity, but it is difficult to see how this might present clinically except that individuals may present with serious conditions such as a perforated gastric ulcer, pancreatitis, or common bile duct or intestinal obstruction but without pain as a symptom. In general nausea is most easily induced by stimulation of the upper rather than lower gastrointestinal tract, whereas pain can be readily induced from all regions. This argues that nausea is more closely related to food intake. In this context it is worth noting the significant involvement of abdominal vagal afferents in regulation of food intake and nausea as well as the digestive motor and secretory patterns and the fact that agonists at several receptors (e.g., CB_1, $GABA_B$, ghrelin) are both antiemetic and promote appetite (Sanger & Andrews, 2006). Nausea could be considered along a spectrum of internal sensations relating to feeding: from hunger to comfortable satiety and pleasant fullness; to nausea, unpleasant fullness, and discomfort; and finally pain (see Chapter 5, in this volume for detailed discussion). This argument is easiest to understand in the context of the gastric distension by food, but the chemical composition (including toxins) of the food should not be forgotten. It is this component that is more likely to be the cause of the nausea than the voluntary ingestion of an excessive volume. There are species, such as the marsupial possum and koalas, whose diet contains plant toxins, and it is argued that this toxic load may be monitored by the genesis of "nausea," which together with conditioned aversions plays an important role in the regulation of food intake (Lawler et al., 1998; Marsh, Wallis & Foley, 2007; De Gabriel et al., 2010; see Chapter 8, in this volume). Thus in some cases "nausea" could be considered to be a normal regulator of food intake.

For both nausea and pain one can ask, "What is the point in knowing?" if nothing can be done to alleviate these unpleasant sensations, bearing in mind the inaccessibility of the organs concerned without surgical intervention. The awareness of these sensations perceived as arising from the gut would allow a human (or other animal) to self-medicate if they had acquired the prior knowledge (see below) and had access to effective treatments. There is evidence that nonhuman primates and some other species self-medicate when suffering visceral malaise (Engel, 2002), although it is unclear how, for example, domesticated dogs and cats "know" to eat grass to induce vomiting. The ingestion of kaolin by laboratory rats given substances that would induce emesis in other species appears to be an innate behavior, and although in an experimental setting the animal only has a choice between food and kaolin, this behavior mimics illness-induced consumption of soil/clay observed in the wild (Mitchell, 1976; Mitchell, Beatty & Cox, 1977).

Although it is likely that responses to pain and the presence of nausea such as a reduction or cessation of food intake and delayed gastric emptying occur via the brain stem and hypothalamus, more complex behavioral responses such as seeking a safe refuge to await recovery (animals showing signs of illness or abnormal behavior are likely to be rapidly predated) or self-medication arguably require conscious decision making. However, studies of rectal distension have shown that even with subliminal levels of stimulation the same regions of the cerebral cortex are activated as when liminal and supraliminal levels of distension are used although at a lower level of intensity (Kern & Shaker, 2002). It is therefore possible that behavior could be affected without the animal being aware of the changed internal state.

The above discussions have focused on nausea originating from ingested substances and centered on the protective roles of nausea in enabling the animal to avoid potentially toxic foods. However, excluding diseases and treatments, nausea originates in humans from one other major cause, namely pregnancy. The nausea in the first trimester of pregnancy is particularly interesting as it is often reported to be the first conscious indication of pregnancy, occurring before the first missed period, and is associated with changed taste perception and dietary preferences, which are argued to be protective of the fetus at the time of development of major organs (see Chapter 12, in this volume). Some describe the sensation as "flu-like" with the symptoms including tiredness, which may encourage energy conservation. It could be argued that the nausea and related symptoms are a way in which the embryo regulates the behavior of the mother to facilitate its own (genes) survival. Menstruation is not universal among nonhuman primates (e.g., Martin, 2007). Even in human females it is not always regular. One in fifteen unselected women in the United States are estimated to be affected by polycystic ovary syndrome, which is associated with a very high incidence of oligomenorrhea/ anovulation (Azziz et al., 2005) and menstruation is sensitive to low body weight and poor diet, which may have been more common among our ancestors. Therefore it is not unreasonable to ask, "How did our female ancestors know that their physiological condition had changed and they were pregnant?" Could protracted nausea be the answer?

Communication

A human or nonhuman primate (e.g., chimpanzee) living in a family group sharing food would be at an advantage if they were able to communicate to others in the group who were eating the same food that they were feeling unwell (e.g., nausea) as this could reduce their ingested toxic load. See Pollick and de Waal (2007) and Chapter 8 in this volume for discussion of communication in apes and other species. Food sharing is common in modern and ancestral human societies and is well documented in chimpanzees. See Jones (2007) for an extensive discussion of why humans share food. Food-induced illness would also be apparent if an individual was curled in a fetal position holding their stomach or vomiting shortly after eating, but arguably nausea would occur sooner and give an earlier indication of a problem. It is also argued that nausea is induced at lower doses of substances than is vomiting (see above). Facial expression and body language provide important indications of illness to other family members, and among primates the neural pathways for face recognition are highly developed (e.g., see Haxby, Hoffman & Gobbini, 2000). Although visual communication is perhaps the most obvious medium to humans, olfaction plays a role in many species including nonhuman primates (for review see Prescott, 2006). The ability to communicate such experiences of food-induced illness would mean that the entire family group would benefit from each individual's experience and such knowledge could be passed to subsequent generations in oral or written form. Although there is evidence that rats have socially induced diet choice mediated by a semiochemical (carbon disulfide) mechanism and naive animals can learn food preferences from demonstrators, it appears that only information on preferences is communicated and not food aversions (Galef & Beck, 1985; Galef et al., 1988; Galef, Attenborough & Whiskin, 1990). Returning to humans, a further aspect of the ability to communicate illness is that it opens the potential for a member of the tribe with specialist knowledge ("doctor") to dispense treatment and in many societies such shamans and medicine men are held in high regard (Frazer, 1922/1998).

FUTURE STUDIES

Humans are the only species in which it is possible to define a sensation as nausea against a set of criteria (including biomarkers such as plasma AVP and the EGG; see Chapters 6 and 7, in this volume) and to ask an individual if they are experiencing that sensation and, if so, to give it some intensity score. This observation would argue that studies of the central pathways and neurotransmitters involved in nausea should be confined to humans although, as discussed above, there are some useful insights that can be gained (with caution) from animal studies. While a variety of techniques are available for imaging of brain function and aspects of pharmacology (e.g., fMRI; Borsook, Becerra & Hargreaves, 2006) as well as for the induction of nausea by ingested (e.g., ipecacuanha; Minton et al., 1993) and injected (e.g., apomorphine; Rowe et al., 1979) substances as well as by the motion sickness pathway, the combination of techniques presents some challenges even assuming that such studies obtain relevant ethical approval. Some of the potential problems, approaches, and questions are outlined below.

Recruitment of Volunteers

Subjects involved in experimental studies (as opposed to clinical trials) of nausea and vomiting have in the main either been military personnel or college students. Arguably volunteers may be self-selecting, undertaking such studies because they know that they are relatively immune to the stimulus or because they see participation as a sign of machismo. The extent to which participation in these and other studies is influenced by financial or other reward (class credits) is not known. The studies have in general investigated a motion stimulus ranging from vection involving an optokinetic drum to rotating chairs, parabolic flights ("the vomit comet"), and amphibious landing craft. A few studies have been performed by contract research organizations recruiting subjects from the general population, and a limited number of other studies have involved pregnant women, patients undergoing clinical investigation, or surgical or chemotherapy treatment for cancer. Overall it would appear possible to recruit subjects to a study of nausea, although the ease of recruitment may depend on the nature of the stimulus the study is intended to investigate (vection, systemically administered drug, brain stimulation) as well as the likely intensity and duration of the nausea and the nature of the measurements to be made (e.g., brain imaging, serial blood samples, EGG). It may be difficult to recruit volunteers to a study requiring exposure to a nauseogenic stimulus on multiple occasions in part because of the induction of learned aversions. There is also an issue of comparing the pathways activated in healthy volunteers by using stimuli selective for the input pathways reviewed above as opposed to studying nausea in patients due to a preexisting condition or treatment.

The Genetics of Nausea Sensitivity

Studies of pain pathways in humans have benefited from studies of individuals with genetic disorders of pain sensitivity. There is at least one report of absence of a vomiting reflex in two male members of a family with hereditary ataxia (McLellan & Park, 1973). The report also includes a description of the response of one of the brothers to ingestion of saturated sodium chloride and subcutaneous apomorphine. In neither case did he vomit or report nausea. The description of the response to apomorphine is particularly revealing as it indicates that he did experience other expected effects of apomorphine:

> At the patient's suggestion, 9 mg of apomorphine was injected subcutaneously. After 10 minutes he became pale and felt unwell; after 15 minutes he yawned and became faint, heart rate fell to 50 beats per minute, and blood pressure fell from 120/80 to 75/55mm Hg. He did not feel localised discomfort and did not retch or vomit. He became drowsy and remained so for one and one-half hours. Recovery was uneventful; at no time did he experience abdominal discomfort, nausea or vomiting (McLellan & Park, 1973, p. 726).

Imaging (and genetic) studies in patients lacking the ability to either vomit or experience nausea would be particularly helpful in identifying the pathways involved, but a prerequisite will be to identify subjects. This may be a difficult task in comparison to identification of subjects with defective pain pathways.

The Stimulus and the Associated Risks

If the aim of the study is to investigate the central nervous system pathways active in subjects reporting nausea, a stimulus should be used that induces nausea alone. It may be relatively easy to produce a state of sustained nausea with a minimal risk of vomiting ensuing when using a motion stimulus (especially vection), but in the case of an ingested or an injected agent this would

depend critically on selection of an appropriate dose, which in turn relies
on the existence of detailed dose-response information in humans. For stimuli
such as apomorphine, the interval between the onset of nausea and ensuing
vomiting may be a few minutes (see Figure 4.2). Hence, under these circumstances, it may be difficult to separate the pathways involved in the two events.
Nausea can also be induced in humans by ingested agents such as syrup
of ipecac (Minton et al., 1993), (-) tryptophan (Greenwood et al., 1975),
L-DOPA (Parkes, 1986), and the partial 5-HT$_{1A}$ receptor agonist buspirone,
which, when given orally, enhanced the nausea induced by intravenous morphine (Oertel et al., 2007). One approach may be to avoid the use of agonist
drugs to induce nausea and to use antagonists. While some of these can induce
nausea when given alone, they reduce the threshold for vomiting and for the
latter to occur requires the administration of an emetic stimulus. For example,
the opioid antagonist naloxone (Kobrinsky et al., 1988) and the CB$_1$ receptor
antagonist Rimonabant (Pi-Sunyer et al., 2006) both induce nausea as a
dose-related side effect.

Apart from being a potentially confounding factor, vomiting is a risk (see
Ladabaum et al., 2001) because of the possibility of aspiration if the subject is
lying down in a scanner with the head restrained as it may not be possible to
remove the subject rapidly. This is likely to be resolved by technical developments in scanner design allowing subjects to be vertical. There is also the issue
of potential contamination of the scanner by aerosolized vomit containing
infectious agents, but this is likely to be less of an issue with the more open
designs of scanners. Nausea is known to be an aversive stimulus, and care must
be taken to minimize the possibility of inducing an aversion by ensuring that
food is not given around the time of administration of the stimulus.

Caloric or galvanic vestibular stimulation provides a readily controlled,
well-studied, discrete experimental stimulus for induction of nausea and
evoking the associated gastrointestinal motor changes (Wolf, 1965; Brandt &
Strupp, 2005); however, it would still be necessary to compare the results
obtained with stimuli acting via the area postrema and the abdominal vagal
afferents.

Direct electrical stimulation of both superficial and deep brain structures
has been used in humans to investigate the potential for various brain regions
to induce motor or sensory responses. More developed techniques such as
deep brain stimulation or the noninvasive transcranial electromagnetic stimulation may prove useful in confirming the involvement in nausea of sites
identified by imaging studies. Although the electrical stimulation techniques
used in the early studies are crude in comparison with current methods, and
hence the results must be interpreted with caution, there are a number of
observations worth pursuing with more sophisticated techniques. Nausea and
a sick-feeling could both be evoked by stimulation of the extreme lateral
portion of the primary somatosensory cortex (S1) (Penfield & Rasmussen,
1950); nausea, vomiting, and epigastric awareness were induced by anterior
cingulate cortex stimulation (Devinsky, Morrell & Vogt, 1995); and two types

of nausea response were evoked by stimulation of the fontal lobe in either cerebral hemisphere (Sem-Jacobsen, 1968; see Figure 4.7): "Nausea I"—in which the subject reported nausea and this was followed suddenly by vomiting and immediate recovery and "Nausea II"—in which the subject reported a more intense response including perspiration and changes in breathing rate and depth. Of particular interest is that the response often outlasted the period of stimulation. It was not possible to change Nausea I to Nausea II by increasing the stimulus strength, suggesting that the nature of the response was site-, not intensity-specific.

Subject Control of the Stimulus

In all human studies where there is a potential for induction of an unpleasant sensation, an ability for the subject to signal his or her immediate desire to withdraw from the study is integral to the experimental design and is usually a requirement of ethical approval. In the case of visceral pain studies and rotating chair motion studies, this can be done by signaling to the investigator. In vection using the optokinetic drum, subjects can terminate the stimulus immediately by closing their eyes. With ingested or injected nauseogenic stimuli, neither the subject nor the investigator has an equivalent degree of control. While an investigator could give an intravenous antiemetic if the nausea became intolerable or if vomiting occurred, there is always the possibility that it may not be effective, especially in the case of nausea. These issues may be a barrier to the study of stimuli other than vection.

It may be possible to investigate patients who have nausea as a preexisting symptom or who may be experiencing nausea as an unmanaged side-effect of treatment, although interpretation may be difficult. One group that may merit investigation are patients with migraine in which nausea is a common symptom. A recent fMRI study demonstrated dysfunction of brain-stem pain modulatory mechanisms in migraine patients (Moulton et al., 2008) illustrating that such techniques now have sufficient resolution to investigate the brainstem pathways likely to be involved in the initial processing of nauseogenic signals from the gut and the area postrema.

What to Measure?

Whatever brain imaging techniques are used, it will be essential to correlate changes in activity in a specific brain region(s)/pathway(s) with the onset, presence, location, magnitude, and cessation of the sensation. Self-reporting of symptoms by the experimental subject is clearly essential, but it will be important to ensure that the temporal resolution is sufficient to enable correlation with imaging data. In addition, a number of biomarkers should be measured to investigate their relationship to changes in brain function. Of particular interest would be the EGG (electrogastrogram), blood pressure, heart rate, skin resistance, swallowing frequency (possibly a surrogate for increased salivation; see Chapter 5, in this volume), and skin color/temperature, all

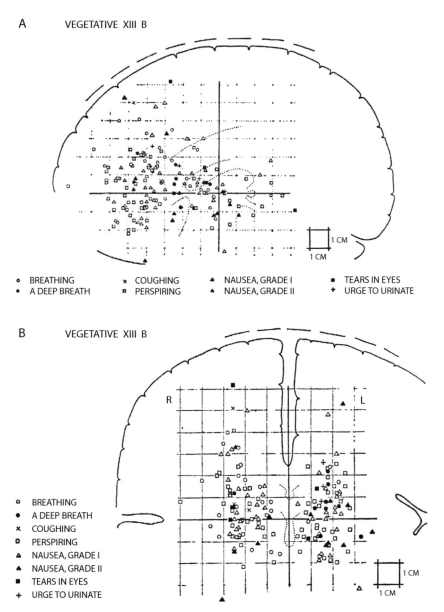

Figure 4.7 Saggital (A) and coronal (B) plane plots of the locations from which nausea (along with other responses) was induced by depth electrographic stimulation in humans. Nausea I is described as "nauseated, sudden vomiting, yawning, fatigue," and Nausea II as "nausea with perspiration, changes in breathing rate and depths." Reproduced with permission from Sem-Jacobsen, 1968.

of which can be recorded continuously, facilitating correlation. Plasma bio-markers of "stress," such as cortisol and adrenaline, as well as of "nausea," such as vasopressin (see Chapter 6, in this volume, for discussion), should also be measured, but the temporal resolution is limited. The constraints imposed by the apparatuses required for different types of brain imaging are likely to be major factors limiting what other measurements may be taken and when they can be taken.

While the focus of future studies is likely to be brain imaging, electroen-cephalography (EEG) may provide additional information and has been used in studies of motion sickness with the authors concluding that there were similarities between the EEG power spectral changes in partial seizures and motion sickness (Chelen, Kabrisky & Rogers, 1993). Increased theta and beta$_1$ activity were recorded and are indicative of drowsiness; however, the imminent vomiting is an arousing stimulus sufficient to wake a sleeping person.

There are probably three types of study that need to be undertaken to be certain that the brain region(s) where activity is changed is involved in the sensation of nausea: (1) activity should be changed (including decreased) in response to any experimental stimulus inducing nausea irrespective of whether it is acting via the vestibular system, the area postrema, or the abdominal vagus; (2) in patients with idiopathic nausea or nausea induced as a result of their disease or treatment, the same region(s) as identified in the experimental study should have modified activity; and (3) pharmacological or other inter-ventions (e.g., acupuncture) with an effect on nausea should also have an effect on the activity in the brain regions identified above. This type of study may be particularly difficult to perform and interpret. For example, it would not be particularly surprising for the nausea and brain activity evoked by a dopamine receptor agonist, such as apomorphine, to be blocked by a dopamine receptor antagonist, such as domperidone, acting to prevent the primary activation of the pathways leading to nausea. However, the real test would be to demonstrate that blockade at a more distal point in the pathway leads to both a reduction in nausea and activity in the brain regions distal to the site of blockade. Such experiments rely on identification of the transmitters in the pathway(s) responsible for the central processing of the "nausea signal."

Where Is Nausea Perceived?

Anecdotally the question, "Where do you feel nausea?" asked of a large group of students will elicit three different responses: head, back of the throat, stomach. Are these individually specific manifestations of the same phenome-non "referred" to different parts of the body or do they represent different pathways by which nausea has been induced? For example, "head nausea" would be more associated with motion sickness, whereas "stomach nausea" would be associated with food poisoning. It is relatively easy to envisage that nausea induced by vestibular stimulation could be primarily perceived as being in the head via the vestibular nerve projections to the cerebral cortex and that the epigastric region would be identified at a conscious level as the source of nausea due to abdominal vagal afferent activation of NTS projections to the insular cortex. But in the case of the area postrema activated by circulating agents, where would the sensation be expected? Should it be the same as the vagal afferent activation because of the inputs of the area postrema to the NTS? The widespread occurrence of disturbances in the electrical activity of the stomach (EGG, see Chapter 7, in this volume) in association with nausea induced by both central (vestibular, area postrema) and peripheral (vagal afferents) pathways if detected by visceral afferents should result in an epigastric sensory component to reports of nausea irrespective of how induced. These aspects require formal investigation as they have implications for how we may envisage the genesis of the sensation and whether we can generalize from one nauseogenic stimulus to another.

CONCLUSIONS

This chapter has reviewed the central nervous system pathways implicated in nausea and vomiting. In the case of vomiting the pathways are relatively well understood; and although the transmitters used in humans may differ in detail from those in the animal species studied, the conserved nature of the brainstem among mammals strongly supports the view that very similar mechanisms operate in humans. Vomiting is a reflex mediated by the brainstem and its occurrence does not require the remainder of the brain, but this is not to say that the brainstem mechanisms are not modulated by more rostral structures. The endocrine, widespread autonomic, and learned aversive responses require projection of information from the brainstem to higher levels of the brain including the hypothalamus, amygdala, anterior cingulate cortex, and insular cortex. Evidence from a variety of animal studies shows that the major inputs by which nausea and vomiting are induced in humans (vagal afferents, area postrema, vestibular system) all have projections to the cerebral cortex and this provides a theoretical substrate for consideration of the pathways likely to be involved in humans. Functional studies (fMRI, EEG) of the brain in humans experiencing nausea are arguably the only way in which we will truly be able to understand the genesis of the sensation of nausea and to discover if there is a "nausea cortex" (possibly the insula and orbitofrontal cortex), but as pointed out above such studies have practical constraints.

Chapter 5

The Autonomic Nervous System and Nausea

If the animal lies down after the injection, it gets up at the onset of nausea. Simultaneously, the pylorus and pyloric part of the stomach contract firmly, the antrum moderately, while the fundus relaxes, the walls becoming flaccid, and the gastric contents are forced into the fundus. There may be unimportant gastric antiperistalsis. The secretion of saliva is markedly increased and the animal stands with the head down and the nose nearly touching the floor. The respiration becomes rapid and irregular, and with increasing nausea the animal makes chewing movements, licks the lips and swallows saliva repeatedly; air is usually swallowed at this time.
—Description by Hatcher (1924, p. 500) of typical prevoming behavior in the dog induced by apomorphine.

Nevertheless, with the more violent stimulation of a rough plane journey there occurred pallor of the face with tachycardia and weak pulse, retching and vomiting of dark bile. Later a smooth journey did not produce such a response.
—Study of gastric function in a "decorticate" man with gastric fistula; Doig, Wolf, and Wolff (1953).

INTRODUCTION

The nervous system classically is divided into central and peripheral divisions, with the latter being subdivided into somatic and autonomic divisions. The somatic division comprises efferent axons to striated muscle and afferent nerves. The autonomic nervous system (ANS), originally defined by J. N. Langley, is comprised of parasympathetic, sympathetic, and enteric divisions and was viewed by him as a motor or efferent system (Langley, 1921). Although the presence of afferent fibers in nerve trunks classified as sympathetic or parasympathetic was known in the early part of the twentieth century from both histological and early electrophysiological studies (Einthoven, Flohil & Battaerd, 1908), the view of a purely efferent system persists in many text books. However, more modern views of the autonomic nervous system encompass afferents by using the names of the trunks in which they travel (e.g., vagal afferent, splanchnic afferent) or using "visceral afferent" as a more general term (Furness, 2006). In this chapter we will include all these components, as it is clear that the "autonomic afferents" play a key role in induction of nausea and vomiting and are a target for antiemetic drugs, while the "autonomic efferents" are responsible for many of the visible and visceral motor phenomena that accompany nausea and vomiting. The ANS regulates diverse bodily functions (see Figure 5.1) and many of these have never been investigated in relation to nausea (or vomiting). For example mobilization of energy stores would be advantageous as would stimulation of the immune system. Also, an inverse covariation between pro-inflammatory cytokines and heart rate variability has been reported in humans (Marsland et al., 2007).

During the experience of nausea and the act of vomiting, arguably all divisions of the nervous system are involved and none of the major bodily systems are unaffected. For simplicity the first part of this chapter will review the involvement of the autonomic efferents in mediating changes in the various body systems that occur prior to the onset of, and during, the presence of nausea. However, it should be noted that the vast majority of studies of the ANS and nausea in humans involve subjects experiencing various forms of motion sickness and hence caution must be exerted in generalizing these observations to nausea induced by other stimuli.

The role of afferents will be discussed in a separate section, which will examine the overall evidence for their involvement in the induction of nausea (and vomiting). Events occurring prior to the onset of retching and vomiting that could be signaled via the afferents and potentially evoke a sensation of nausea will also be reviewed. There has been a considerable body of work that attempts to use either baseline measures of autonomic function or provocative tests usually of cardiovascular function to predict sensitivity to emetic stimuli. Such studies will not be discussed, and the reader is referred to Muth (2006) for a discussion of this topic.

AUTONOMICALLY MEDIATED CHANGES IN BODY SYSTEMS DURING NAUSEA

Skin

In human tribes and families where food sharing is common, a sudden change in the appearance of the facial skin (e.g., color or sweating in the absence of a thermal stimulus) in one member shortly after eating could have survival value for the other members in the absence of specific verbal or other form of communication.

Physiological changes in the skin are probably one of the only outward signs in some people that they may be experiencing nausea, with descriptions of people who are seasick looking green ("green around the gills") or pallid and feeling cold and clammy to the touch (but see below). However, such changes in appearance are not specific, may not be apparent in all subjects, and when present have a variable temporal relationship to nausea, with some authors reporting occurrence prior to nausea and others coincident with nausea. In addition, in studies of motion sickness some subjects exhibited skin flushing prior to the onset of pallor or showed either pallor or flushing

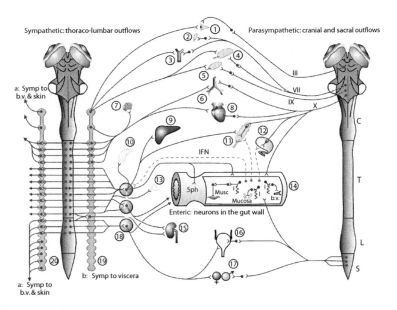

Figure 5.1 Schematic representation of the efferent (motor) pathways of the ANS, including illustration of some peripherally confined afferent neurons. Autonomic visceral afferent neurons relaying signals to the CNS have been omitted to simplify the diagram. The brain stem and spinal cord are represented twice, on the left to show sympathetic connections and on the right to show parasympathetic connections. The enteric division is represented by neurons within the gut wall (center of diagram, 14). *Sympathetic outflows.* a: To the left side of the spinal cord, sympathetic chain (paravertebral) ganglia are represented; some neurons of these ganglia supply blood vessels (b.v.) throughout the body and effectors in the skin (sweat glands pilomotor muscles). These pathways have synapses in the paravertebral ganglia. For simplicity of illustration, pathways that run rostrally and caudally within the sympathetic chains are not illustrated. b: On the right side of the cord are the connections that pass first through the sympathetic chains and then through prevertebral ganglia and plexuses (18) to supply visceral organs, as well as pathways that supply structures in the head and neck and intracranial arteries. Synapses occur in either prevertebral or paravertebral ganglia. *Parasympathetic outflows.* These emerge from cranial and sacral levels and innervate structures in the head, neck, abdomen, and pelvis, but not in the limbs. *Enteric neurons.* These are represented within the outline of the intestine (14). The enteric reflex circuits contain intrinsic primary afferent neurons (IPANs, I), interneurons, and motor neurons. As illustrated, these control muscle (musc), the secretory epithelium of the mucosa, and blood vessels (b.v.). *Sph.* This indicates the sphincter regions of the intestine that are controlled by enteric and extrinsic neurons. *Peripherally confined neural connections between organs.* (------). One of the neurons that contributes to these circuits is the intestinofugal neuron (IFN) that projects from the intestine to prevertebral ganglia. *Target tissues and organs.* (1) Eye, (2) Lacrimal glands, (3) Intracranial arteries, (4, 5) Salivary glands, (6) Airways, (7) Brown fat, (8) Heart, (9) Liver, (10) Spleen, (11) Pancreas, (12) Gallbladder, (13) Adrenal gland, (14) Tubulara gastrointestinal tract, (15) Kidney, (16) Urinary bladder, (17) Genital organs, (18) Prevertebral ganglia and plexuses, (19, 20) Sympathetic chains (paravertebral ganglia and their interconnections). *Spinal cord levels.* C, cervical; T, thoracic; L, lumbar; S, sacral. Modified and used with permission from Furness, 2006.

(Harm, 1990) and in patients undergoing chemotherapy, Morrow, Angel, and DuBeshter (1992) reported facial (cheek) pallor reached a maximum 40–50 minutes before emesis, but that 10–20 minutes before emesis a blush was apparent. Facial skin temperature decreased during nausea and reached its maximum 55–65 minutes prior to the onset of vomiting, although it decreased further during vomiting. With the exception of the Morrow, Angel, and DuBeshter (1992) study, all studies of cutaneous physiology in this area appear to have used stimuli evoking some form of motion sickness (e.g., parabolic flights, cross-coupled motion, caloric vestibular stimulation, oscillating video) and hence it is difficult to generalize about the skin changes that accompany nausea. In addition, there may be regional differences in effects, as while forehead (metopic) sweating was seen in response to nausea evoked by an oscillating video stimulus, palmar sweating did not increase (Himi et al., 2004) (see Figure 5.2). The changes in the electrogastrogram (EGG) recorded during the same time periods are also shown in Figure 5.2 to illustrate the temporal coincidence between the increase in EGG power and metopic perspiration.

Sweating, indicated by changes in galvanic skin response, has been reported in regions associated with thermal and emotion-induced sweating responses during motion sickness (McClure & Fregly, 1972). However, it was concluded that the sweating from the thermal sweat areas on the dorsal surface of the hand and the forearm were more likely to be specific for nausea than the induction of sweating in the palm, which was more associated with any form of arousal.

Overall, pallor and cold sweating are commonly reported in patients experiencing nausea from several causes but they also occur in many other clinical settings. However, in studies of motion sickness Reason and Brand (1975) argued that pallor was a more reliable indicator of nausea than was cold sweating.

It is worth noting that some of the changes described above are very similar to those commonly reported in patients with migraine. While facial pallor is common, some patients exhibit flushing of the forehead in association with pain, and clammy hands and feet are reported, as is profuse sweating in some patients (Davidoff, 1995).

The control of the facial circulation is complex and is regionally specialized (see Janig, 1990; Levick, 1991; Appenzeller & Oribe, 1997; Collins, 1999; Drummond, 1999, for reviews and references covering the following paragraph).

Sympathetic vasoconstrictor fibers originating from the upper thoracic spinal cord supply the nose, lips, eyes, and ears in particular, and these effects are mediated by noradrenaline acting on α-adrenoceptors. These areas have a high density of arteriovenous anastomoses (AVAs), which function to divert blood to and from the capillary loops in the more superficial layers of the skin and are involved in thermoregulation via control from the hypothalamus. Elevated sympathetic tone will lead to constriction of the AVAs, producing reduced blood flow and heat loss (net heat conservation). However,

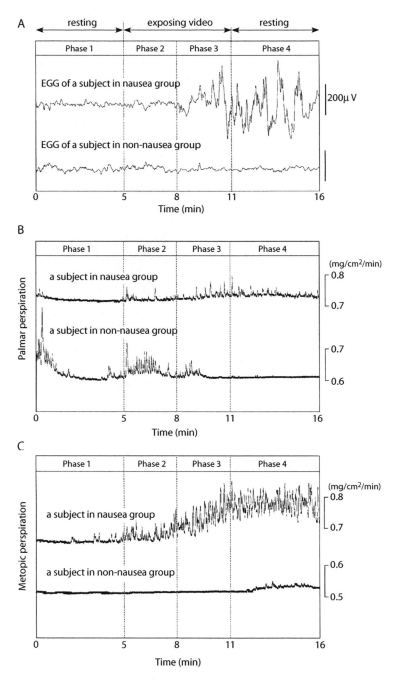

Figure 5.2 Electrogastrogram (EGG) and sweating responses to watching an irregularly oscillating video. Phase 1—resting (0–5 min); Phases 2 and 3—exposure to the video (5–11 min); Phase 4—resting following exposure to the video (11–16 min). Upper panel A. Typical EGG records of subjects in the nausea and non-nausea groups. Lower panels B, C. Typical examples of the changes in palmar (B) and metopic (C) perspiration of subjects in the nausea group and the non-nausea group. Figure and legend modified with permission from Himi et al., 2004.

the face is also supplied by sympathetic vasodilator fibers, which have been shown to be activated by psychological stimuli (e.g., mental stress, arousal stimuli, emotional stress). As vasodilation and emotional sweating often occur together it has been argued that they may be coupled via the action of the neurotransmitters vasoactive intestinal peptide (VIP) and acetylcholine (ACh). In contrast to the AVAs described above, which are regulated from the hypothalamus, these sympathetic vasodilator fibers are likely to be regulated from the forebrain. Finally, the lips and forehead are also supplied with parasympathetic vasodilator fibers using acetylcholine and VIP as neurotransmitters. It is notable that parasympathetic dilator fibers also supply nasal, lachrymal, and salivary glands, and that both sets of fibers originate from the inferior and superior salivatory nuclei in the brain stem. Salivation, lacrimation, and forehead vasodilation are all induced by noxious stimulation of the buccal cavity and may all be part of an orofacial defensive reflex (Drummond, 1999). The sweat glands are innervated by sympathetic nerves using acetylcholine as a neurotransmitter (Janig, 1990).

Both pallor and sweating would be caused by an increase in activity of the sympathetic adrenergic and cholinergic efferents respectively, with the pallor perhaps being contributed to by circulating vasopressin (see Chapter 6, in this volume). Facial flushing requires withdrawal of sympathetic constrictor tone and an increase in activity in vasodilator efferents (Drummond, 1999).

A number of techniques (Harm, 1990; 2002) are available for real-time recording of skin color, temperature, blood flow, resistance/conductance, and sweating and offer an opportunity to investigate the temporal relationship between changes in skin physiology, the onset of reported nausea, and other physiological variables in settings other than motion sickness. For example, subjects given apomorphine commonly report feeling hot and sweaty (Cannon et al., 1983), but this may not necessarily be related to nausea.

Skeletal Muscle

Vasodilation is seen in the forearm but not calf muscle during acute mental stress (Levick, 1991), and such a response might be expected in subjects experiencing nausea, although this has hardly been investigated. In subjects given apomorphine, evidence for forearm vasodilation was obtained indirectly from venous oxygen saturation (Ehrlich & Wallisch, 1943, cited in Barcroft & Swan, 1953), and plethysmography showed an increase in forearm blood flow during motion sickness (Stott, 1986). The mechanism is likely to be due to a decrease in adrenergic sympathetic vasoconstrictor tone, which is relatively high, but there is also evidence that, as is well established in carnivorous animals, sympathetic cholinergic vasodilator nerves are also present in humans (Levick, 1991). The vasodilation may also involve the sympathetically mediated stimulation of adrenaline secretion from the adrenal medulla, as adrenaline causes vasodilation in the myocardium, liver, and skeletal muscle via β-adrenoceptors (Broadley, 1996).

Respiratory System

Airway muscle tone and submucosal gland secretion are both regulated by vagal efferents with the sympathetic innervation having an indirect effect on tone, via modulation of the parasympathetic effect on tone in humans, and an effect on mucus secretion and bronchial blood flow (Barnes, 1999). The airways are also sensitive to circulating adrenaline and a degree of broncho-constriction may occur during nausea via this mechanism. As far as we are aware there have not been any published studies of airway function during nausea, and even ventilation itself although not controlled by autonomic efferents has hardly been studied. Gastric distension has been reported to increase airway secretion in cats via a pathway dependent on an intact abdominal vagus (German et al., 1982), and although the functional significance is unclear it is proposed that this a gastrotracheal vagally mediated secretory reflex that could serve to protect the airways and lungs against aspirated vomitus (German et al., 1982).

Mechanical factors protecting the airways during retching and vomiting have been investigated in dogs by Lang et al. (2002). It is worth noting that ipecacuanha syrup has been used as both an emetic and an expectorant with the latter effect perhaps being a consequence of a reflex stimulation of airway secretion secondary to stimulation of gastrointestinal vagal afferents. In motion sickness some hyperventilation resulting in a reduction in end-tidal carbon dioxide percentage has been reported (Sinha, 1968), and a small increase in respiration rate was recorded while watching an irregularly oscillating video (Himi et al., 2004). Lang (1990) reported an increase in respiratory rate in dogs at both subemetic and emetic doses of apomorphine in the period prior to the initiation of the retrograde giant contraction in the small intestine (see below). Interestingly, the peripherally acting emetic cholecystokinin octapeptide (CCK-8) did not evoke similar changes in respiratory rate although the gastrointestinal effects were similar to apomorphine.

Yawning or sighing, both modifications of respiration, are frequently reported as prodromal signs (Reason & Brand, 1975), but the underlying reason why they occur is unclear although they may be linked to the beneficial effect of controlled breathing on the sensation of nausea (Yen Pik Sang, Golding & Gresty, 2003). Hiccups have been reported in some subjects given apomorphine at emetic doses (Cannon et al., 1983).

Cardiovascular System

The cardiovascular changes associated with nausea are the physiological changes most studied, probably because of the ease with which they can be measured continuously in humans and the underlying autonomic changes deduced. An early study by Wolf (1943) using caloric vestibular stimulation showed tachycardia at the time nausea was reported with a gradual decline as the nausea resolved (see Figure 5.3) and tachycardia was also reported in a decorticate man during a turbulent flight (Doig, Wolf & Wolff, 1953).

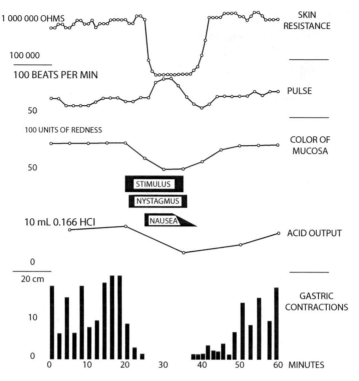

Figure 5.3 Changes in autonomic functions associated with nausea induced by caloric stimulation of the vestibular apparatus in a subject with a gastric fistula. Nausea was accompanied by decreased skin resistance, increased heart rate, blanching of the gastric mucosa, decreased gastric acid secretion, and decreased gastric motility. Reproduced with permission from Wolf, 1943.

Tachycardia has also been reported in humans during vection (Hu et al., 1991). In ferrets and piglets following radiation and cisplatin respectively (Tuor, Kondysar & Harding, 1988; Milano et al., 1995) tachycardia occurs, and it has also been reported following the administration of apomorphine in dogs (Lang, 1990). The increase in heart rate was not dependent on the occurrence of vomiting, with tachycardia observed in animals treated with atropine. The latter supports an involvement of sympathetic activation in mediating the tachycardia rather than withdrawal of vagal drive, although this needs to be investigated in humans. The peripherally acting emetic agent CCK-8 was without significant effect on the heart rate, showing that in the period immediately prior to the onset of emesis tachycardia is not inevitable.

Tachycardia is perhaps not surprising because of the generally stressful nature of nausea but generalization is unwise as in humans the onset of

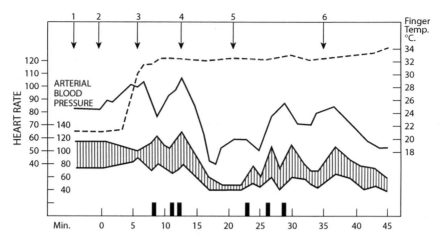

Figure 5.4 Experiment showing the likeness of the effects of apomorphine to those of the vaso-vagal syndrome. There is bradycardia, precipitate fall in blood pressure, and vasodilation in muscle as shown by a rise in the oxygen saturation of the venous blood from the arm vein.1: Oxygen saturation 22 percent. 2: 10mg. apomorphine. 3: Yawning feeling of fatigue. 4 and 5: Oxygen saturations 49 and 50 percent respectively. Vomiting is denoted by the solid rectangles. Reproduced with permission from Barcroft and Swan, 1953.

vomiting induced by apomorphine is accompanied by bradycardia and a marked fall in blood pressure (see Figure 5.4) (Ehrlich & Wallisch, 1943, cited in Barcroft & Swan, 1953). The authors drew attention to the likeness of the effects of apomorphine to the vaso-vagal syndrome, and this may account for reports of dizziness and lightheadedness in subjects given apomorphine (Cannon et al., 1983).

In patients undergoing chemotherapy, Morrow, Angel, and DuBeshter (1992) reported a bradycardia coincident with nausea and a tachycardia with the onset of emesis. Swallowing is accompanied by a transient tachycardia (Appenzeller & Oribe, 1997) and as nausea is often accompanied by an increase in swallowing (probably secondary to increased salivation) tachycardia may be a secondary effect. Extensive studies of heart rate and blood pressure associated with motion sickness failed to identify any consistent changes (Reason & Brand, 1975) but this requires detailed investigation using more modern techniques with high temporal resolution.

More recent studies have tended to focus on measurements of heart rate variability and respiratory sinus arrhythmia, which have variously been measured during motion sickness and cancer chemotherapy–induced nausea and vomiting. Before describing the results, the significance of each measure commonly used in the clinic to asses autonomic function will be outlined (Appenzeller & Oribe, 1997).

Heart Rate Variability

Heart rate variability (HRV) is derived from recordings of the electrocardiogram (ECG), and one way in which it is assessed is by measuring the standard deviation of successive R-R wave differences (SDSD) (Morrow et al., 2000). HRV is proposed to reflect activity in the vagal (parasympathetic) supply to the heart and has been used as an indicator of overall parasympathetic system activation including that to the gut although this may be an erroneous conclusion (see section below on the stomach). An increase in SDSD is indicative of an increase in cardiac vagal efferent activity.

Respiratory Sinus Arrhythmia

Respiratory sinus arrhythmia (RSA) is another measure of cardiac parasympathetic activity and measures the respiratory modulation of the cardiac interbeat interval. An increase in RSA indicates an increase in cardiac vagal efferent activity.

Morrow et al. (2000) recorded the SDSD continuously in ovarian cancer patients following the administration of chemotherapy, with recordings including the time prior to and during the onset of reported nausea. A progressive increase in the SDSD was recorded following administration of chemotherapy, but the onset of nausea occurred consistently after the SDSD had peaked (see Figure 5.5). The rise in SDSD indicates a steady increase in cardiac vagal efferent activity, but it is clear that at the time nausea is first reported this activity is returning to, but has not reached, pre–chemotherapy administration levels. The onset of the report of nausea is occurring at a time when there is a withdrawal of an elevated level of cardiac vagal efferent activity. A subsequent study of cancer patients undergoing chemotherapy revealed a trend for the RSA to decrease over the hour preceding the onset of nausea, but this effect was not statistically significant (Gianaros et al., 2001). In a similar study Morrow et al. (1999) reported a higher number of "abnormal" tests of ANS function (e.g., cold pressor, Valsalva ratio, max–min heart rate) in the two hours following chemotherapy in patients who would subsequently go on to develop "high" as opposed to "low" levels of nausea.

A decrease in heart rate variability indicative of a withdrawal of cardiac vagal efferent activity was reported during the development of motion sickness induced by vection (Hu, Stern & Koch, 1991). These changes were accompanied by an increase in skin conductance, which was negatively correlated with the mean of the difference between successive heartbeats. Further support for a withdrawal of cardiac parasympathetic activity during vection comes from a study by Gianaros et al. (2003) showing a progressive decrease in RSA with vection.

Attention has focused on the cardiac rhythm changes that may accompany the onset of nausea primarily because of the noninvasive nature of the measurements and the insights they may provide into the autonomic nervous system changes that accompany nausea. However, with this focus it is easy to

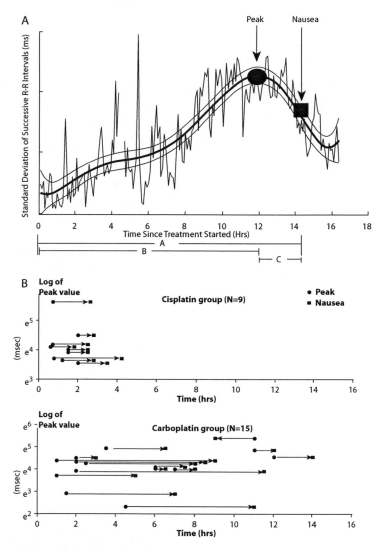

Figure 5.5 Upper Panel A. The relationship between the time after the start of administration of carboplatin and cyclophosphamide and the standard deviation of successive R-R intervals measured over > 16 hrs in an individual patient with ovarian cancer. The solid line is an eighth-order polynomial used to smooth the data, and the thin lines to each side of the solid line represent the standard error of the mean for the values. Three measurements were defined for each patient from such plots: A = the time from the start of cytotoxic drug administration until patients first reported nausea; B = the time from the start of cytotoxic drug administration until the peak value of SDSD was reached (SDSD peak latency); C = the time from peak SDSD value to the first report of nausea (SDSD peak–nausea interval). Lower panels B. Solid circles show the time in hours after drug administration (time 0) when the peak SDSD occurred for individual patients given cisplatin (upper panel, $n = 9$) or carboplatin (lower panels, $n = 15$). The solid square for each of the patients shows the time after chemotherapy administration when they first reported nausea. Reproduced with permission from Morrow et al., 2000.

forget that there may be changes in blood flow to internal organs mediated by sympathetic vasoconstrictor neurons or circulating hormones such as vasopressin. The changes in blood flow to the gastrointestinal tract would be of particular interest as, in a subject with a gastric fistula, Wolf (1943) reported gastric mucosal pallor during nausea evoked by caloric vestibular stimulation and this was associated with a decrease in gastric contractions and acid secretion. Pallor and reduced gastric acid secretion also accompanied nausea induced by ipecac or cigarette smoking (Wolf, 1965).

A reduction in middle cerebral artery blood flow velocity was seen one ($-22 \pm -5\%$) to two ($-13 \pm -4\%$) minutes prior to the onset of nausea in subjects during centrifugation (Serrador et al., 2005), but no change was observed in subjects who did not report nausea. This observation needs to be pursued using other nauseogenic stimuli. The cerebral arteries receive a dense sympathetic constrictor innervation using primarily neuropeptide Y (NPY) and 5-hydroxytryptamine (5-HT) as transmitters with a minor contribution from noradrenaline (N-Ad). There are also vasodilator fibers using VIP and ACh (see Goadsby, 1990 for review of cerebral circulation).

Adrenal Gland

The adrenal medulla is innervated by splanchnic efferents that when activated stimulate secretion of catecholamines and in particular adrenaline. Such a sympathetically mediated secretion of adrenaline could contribute to the genesis of the sensation of nausea (directly or indirectly; see Chapter 6, in this volume) associated with psychological stress, pain, and several centrally acting stimuli (e.g., apomorphine, motion).

Gastrointestinal Tract

Salivary Secretion

An increase in salivary secretion has been reported in macaque monkeys, dog, cat, ferret, and house musk shrew (*Suncus murinus*) prior to the onset of vomiting and is accompanied by an increase in swallowing. Salivation is one of the measures used in a motion sickness rating scale in the cat (Suri, Crampton & Daunton, 1979). The salivary glands are predominantly under parasympathetic control (Proctor & Carpenter, 2007), with an involvement of acetylcholine as well as other transmitters including VIP and Substance P (SP) Although salivation indicates that the parasympathetic supply is active, it is unlikely that salivation itself is an indicator of the onset of nausea as this response can be evoked by emetic stimuli even in anesthetized and decerebrate animals (e.g., Furukawa & Okada, 1994; Furukawa et al., 1998). However, the sudden presence of large amounts of saliva in the mouth is probably perceived and may have behavioral consequences (e.g., mouth scratching reported in ferrets; see Chapter 8, in this volume). In the cat exposed to motion, Lang, Sarna, and Shaker (1999) showed that the incidence of licking (46%) was greater than that of overt salivation (34%) suggesting that the two events are not necessarily causally linked. It is of note that only about half of the cats had overt salivation, but additionally it was demonstrated that salivation also occurred in animals that did not vomit during vertical oscillation. While salivation is increased prior to the onset of emesis, studies in the dog show that it is reduced during episodes of retching (Furukawa & Okada, 1994). Although humans may report increased salivation prior to the onset of vomiting, this is not a universal finding, and some report a dry mouth. One of the formal studies of salivation indicates that there may be a mismatch between actual salivation and the perception. For example, in a field study of seasickness, while eight subjects reported an increase in salivation in fact in six there was a measured decrease (Gordon et al., 1989). A buildup of saliva in the mouth due to a stress-related decrease in swallowing could account for the difference in perception in this setting. In Tom, the patient with a gastric fistula, Wolf (1965) reported salivation on the instillation of ipecac directly into the stomach and also during caloric vestibular stimulation. It is clear that further well-controlled studies are required using the minimally invasive techniques that are available for the measurement of salivation in humans.

Gastrointestinal Motility and Secretion

The following quote about the relationship between nausea and gastrointestinal motility from Sarna (1989) is unfortunately still correct: "there is no known abnormal gastrointestinal motor pattern that lasts for hours or that correlates with this subjective response." Despite this there are a number of motility changes that occur prior to vomiting, and while they are unlikely to be causally related to nausea a discussion of them provides a snapshot of the events occurring when nausea is probably present and prior to the onset of retching and vomiting.

The gastrointestinal motility changes occurring prior to the onset of retching and vomiting are well characterized especially in the dog, and as far as can be ascertained similar changes also occur in humans. As aspects are similar to those reported in humans reporting nausea they will be reviewed here. In addition, as there is some evidence that these motor changes can be evoked by doses of agents that evoke emesis when given at higher doses it is possible that they may also occur in association with nausea, which itself can also be evoked at lower doses than are required to induce retching and vomiting.

Swallowing   Although not strictly mediated by the ANS, swallowing can be both initiated and increased in frequency by emetic stimuli in conscious, anesthetized, and decerebrate animals (Andrews et al., 1990b; Lang, Sarna & Dodds, 1993; Smith, Paton & Andrews, 2002). Gastric antral distension in the anesthetized cat at levels higher than those required to evoke reflex corpus relaxation evoked swallowing (Abrahamsson, 1973). An increase in swallowing frequency was reported in dogs given a subemetic dose of apomorphine, and at an emetic dose swallowing increased prior to the onset of vomiting

(~ 1 min vs. ~ 2.5 min) (Lang, Sarna & Dodds, 1993). Cervical vagal blockade in the dog prolonged the swallowing response to apomorphine as well as increasing the peak frequency without affecting the emetic response (Lang, Sarna & Dodds, 1993), but the mechanism is unclear. Lang et al. (1993) make an important point that swallowing may be a "good index of the intensity of the emetic stimulus" as they showed a relationship between the frequency of swallowing and the subsequent number of vomits. Further studies are required to examine the relationship between the intensity of salivary secretion (particularly marked in the dog), swallowing frequency, and magnitude of the subsequent emetic response.

Gastric Motility   An absence of gastric peristalsis and low tone in the proximal stomach was an early finding from radiographs of subjects experiencing nausea (Barclay, 1936; Lumsden & Holden, 1969) and in studies of cats given emetic stimuli (Cannon, 1898; Smith & Brizzee, 1961). Relaxation of the proximal stomach is probably the earliest event reported following administration of emetic and some subemetic doses of centrally acting agents such as apomorphine, morphine, and an α-adrenoceptor agonist (Abrahamsson, 1973; Blancquaert et al., 1982; Lefebvre, Willems & Bogaert, 1981; Willems & Lefebvre, 1986; De Ponti et al., 1990) (see Figure 5.6).

In the cat, relaxation of the proximal stomach has also been observed in response to stimulation of the pharynx, esophagus, and cardiac vagal afferents (Abrahamsson & Jansson, 1969; Abrahamsson, 1973), all stimuli capable of inducing retching and vomiting. In both the cat and the dog, the recovery of gastric tone following vomiting induced by apomorphine is protracted, taking 1–2 hours (Abrahamsson, 1973), and in humans gastric contractions are suppressed for 50–90 minutes following induction of nausea (Wolf & Wolff, 1948). Swallowing itself is associated with gastric relaxation, and it is possible that the increased salivation and swallowing often reported in subjects experiencing nausea further contribute to this effect. In humans a reduction in gastric tone and/or inhibition of contractile activity has also been reported accompanying nausea induced by motion, vection, caloric vestibular stimulation, tobacco smoking, and apomorphine (Wolf, 1965; Reason & Brand, 1975; Faas et al., 2001) (see Figures 5.3 and 5.7).

Dose response studies with apomorphine in humans (Ramsbottom & Hunt, 1970) have shown that a delay in gastric emptying occurs at sub-nausea-inducing doses, providing further supporting evidence that vagally mediated gastric relaxation may be the earliest GI tract indication of activation of emetic pathways. It also indicates that nausea is not an inevitable consequence of slowed gastric emptying and that abdominal visceral changes occur prior to the conscious awareness of nausea. The relaxation is mediated by the vagus and is most likely mediated by the same mechanism as is involved in proximal gastric accommodation following a meal; namely, increased activity in the vagal efferents supplying the postganglionic fibers using nitric oxide (NO) and VIP as inhibitory transmitters, and a reduction in the cholinergic efferent pathway.

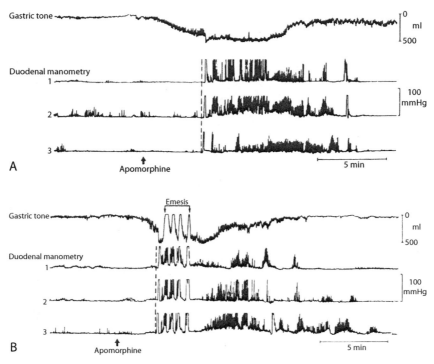

Figure 5.6 Upper panel A. Effect of a subemetic dose of apomorphine (0.01 μg/kg i.c.v.) on gastric tone and duodenal motility. Note gastric relaxation (intragastric volume increase) and a duodenal RPC, followed by post-RPC phasic contractions. Lower panel B. Effect of emetic dose of apomorphine (0.03 μg/kg i.c.v.) on gastric tone and duodenal motility. Note emesis preceded by gastric relaxation and a duodenal RPC and followed by post-RPC phasic contractions in the duodenum. During emesis, note four episodes of intra-abdominal pressure increase recorded simultaneously as retching artifacts by barostat and manometry. Reproduced with permission from De Ponti et al., 1990.

The inhibition of ongoing contractile activity is likely to be mediated by the same type of mechanism. The relaxation of the proximal stomach and inhibition of gastric contractions particularly in the distal stomach will delay gastric emptying and hence reduce the delivery of toxins ingested with the food into the intestine, where the risk of absorption into the blood is higher. The reduced rate of emptying would also serve to "flatten" the rise in the plasma concentration of any toxin absorbed, which may reduce its toxicity and reduce the likelihood of the hepatic detoxification mechanisms being overwhelmed. The relaxed proximal stomach also acts as a receptacle for the intestinal contents propelled to the stomach by the retrograde giant contraction (RGC, see below). It is worth noting that Abrahamsson (1973) reported that dogs postured to vomit during gastric relaxation, suggesting that the animal became

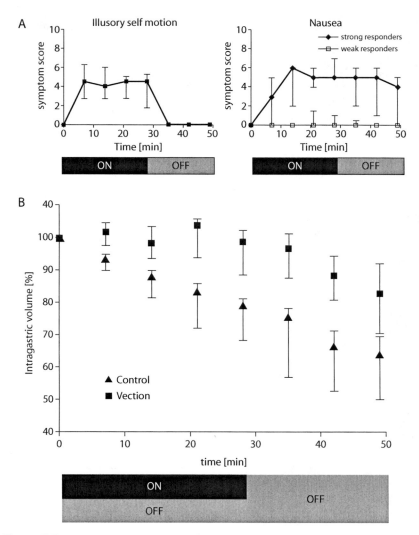

Figure 5.7 Upper panel A. Scores for illusory self-motion *(left)* and nausea *(right)* as rated by the subjects in *study part 1*. Self-motion was perceived by all subjects under vection (on) and disappeared upon withdrawal of the stimulus (off). Subjects fell into the following two groups with respect to their nausea ratings: strong responders ($n = 5$, score ≥ 4) and weak responders ($n = 7$, score ≤ 2). Data are medians (interquartile ranges). Lower panel B. Gastric emptying profiles obtained in *study part 1* during the vection and control days. Vection significantly delayed gastric emptying compared with control. Data are medians (interquartile ranges). Reproduced with permission from Faas et al., 2001.

aware of the imminence of vomiting although the origin of the signal is unclear.

The changes in the frequency (tachygastria/bradygastria) and pattern (dysrhythmia) of the electrogastrogram (EGG) recorded in subjects experiencing nausea induced by a number of stimuli are reviewed in detail in Chapters 7, 9, 14, and 15 in this volume. There is some evidence that gastric dysrhythmia precedes the onset of reported symptoms of nausea and the rise in plasma vasopressin. As the separation between the symptom reports was about one minute (Koch et al., 1990; Chapter 7, in this volume), there is clearly a need for additional studies using high temporal resolution techniques and a range of stimuli to confirm this important sequence of events. Using a vection stimulus, Hasler et al. (1995a) reported that measurable increases in tachygastric activity preceded the onset of symptom reports and in addition the maximal changes in tachygastria (% of signal > 4.5 cpm) preceded the report of maximal nausea by 40 seconds. The observations are consistent with the hypothesis that nausea itself does not "cause" the EGG changes.

The motor correlate of the tachygastria/tachyarrhythmia is a reduction of antral motility, and while this may have an endocrine origin (see Chapter 6, in this volume) it has been proposed that this is due to an increase in sympathetic activity with a reciprocal decrease in parasympathetic activity (Stern et al., 1994), with some support for this coming from studies of vection in humans showing that the α-adrenoceptor antagonist phentolamine reduced both gastric dysrhythmia and nausea (Hasler et al., 1995a). In addition, in cats exposed to vertical motion, supradiaphragmatic vagotomy abolished the RGC (see below) but bradygastria, decreased GI motility, and vomiting still occurred. Both vomiting and bradygastria also occurred in vagally intact animals treated with atropine (Lang, Sarna & Shaker, 1999). The order of onset of the various GI events (when present) following the onset of motion in the Lang, Sarna, and Shaker (1999) study was: Decrease GI motility (1.6 ± 0.3 min) > Bradygastria (2.2 ± 0.4 min) > Salivation (4.3 ± 1.0 min) > RGC (6.6 ± 1.3 min) > Vomiting (7.2 ± 1.3 min). Interestingly, when emesis was induced at a much shorter latency (2.4 ± 0.3 min) than with motion by using a drug (UK-14304, an α_2 receptor agonist), the mean latency to the onset of each event occurred in the same rank order.

Both of the above studies support an involvement of sympathetic efferent nerves in bradygastria/dysrhythmia, but do not exclude an involvement of vagal efferents driving postganglionic inhibitory (NO, VIP) neurons. It would be of interest to undertake studies using an inhibitor of nitric oxide synthase (NOS).

Gastric Secretion

Gastric secretion has not been systematically studied in subjects experiencing nausea. In Tom, the patient with a gastric fistula, Wolf (1949, 1965) described the effects of several "nauseogenic" stimuli on gastric secretions collected by aspiration. During caloric vestibular stimulation it was observed that the gastric mucosa became pallid and there was a decrease in titratable acid, but, significantly, it was also noted that there was an apparent increase in mucus secretion and gastric juice samples were viscid. A similar effect was reported following ingestion of ipecac (Wolf, 1949), and in addition bile was present in the secretion at a time coincident with the onset of nausea. In dogs with either vagally denervated stomachs or transplanted fundic pouches (with and without abdominal sympathectomy), distension in the region of the esophago-duodenal anastomosis sufficient to induce "nausea and retching" reduced both the volume and titratable acidity of histamine-stimulated gastric secretion (Grossman et al., 1945). In the same study, apomorphine was reported to have a similar effect. Although it is difficult to ascribe the effects on secretion to nausea as opposed to retching, the study is of interest because the effect appears to be relatively prolonged, lasting from 30 to 60 minutes after the stimulus. In addition, because the pouches are extrinsically denervated, the effect must be mediated by a circulating factor. While the main physiological mechanism for release of gut hormones is via the sensing of the luminal environment, it is likely that the mechanical stimulus used in the above study will have evoked release. Of the major gut hormones located in the duodenum and which have been shown to inhibit gastric secretion, the main candidates are secretin and somatostatin. Other candidates include GLP-1, GLP-2, and oxyntomodulin, but these have a more distal location in the intestine (Chaudhri, Small & Bloom, 2006). Vasopressin secreted from the posterior pituitary in response to abdominal vagal afferent activation by duodenal distension is clearly another candidate, with studies on Tom (Wolf, 1965) showing gastric mucosal pallor and reduced acid secretion.

Although the evidence is relatively weak, a reduction in gastric acid secretion with a concomitant increase in mucus production presumably accompanied by an increase in bicarbonate ion secretion is what would be expected in advance of vomiting to reduce the impact on the esophageal, pharyngeal, and buccal mucosa and dentition. Although there is indirect evidence to show that the reduction of gastric acid secretion could be due to a hormone, an effect of the extrinsic autonomic nerves should not be excluded until well-controlled studies have been undertaken using more modern methods for assessment of gastric secretion and blood flow.

Retrograde Giant Contraction (RGC)   Large-amplitude contractions, apparently traveling in and oral (i.e., towards the mouth) direction in the small intestine and sometimes the distal stomach and occurring prior to the onset of vomiting, have been reported in studies over the last 100 years in several species with an emetic reflex (e.g., dog and cat; see Alvarez, 1925). The ability to override the normal oro–anal direction of peristaltic contractions and propulsion of contents may be a highly conserved mechanism as, as far as can be ascertained, vomiting in fish involves a retrograde contraction of the stomach that forces gastric contents into a relatively short and wide esophagus from where it is then expelled (Andrews & Young, 1993). Retrograde contractions in the stomach of the small shark *Scyliorhinus canicula* can be evoked by stimulation of the splanchnic efferents (Andrews & Young, 1993).

It is important to distinguish "retrograde contractions" in the gut from *the* retrograde giant contraction (RGC), which has a particular set of characteristics; the list below is based primarily on data from the dog, the species in which this event has been studied most extensively (Lang, 1990; Lang & Marvig, 1989; Lang, Marvig & Sarna, 1988; Lang et al., 1986; Lang, Sarna & Shaker, 1999) (see Figure 5.8). A video-recording of a radiographic study of the RGC in the dog undertaken by Ehrlein and Schemann can be found at www.wzw.tum.de/humanbiology/data/motility/.

The main characteristics of the RGC are listed below.

- Onset of the RGC is preceded by suppression of ongoing phasic contractions in the small intestine with the effect occurring almost synchronously in all regions. This occurs in the presence of atropine, so is unlikely to be due to withdrawal of vagal cholinergic (muscarinic) drive and therefore likely to be due to vagal activation of intrinsic inhibitor neurons (e.g., NO, VIP).
- Originates in the mid-part of the small intestine and progresses from the point of origin toward the stomach and may involve the gastric antrum.
- A single, large-amplitude contraction that in the small intestine is up to ~ 80% larger than phase III of the migrating motor complex. The amplitude of the RGC is unrelated to the dose of emetic agent used.
- Mediated by the vagus and blocked by muscarinic receptor antagonists (e.g., atropine).
- Can occur spontaneously but is usually evoked by an emetic agent at both fully emetic and subemetic doses.
- When doses of an emetic agent are used that result in retching and vomiting the retching does not begin until the RGC has progressed to the stomach.
- The RGC is followed by a burst of phasic contractions, of smaller amplitude than the RGC, that propel small intestinal contents in an aboral direction. In vagally intact animals while the RGC is blocked by atropine, post-RGC contractions still occur in the correct temporal relationship to the onset of vomiting induced by apomorphine.
- The RGC is not essential for retching and vomiting to occur.

The RGC in mammals has two main functions. First, it will return any toxin–containing gastric contents that have entered the small intestine to the stomach, from where they can be ejected, and second, alkaline intestinal contents entering the stomach will help buffer the acidic gastric contents prior to ejection. The RGC is probably responsible for the presence of bile in vomitus, although bile can enter the stomach when antral motility is reduced relative to that in the duodenum (Code et al., 1984). Furthermore there is evidence for

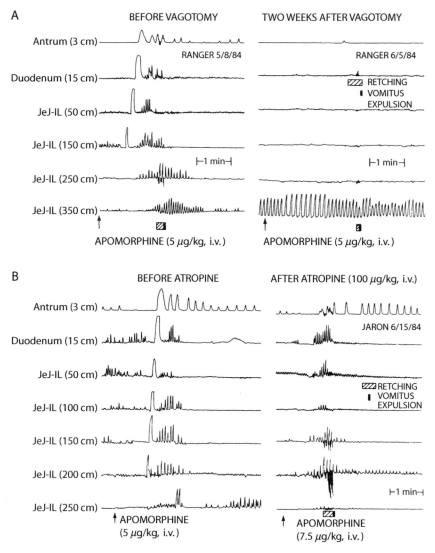

Figure 5.8 Upper panel A. The gastrointestinal motor correlates of vomiting and the effect of supradiaphragmatic vagotomy. The retrograde giant contraction (RGC) begins at about mid–small intestine and propagates through the gastric antrum. The post-RGC phasic contractions occur after the RGC primarily in the lower half of the small intestine. Supradiaphragmatic vagotomy blocked both motor correlates of vomiting but did not block retching or vomitus expulsion (JeJ-IL, jejunoileum). Numbers in parentheses indicate the distance in centimeters of the strain gauge transducers from the pylorus. Lower panel B. The effect of atropine in the gastrointestinal motor correlates of vomiting activated by apomorphine. Atropine blocks the retrograde giant contraction (RGC) but not the post-RGC contractions. Definitions as in upper panel. Reproduced with permission from Lang, Sarna, and Condon, 1986.

contraction of the gall bladder prior to the onset of vomiting (Qu, Furukawa & Fukuda, 1995). Bile is known to be a mucosal irritant, and its presence in the stomach may provide an additional nauseogenic or emetic stimulus.

The RGC-like activity has been recorded in humans (e.g., Thompson & Malagelada, 1982; Davidson & Pilot, 1993), although it is not as well characterized as in the dog. Figure 5.9 shows a rare recording of the RGC in a healthy volunteer, where nausea was induced using an infusion of the macrolide antibiotic erythromycin.

Although there is no direct evidence that the RGC contributes to the sensation of nausea per se, Sarna (1989) has suggested that the "brief nausea and abdominal discomfort" felt immediately prior to vomiting may be related to the RGC and entry of intestinal contents into the stomach. Although the proximal stomach is relaxed at this time and antral motility reduced, this sudden distension of the stomach by the arrival of intestinal contents could theoretically give rise to nausea and abdominal discomfort via vagal afferent activation. Some subjects report a "sinking sensation in the stomach (epigastrum)" immediately prior to vomiting that could be related to these mechanical changes, but this has not been investigated directly. The RGC is also of interest because, as we saw with gastric relaxation, it can be evoked by subemetic doses of both centrally (e.g., apomorphine) and peripherally (e.g., copper sulfate, CCK-8) acting emetics (Lang, 1988; 1990), and the threshold for its induction by several emetic stimuli can be lowered by naloxone (Lang & Marvig, 1989). As nausea can be induced by "low intensity" stimulation of pathways that, when more intensely activated, evoke retching and vomiting, detailed investigation of the central pathways by which these preemetic events

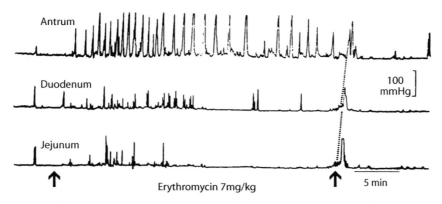

Figure 5.9 Retroperistaltic contraction in human GI tract induced by erythromycin (EM). EM (7 mg/kg) was given for 30 minutes (shown by the arrows). During the infusion high amplitude contractions occurred in the stomach, while the small bowel appeared to be quiescent. The retroperistalsis occurring at the end of the EM infusion was accompanied by nausea. Used with permission from Davidson and Pilot, 1993. Copyright Hodder Arnold, 1993..

are produced may help better differentiate the signals for nausea as opposed to vomiting. The occurrence of sudden onset gastric relaxation and the RGC may mark the transition point from nausea to vomiting.

The neural correlates of the gastrointestinal motor and secretory changes that accompany nausea and vomiting have been little investigated. However, a study by Blackshaw, Grundy, and Scratcherd (1987) in the anesthetized ferret showed an increase in vagal efferent discharge coincident with the onset of lip-licking and retching induced by hypertonic saline in the stomach (see Figure 5.10). This observation supports the view outlined above that it is unwise to extrapolate about the abdominal vagus from data derived from studies of heart rate variability.

THE ROLE OF AFFERENTS IN THE AUTONOMIC NERVOUS SYSTEM IN NAUSEA

Robert Boyle's statement, "Tis profitable for a man that his stomach should nauseate and reject things that have a loathsome taste or smell," implies that the stomach is the seat of the sensation of nausea and that in response to the adequate stimulus it should "reject" (i.e., vomit) the cause (Boyle, 1996/1686,

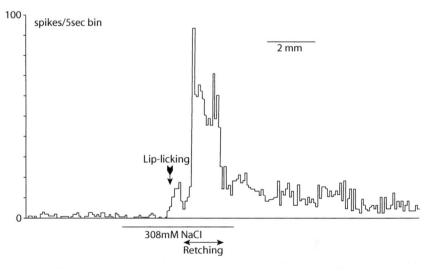

Figure 5.10 Histogram of efferent fiber discharge (in impulses/5 s) against time in minutes before, during, and after retching induced by duodenal perfusion with hypertonic saline (308 mM). Efferent discharge increased approximately 90 s after the rise in duodenal osmolarity coincident with prodromata such as lip-licking (shown by the arrow) and increased further during retching. On reverting back to perfusion with isotonic saline (end of bar), the frequency of efferent discharge gradually returned to its original level. Reproduced with permission from Blackshaw, Grundy, and Scratcherd, 1987.

Sect. V., p. 74). For both events to occur, the stomach and other gut regions must have a detection system that connects to the central nervous system, and the afferents supplying the gastrointestinal tract and selected other organs are in an ideal position to provide such an input. This section will review the evidence for the involvement of the visceral ("autonomic") afferents in providing an input signal to the central nervous system that will subsequently give rise to the sensation of nausea. The autonomic nerves of primary interest are the abdominal vagus and the greater splanchnic, which supply the upper GI tract, the site often associated with the location of the sensation of nausea and also a site from which it can be evoked. It must be emphasized that in most cases direct evidence for an involvement of a specific set of afferents in nausea or vomiting in humans is lacking because of a paucity of human studies and an absence, for obvious reasons, of studies where nausea has been studied under controlled conditions before and after selective nerve lesions. Thus the involvement of the vagus in particular is based upon a combination of experimental animal data and studies in humans showing that similar stimuli evoke nausea or vomiting and that they can be blocked by drugs that affect the same pathway in animals.

Vagal Afferents

The vagus is often called the "wandering nerve," and this is an accurate reflection of the extensive territory it supplies. Afferents in the vagus supply the posterior pharynx and epiglottis (via an internal branch of the superior laryngeal nerve) and the gastrointestinal tract from the upper esophagus to the transverse colon, collecting information on the luminal environment and muscle tension and conveying it primarily to the nucleus tractus solitarius (NTS) in the dorsal brain stem. It is important to note that in the common laboratory species ~ 80–90% of the abdominal vagal nerve fibers are afferent, suggesting that its major role is monitoring the gastrointestinal tract (Andrews, 1986). The subsequent processing and projection of this input is discussed in Chapter 4 (in this volume). There is a body of evidence from lesion studies (abdominal vagotomy), afferent recording, and electrical stimulation of the cut central end of the vagus implicating the abdominal vagal afferents in the induction of retching and vomiting and also prodromata such as licking and swallowing, and less extensive evidence that vomiting can also be evoked by cardiac vagal afferents.

Afferents from the posterior pharynx are capable of evoking the gag reflex, which has some similarities to both a retch and a cough. Although the rat does not vomit it does have a gag reflex evocable by mechanical stimulation of the pharynx (Andrew, 1956), perhaps suggesting that the vomiting reflex is degenerate or incomplete rather than absent. Curiously, the pulmonary and airway afferents do not appear to be capable of evoking vomiting and indeed may have an inhibitory effect (Zabara, Chaffee & Tansy, 1972) although they are capable of evoking the cough reflex, which is also mediated via the NTS and involves the diaphragm and abdominal muscles in the motor output.

Despite the wealth of evidence that the abdominal and selected other vagal afferents (e.g., cardiac) are involved in induction of vomiting, direct evidence that the same afferents are involved in the genesis of nausea in humans is lacking perhaps with the exception of a comment by Lewis (1942) that vagal stimulation in humans can evoke nausea. In animals the evidence is indirect for reasons discussed extensively in Chapter 8 (in this volume). As abdominal vagal afferents are broadly classified as either mechano- or chemoreceptors, the discussion below is based on evidence that either mechanical or luminal chemical stimuli evoke nausea although this division is somewhat artificial.

Mechanical Stimuli

Early studies by Payne and Poulton (1927) using themselves as subjects reported nausea and, "an uneasiness in the pit of the stomach" in response to balloon distension of the esophagus. They also noted that as distension increased, "there was a transition in the sensation from nausea through painful nausea to pain alone; so the sensations recorded were really mixed, with nausea or pain predominating as the case may be." It is interesting to note that pain replaced nausea and that they did not experience both at the highest levels of distension. Similar studies confirmed that nausea could be induced from the esophagus and showed that it was more readily induced by distension of the stomach and duodenum (Ivy & Vloedman, 1925; Bloomfield & Polland, 1931; Polland & Bloomfield, 1931). Nausea was not reported on distension of the descending colon or sigmoid. In several cases retching and vomiting ensued, and Bloomfield and Polland (1931) comment, "It was of interest to observe how violently sick the subject could be as the result of a purely mechanical stimulus." More recent, better-controlled studies using distension showed that nausea can be induced by distension of the distal but not the proximal stomach (see Figure 5.11) with a balloon at levels below those evoking pain (Ladabaum et al., 1998) arguing for an involvement of vagal rather than splanchnic afferents. In obese patients implanted with a gastric balloon to facilitate weight loss, nausea was a common initial side effect (Ramhamadany, Fowler & Baird, 1989).

The above studies are all experimental and were intended to investigate the possible sensations that could be evoked from the upper gastrointestinal tract by distension. It is questionable whether such levels would be reached in the course of normal feeding in humans except perhaps in gurgitator (rapid eating) contests.

There is evidence that the sensory response to gastric distension is not fixed but can be altered by the presence of lipids in the duodenum. For example, levels of gastric distension that evoked very low nausea scores when the duodenum was infused with saline, induced substantially higher scores when lipid was present in the duodenum (Feinle et al., 2001). Intraduodenal administration of the local anesthetic benzocaine reduced the sensation of nausea in the presence of lipid by 36%, implicating small intestinal nerves in this effect; but, as the plasma level of cholecystokinin (CCK) was also reduced,

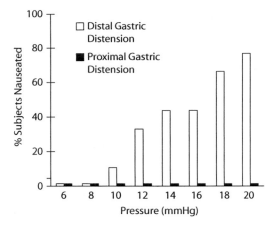

Figure 5.11 Percentage of subjects reporting nausea during gastric balloon distension. A significant number of subjects developed nausea in a pressure-dependent fashion with distal gastric distension, whereas no subject reported nausea with proximal distension. $P < 0.01$, x^2 test for overall proportion of subjects nauseated with distal vs. proximal distension.Reproduced with permission from Ladabaum et al., 1998.

it was not possible to differentiate between direct as opposed to indirect effects. The hypothesis that small intestinal afferents modulate gastrointestinal sensations and visceral perception is further supported (although not conclusively demonstrated) by a study showing that the susceptibility to vection and the intensity of the nausea was increased by a high-fat meal, provided that time was allowed for it to pass into the intestine (Feinle, Grundy & Read, 1995).

Fat has long been known to have the potential to induce nausea, as we see in this quote from Sir Hans Sloane (1660–1753), who found chocolate "nauseous and hard of digestion which came from the great oiliness" (quoted in Rice, 2000). Although the above study by Feinle, Grundy, and Read (1995) used lipid infusion into the duodenum, it would be interesting to know if a similar modulation of gastric sensation could be evoked by a range of "noxious" stimuli. It is known that noxious stimulation of the duodenum can produce a reflex delay in gastric emptying and this has been argued to be protective (Davis et al., 1986), so an increase in the sensitivity of the stomach would be consistent with this role.

Although the focus is on distension, it is important to recall that what is being signaled is intramural tension and that alterations in the wall tension will result in a change in the nature of the afferent signal (and arguably, sensation) in response to a given volume of distension. For example, impaired gastric accommodation (due to a defect in the vagal inhibitory innervation) will lead to an elevation of wall tension at a given volume and an enhanced vagal afferent discharge. The above studies provide a consistent body of evidence that distension of the upper gut can induce the sensation of nausea at a lower level of distension than that required to induce pain. This argues that in the

above cases nausea results from activation of the vagal afferent mechanoreceptors located in the muscular wall of the esophagus, stomach, and duodenum
and which respond to distension of the viscus. The abdominal vagal afferent
axons have conduction velocities in the range for small myelinated (Aδ) or
unmyelinated (C) nerve fibers, with information in the latter fibers taking
perhaps half a second or more to reach the brain stem from the gut. A review
of the detailed physiological properties of these afferents is outside the scope
of this chapter, and the reader is referred to recent reviews and specific papers
on the topic (Page & Blackshaw, 1998; Ozaki, Sengupta & Gebhart, 1999;
Phillips & Powley, 2000; Brookes, Zagorodnyuk & Costa, 2005). However,
three properties of these afferents require comment, as they are of relevance to
the genesis of the "nausea signal":

- In addition to being sensitive to distension of the stomach or other
  viscus, the mechanoreceptors are also capable of responding to
  contraction of the gut muscle, and recordings from the afferents
  show that they detect even the small-amplitude gastric antral contractions present in the absence of an overt stimulus (Andrews et al.,
  1980).
- Studies of vagal afferent mechanoreceptors in a number of locations
  (e.g., esophagus, stomach, jejunum) and a variety of species (e.g., cat,
  dog, ferret, rat, mouse) have not provided any evidence for the existence of afferents with a "high" threshold for activation by distension.
  What is meant by this is that the afferents can be activated by levels of
  distension below those considered noxious, the latter often designated
  as those producing a reflex increase in blood pressure (Cervero, 1982).
  This distinguishes the vagal afferents from some types of spinal
  (splanchnic) afferents involved in nociception. Gastric vagal afferents,
  which encode the degree of distension, up to and including noxious
  levels of distension have been described but their threshold for
  activation is still "low," so although they may be involved in nociception they still operate over the physiological range. In the distension
  studies described above, nausea is always induced at a lower level of
  distension than pain supporting the proposal that the vagal rather
  than splanchnic mechanoreceptive afferents provide the peripheral
  signal for nausea.
- The sensitivity of the mechanoreceptors is not fixed but can be altered
  by a number of chemicals including adenosine triphosphate (ATP, a
  product of inflammation), prostaglandins, glutamate, nicotine,
  γ-aminobutyric acid (GABA), and bradykinin (Beyak & Grundy,
  2005; Brookes, Zagorodnyuk & Costa, 2005). In addition, the mechanoreceptors can be activated by chemicals such as platelet activating
  factors, which does not sensitize the afferents (Ozaki, Sengupta &
  Gebhart, 1999), by bile, and by 5-hydroxytryptamine. Thus in clinical
  settings where the gastrointestinal tissue may be irritated, inflamed, or

be recovering from an infection, the properties of the mechanoreceptors may be altered.

Chemical Stimuli

The gastrointestinal mucosa is also supplied with vagal afferents. These monitor various chemical features of the luminal environment (e.g., glucose,
fats, osmolarity, pH) with the precise properties depending on their exact location. They are also able to respond to mechanical stimulation of the mucosa
such as the brushing of a bolus. These afferents are proposed to be involved
in the vomiting induced by intragastric hypertonic solutions, copper sulfate,
ipecacuanha, and enterotoxins as studies in laboratory animals have shown
that the normal emetic response to these agents is abolished or markedly
reduced by abdominal vagotomy (Andrews et al., 1990b). As these stimuli can
also evoke nausea and vomiting in humans, by extrapolation they are implicated in the responses in humans. However, in contrast to the studies using
distension as a stimulus to induce nausea, similarly controlled studies using
graded chemical stimuli are relatively lacking in humans. One exception is
studies on the effect of ingestion of copper solutions related to measurement
of the "No Observed Adverse Effect Level" (NOAEL) used in the determination of acceptable levels in beverages, food, and water (Araya et al., 2001). The
incidence of nausea is related to the concentration of copper (given as copper
sulfate, as is the case in animal studies), the reporting of nausea was most
frequent within 15 minutes of ingestion, and nausea was evoked at lower concentrations than required to evoke vomiting (when it occurred) (Araya et al.,
2001; Olivares et al., 2001) (Figure 5.12). Ingestion of copper containing

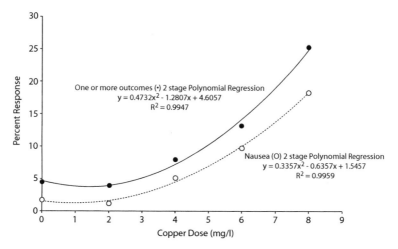

Figure 5.12 Subjects that reported one or more adverse gastrointestinal outcomes (•)
or nausea alone (O) as a function of the ingested copper concentration. Reproduced
with permission from Araya et al., 2001.

solutions may provide a method for induction of nausea via activation of gastrointestinal afferents in human MRI studies (see Chapter 4, in this volume).

There is a body of evidence from animals implicating the mucosal afferents in the acute nausea and vomiting induced by systemic cytotoxic anticancer drugs, the most extensively studied of which is cisplatin. Furthermore, the efficacy of 5-HT$_3$ receptor antagonists against acute vomiting in patients treated with the cancer chemotherapy agent cisplatin again implicates the vagus, as in animals the abdominal vagal afferents are involved in the acute phase of cisplatin-induced emesis (see Rudd & Andrews, 2005, for review).

The proposed anatomical substrate for these afferents accounts for the diversity of stimuli to which they can respond and has a number of morphological and molecular features in common with the taste buds. It is proposed that the detector cell is an enteroendocrine cell in the epithelium particularly of the stomach and small intestine. In response to particular chemicals, which can access the cell either from the lumen or from the blood (e.g., cisplatin), the enteroendocrine cell releases one or more mediators locally, and these act on receptors located on the terminals of vagal afferents (Andrews, Rapeport & Sanger, 1988; see Andrews & Rudd, 2004, for review). Some of these mediators may also enter the circulation to act at another site (e.g., the CNS), where they may be involved in signaling satiety (e.g., median eminence), regulating metabolism, or modulating gut motility.

Of the mucosal afferents the relationship between the 5-hydroxytryptamine-containing small intestinal enterochromaffin cells (EC) and the vagal afferents is probably the most extensively studied because of their involvement in the acute phase of chemotherapy-induced emesis. In brief, it is proposed that cisplatin (and other cytotoxic drugs), via the generation of reactive oxygen species and influx of calcium ions, release 5-HT by exocytosis and that it acts on the ligand-gated ion channel 5-HT$_3$ receptor located on the peripheral terminal of the abdominal vagal afferents (see Figure 5.13).

Recordings from these vagal afferents indicate that they begin to respond within a few minutes of intravenous administration of cisplatin given at doses known to produce behavioral effects in the same species and that the response is immediately curtailed by administration of selective 5-HT$_3$ receptor antagonists known to block emesis (e.g., Horn et al., 2004). Although 5-HT is probably the main messenger involved in the EC cells (Zhu et al., 2001), there is evidence implicating substance P (see Andrews & Rudd, 2004, for review) and it is likely that these and other (e.g., prostaglandins) substances interact, with some acting as activators and others as sensitizers of the afferents. It must be emphasized that in the case of 5-HT it is not proposed that it is released systemically to act at a distant site, although for other enteroendocrine cells this is the case (see below).

The similarity between the EC cell/vagal afferent unit and the structure of the taste buds was recognized following early electron microscopic studies of the intestinal mucosa (e.g., Newson et al., 1979; 1982), and this analogy

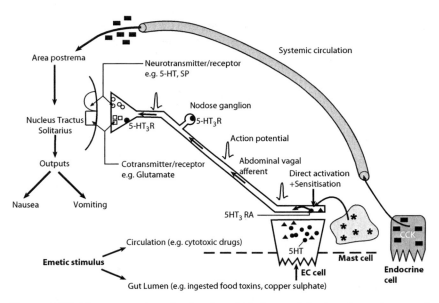

Figure 5.13 The proposed mechanism by which ingested food toxins and mucosal irritants and systemically administered cytotoxic drugs (e.g., the anticancer agent cisplatin) can drive the nucleus tractus solitarius (NTS) in the dorsal brain stem and hence access pathways responsible for the induction of nausea and vomiting. It is proposed that the enterochromaffin cell (EC) responds to the stimulus by releasing 5-hydroxytryptamine (5-HT, granules) by exocytosis to act locally on 5-HT$_3$ receptors (5-HT$_3$R) located on the peripheral terminal of the abdominal vagal afferent. 5-HT$_3$ receptors are also found in other locations on the vagal afferent as well as in the NTS, but the peripheral site is considered to be the main one at which 5-HT$_3$ receptor antagonists act against chemotherapy-induced emesis. The 5-HT can not only stimulate activity in the afferent but can also sensitize the terminal to the action of other locally released agents. Other substances have been implicated, including Substance P (▲) from the EC cell, CCK from enteroendocrine cells (see Chapter 6, in this volume) and histamine (∗) and prostaglandins from mucosal mast cells. In some cases (e.g., CCK, ■), the mucosal released substances enter the systemic circulation and could act via the area postrema. The neurotransmitter(s) used by the abdominal vagal afferent is not known, although glutamate has been implicated and is likely to be a cotransmitter with both 5-HT (5-HT$_3$ receptor) and substance P (NK$_1$ receptor) implicated. However, this has not been studied in detail in species with an emetic reflex. See text for details and references.

was further supported by neurophysiological studies showing that 5-hydroxytryptamine had a paracrine signaling role in the taste buds, with 5-HT$_3$ receptors implicated in gustatory afferent activation (Kaya et al., 2004; Huang et al., 2005). Furthermore, when molecular studies investigating the detection and transduction mechanisms in the tongue were applied to the gut epithelium they showed in essence that "taste receptors" in one form or another are located in the epithelium from the tip of the tongue to the end of the gut. These studies were largely driven by an attempt to understand the way in which the gut senses the major nutrients, but the findings have wider implications. Gut enteroendocrine cells possess taste receptor molecules able to respond to sweet and bitter tasting substances and as a result release their mediators locally to act, for example, on afferent terminals (intrinsic and extrinsic) or to enter the circulation to have distant (endocrine) effects. Of most relevance to nausea is the T2R family of G protein–coupled receptors (GPCR) and the G proteins $G\alpha_{gustducin}$ and $G\alpha_{transducin}$ involved in the detection of bitter-tasting substances, and which are expressed in populations of gastric and intestinal epithelial cells (see Rozengurt, 2006, and Sternini, 2007, for reviews). Bitter tastants are proposed to interact with the above signaling molecules and to induce an influx of Ca^{++}, which in turn mediate the exocytotic release of the peptide (e.g., CCK, PYY, GLP-1) and other mediators (e.g., 5-HT) stored in the cells. Bitter tastants given directly into the stomach are capable of inducing activation of the nucleus tractus solitarius (presumably via vagal afferent activation), a delay in gastric emptying, and conditioned aversion (Sternini, 2007; Hao, Sternini & Raybould, 2008; Glendinning et al., 2008), although as far as we are aware the emetic potential of ultrapotent agonists of the bitter-taste receptor such as denatonium has not been investigated. Cycloheximide is a bitter tastant able to induce an influx in Ca^{++} in enteroendocrine-like cell lines and for which a receptor has been located in human STC-1cells (mT2R105) and rat GI tissues (rT2R9). However, cycloheximide is also a cytotoxic agent with emetic effects, and by analogy with other agents it is likely that this is at least partly via an effect on enteroendocrine cells and the vagus (Andrews et al., 1990b). Many alkaloids used by plants to defend themselves are both bitter tasting and emetic so may act via a similar mechanism, but it should also be borne in mind that some could also act directly on the afferent nerve terminal or the enteroendocrine cells via the well-known effects on ion channels (e.g., veratridine on the Na^+ channel, nicotine on the NAChR). It is also worth noting that patients undergoing chemotherapy report a bitter taste lasting ~1 hour following systemic administration of cyclophosphamide, methotrexate, and 5-FU (Fetting et al., 1985). It is clear that studies are needed to investigate the binding properties to the family of bitter taste receptors of substances known to produce nausea or vomiting and also to identify the presence or absence of such receptors in other tissues, such as the area postrema, from where aversions and emesis can also be evoked.

Although the focus has been on the bitter detection system, the gut also has similar detection systems for salts, lipids, and sugars and hence inappropriately high luminal levels could evoke nausea and vomiting via vagal afferent activation. In addition, all the enteroendocrine and related cells are involved in the physiological motor (e.g., modulation of gastric emptying), secretory (modulation of gastric acid secretion), metabolic (e.g., glucose homeostasis), and behavioral (e.g., satiety) responses to nutrient ingestion in addition to their proposed involvement in induction of nausea and vomiting.

Splanchnic Afferents

In contrast to the abdominal vagal afferents, electrical stimulation of the splanchnic "sympathetic" afferents fails to evoke either retching and vomiting or any of the emetic prodromata in anesthetized animals (Andrews et al., 1990b) although ipsilateral abdominal muscle contraction is evoked. Lesion studies in animals show that under some circumstances (particularly with intraperitoneal administration of toxins) while greater splanchnic nerve section fails to affect the emetic response, lesion of the greater splanchnic nerve at the same time as the abdominal vagi appears to enhance the effect of vagotomy alone (Andrews et al., 1990b; Andrews, Bhandari & Davis, 1992; Hawthorn, Ostler & Andrews, 1988). In addition, neurophysiological studies have shown changes in the properties of the splanchnic afferents in response to abdominal vagotomy (Hillsley & Grundy, 1999). However, none of these studies provides direct evidence for an involvement in induction of emesis in intact animals. It is worth noting that intraperitoneal lithium chloride, which is often used as the noxious unconditioned stimulus intended to induce nausea/visceral malaise in studies of conditioned taste aversion (CTA, see Chapter 8, in this volume), in the rat increases activity in both gastric vagal and splanchnic afferents (Niijima & Yamamoto, 1994) with the effect on the splanchnics being proportionately greater.

In humans, the major sensation evoked by splanchnic afferent activation is pain, and splanchnic nerve block is one of the treatments for intractable upper GI tract pain. In the above section it was also argued that because the primary role of the splanchnic afferents is nociception and because nausea was evoked at levels of distension lower than those producing pain, then it was likely that the vagal rather than the splanchnic afferents were involved in the genesis of the sensation of nausea.

Although the evidence for a direct involvement of the splanchnic afferents in the genesis of nausea is weak, there is no doubt that nausea is associated with severe pain in many parts of the body including the gut (e.g., biliary tree). The mechanism has not been studied, but it may be associated either with high circulating levels of adrenaline or other endogenous mediators released during trauma or with a lowering of the threshold for the induction of nausea by other inputs secondary to activation of nociceptive inputs to the nucleus tractus solitarius. For example, the incidence of postoperative nausea and vomiting (PONV) is increased in patients experiencing pain following abdominal surgery and treatment of the pain dramatically reduced the incidence of nausea (Andersen & Krohg, 1976).

Although pain is the sensation most associated with activation of visceral (sympathetic) afferents terminating in the dorsal horn of the spinal cord, there is a growing body of evidence from studies in primates that the lamina I spinothalamocortical pathway has an involvement in "interoception" beyond pain via projections to the right anterior insula (Craig, 2002; 2003; 2009b; Chapter 4, in this volume). Studies are required in patients with anterolateral cordotomy to investigate the sensation of nausea in response to abdominal visceral stimulation. Irrespective of a direct involvement in the genesis of nausea, the splanchnic afferents can have an indirect role via the ascending spinothalamic pathway, which sends collaterals to the nucleus tractus solitarius and the parabrachial nucleus (Saper, 2002). These collaterals could either modulate the sensitivity of the vagal projection pathways or because of the convergence could activate the same nuclei receiving a vagal afferent (NTS, parabrachial) and which are involved in rostral projection of information from abdominal vagal afferents.

WHAT IS THE NATURE OF THE SIGNAL(S) FROM THE GASTROINTESTINAL TRACT?

Two situations need to be addressed. The first is the case of when the stimulus for induction of nausea is itself present in the gut as in the case of a luminal irritant, gastric distension, and delayed gastric emptying or in the extreme case of direct stimulation of abdominal or other vagal afferents. This is arguably the biologically most relevant origin of a nausea signal, as together with vomiting it forms a part of the defensive system against ingested toxins. The second is the more general case of the signaling of the motility (or other) changes associated with modifications in the EGG frequently reported to be correlated with the presence of nausea induced by a range of stimuli (see Chapter 7, in this volume). The post-NTS processing of the vagal and other inputs is reviewed in Chapter 4 (in this volume).

To return to the first issue, there is little doubt that appropriate activation of vagal afferents and especially those from the gut can evoke the sensation of nausea and that these afferents are also involved in signaling hunger and satiety. The vagal afferents are also involved in vago-vagal and vago-splanchnic reflexes regulating gut function as well as reflexes such as vomiting involving autonomic and somatic efferents. An obvious question is how the afferent signal is encoded to evoke the required sensory (e.g., nausea, satiety), behavioral (e.g., feeding), or reflex (e.g., gastric accommodation, vomiting) response. Limited data from afferent recording and electrical stimulation as well as more circumstantial evidence from behavioral studies and analogies with other systems suggest that the response is determined by the intensity of afferent activation and that the various responses exist along a continuum. For example, the threshold of gastric distension to evoke pleasant satiety in humans is lower than that required to evoke nausea (note that some satiety signals such as CCK can also evoke nausea and aversive responses; see Chapter 8, in this volume). "Low" frequency electrical stimulation of abdominal vagal afferents evokes a reflex gastric relaxation, whereas "high" frequency stimulation evokes licking and swallowing followed by retching and vomiting. Afferent recording studies have focused on the relationship between the intensity of a stimulus and the frequency of discharge in an individual afferent axon. But it is likely that encoding the signal for a reflex as opposed to nausea is more complex, with the number of axons activated, the duration of activation, and the location of the afferents also being important. Although it is possible using electrical stimulation of the central cut end of an abdominal vagal trunk in anesthetized or decerebrate animals to identify the minimum frequency and duration of stimulation to induce emesis (~30 Hz for 15 s in the ferret), there is no comparable information about induction of nausea. The signal for induction of vomiting must be clearly differentiated from that for either nausea or a reflex change in motility because of the possible metabolic consequences of vomiting, which may be substantial in a small mammal (Andrews et al., 2005). Accidental triggering of vomiting would be maladaptive. However, although the immediate consequences for inappropriate induction of nausea are less dramatic (cessation of feeding), the subsequent formation of a conditioned aversion to a dietary constituent could have a long-term impact on survival if the food range became restricted. In species with a very narrow dietary range and a reluctance (neophobia) to switch diet it could be disastrous. Consider a giant panda that developed an aversion to bamboo! This raises the question of how long it is necessary to stimulate an emetic input to induce a learned aversion? Studies in the house musk shrew (*Suncus murinus*) show that 10 minutes' motion exposure is sufficient to induce conditioned food avoidance, although it is not possible to determine for what portion of this time (or subsequently) the animal is experiencing nausea (or an equivalent; see Chapter 8, in this volume).

The above speculative discussion illustrates the paucity of detailed knowledge about the nature of the afferent signals in the vagus. It is clear that both mucosal chemoreceptors and muscle mechanoreceptors are capable of inducing both nausea and vomiting. Although simple stimulus intensity-frequency coding in the afferents could account for many of the experimental observations by analogy with gustatory and olfactory signaling, it appears likely that it is the discharge in a number of neurons—population coding—that provides the nucleus tractus solitarius with the information required to produce the appropriate sensory, behavioral, or reflex response. Telemetric and analytical (e.g., principal component analysis) techniques are now sufficiently developed to permit studies of vagal activity in unrestrained animals so that activity patterns could be correlated with behavior. In addition, the development of techniques for blocking the abdominal vagus in humans as a treatment for obesity may provide an opportunity for a study of the role of the vagus in the genesis of nausea (Camilleri et al., 2008).

To return to the second issue, conceptually it is easy to understand that incremental stimulation of a population of abdominal vagal afferents could evoke a range of sensory, behavioral, and reflex responses. The hierarchical defense model (Davis et al., 1986) would argue that the ability of the vagal afferents to detect toxic food in the upper gut and to evoke nausea and vomiting is a phylogenetically ancient defensive mechanism and may be the earliest and most important postingestive mechanism. The ability to signal to the central nervous system information about the fate of food postingestion and preabsorption would be advantageous not only from the aspect of defense but also by enabling an animal to make short-term decisions about predatory or foraging behavior. The high ratio of abdominal vagal afferents to efferents in a range of mammals (Andrews, 1986) supports the argument that the afferents have a significant function, and such an argument would be strengthened if similarly high ratios were found throughout the vertebrates, but such data are lacking, although it is known that vagal afferents are present in fish, amphibians, reptiles, and birds.

However, nausea can be induced by diverse stimuli acting outside the gastrointestinal tract (e.g., area postrema, vestibular system) and these stimuli as well as those acting via the vagal afferents induce changes in the electrical activity of the stomach (the electrogastrogram [EGG] is reviewed in Chapter 7, in this volume), which appear to correlate with gastric (antral) motor quiescence (Chen & McCallum, 1993). These EGG changes can be induced by systemic agents as well as extrinsic autonomic efferents and are a common (but not universal) finding in humans experiencing nausea, with preliminary evidence that similar changes can occur in animals such as the ferret and *Suncus* prior to the onset of emesis (Percie du Sert, Rudd & Andrews, 2007; Percie du Sert et al., 2009). The question arises that if such changes in the EGG and the related motor quiescence (You & Chey, 1984) constitute a signal for nausea via the vagal afferents, how is this detected? If the signal is indeed the motor quiescence (i.e., the absence of contractile activity and perhaps a reduction in tone), this is reminiscent of the following quote from *Silver Blaze* by Arthur Conan Doyle (1859–1930).

> Is there any point to which you would draw my attention? To the
> curious incident of the dog in the night-time. The dog did nothing in
> the night-time. That was the curious incident remarked Sherlock Holmes.
> (*The Memoirs of Sherlock Holmes*, 1896, p. 23, quoted in Cohen and
> Cohen, 1972)

In vivo and in vitro recordings of antral motility show that some rhythmic contractile activity and tone is normally present, and it is this level of activity that is modulated by nerves, hormones, and local factors. Single-fiber recording from abdominal vagal afferents with receptive fields in the antrum shows that even these low levels of motility are signaled (Andrews, Grundy & Scratcherd, 1980). Thus it is conceivable that silence in the mechanoreceptive gastric vagal afferents (particularly in the antrum) is an abnormal state and this *absence* of input constitutes a signal. Silence in splanchnic afferents could of course also contribute. The relaxation of the proximal stomach would also lead to a reduction in the discharge of mechanoreceptors located there. While this is a possible mechanism, it would predict that blockade of vagal afferent transmission or surgical vagotomy (in the absence of the induction of secondary effects such as dumping syndrome) would induce nausea, but the evidence does not support this proposal. In addition, the vection study of Faas et al. (2001) failed to find a relationship between the severity of nausea and either the inhibition of antral contractile activity or reduction of gastric emptying. This observation does not exclude these events being signaled as "nausea" or "no nausea" once a threshold is achieved, which may be different among individuals. In their model of vection-induced nausea, Stern and Koch (1994) proposed that gastric tachyarrhythmia resulted in an increase in both vagal and splanchnic afferent activity, although the underlying mechanism was not discussed. An increase in vagal afferent activity would be conceptually simpler to understand, but the link between the EGG changes and afferent activity remains to be elucidated.

If the mechanism by which the sensation of nausea is induced is via a specific modification of upper gastrointestinal tract function resulting in activation of vagal afferents, irrespective of the input pathway activated (i.e., vestibular system, area postrema, vagal afferents), then the question remains how are they activated? Among several possibilities worthy of investigation are signaling of the reduced gut blood flow (particularly the mucosa; Wolf, 1943) which is presumed to occur in association with nausea, activation of vagal afferent terminals by systemic agents known to be elevated in subjects with nausea (e.g., vasopressin, adrenaline), or modification of the normal signaling properties of the vagal afferents by systemic or locally released substances. It is possible that splanchnic afferents could also detect these stimuli, but this needs further investigation by afferent recording.

In both of the above scenarios it is relatively easy to envisage that transmission of vagal afferent information to the brain stem and subsequent projection to higher regions of the brain could give rise to a sensation described as nausea, which is perceived as originating from the upper abdominal viscera. However, how nausea is induced and linked to the upper abdominal viscera in the case when there is no stimulus originating from the gut is unclear (see Chapter 4, in this volume).

EXTRA-GASTROINTESTINAL AFFERENTS INVOLVED IN NAUSEA

The above sections have rightly concentrated on the gastrointestinal tract as the source of visceral afferent signals for nausea. However, nausea occurs in ~13% of patients with myocardial infarct, and nausea and vomiting in ~26% (Gnecchi Ruscone et al., 1986); but, because of the dyspeptic-like symptoms and the reflex gastric relaxation that occurs in response to activation of some cardiac afferents (Abrahamsson & Thoren, 1973; Johannsen, Summers & Mark, 1981), it is difficult to argue that the afferents responsible for the sensation arise from the heart, although it seems likely. Evidence for induction of nausea (and vomiting) from the carotid sinus comes from nausea and dizziness and nausea reported as prodromes to syncope in carotid sinus syndrome (e.g., see Toorop et al., 2007) and the modulatory effects of carotid chemo- and baroreceptors on the emetic reflex (Uchino et al., 2006). Furthermore prevention of the hypotension associated with spinal anesthesia reduced the incidence of nausea and vomiting from 66% to 10% (Datta et al., 1982).

Clinical observations show that trauma to the testicles, renal pelvis, urinary bladder, and uterus, as well as raised intracranial pressure, can induce nausea and vomiting in humans. Although not formally investigated, all these structures have an "autonomic" afferent innervation, which could be involved in addition to the mechanisms outlined at the end of the section above.

OUTSTANDING ISSUES AND CONCLUDING COMMENTS

While events mediated by the autonomic nervous system occurring prior to the onset of vomiting, and hence which could be contemporaneous with the presence of nausea, are relatively well described, with perhaps the exception of the decrease in gastric motility, their causal linkage to the genesis of the sensation of nausea is unlikely. Although sweating, pallor, and salivation all contribute to the clinical picture of a human with nausea, each of the changes occurs in other settings without the sensation of nausea (cf. James-Lange and Cannon-Bard theory of emotion).

The sections above have identified a number of physiological functions altered prior to the onset of vomiting in animals (particularly the dog) and associated with the onset or occurrence of nausea in humans. Some of these changes such as rise in blood pressure, cutaneous vasoconstriction, and tachycardia can be ascribed to general arousal associated with a stressful event and may also help buffer the cardiovascular system against the physical effects of vomiting. These changes are likely to involve the hypothalamic or higher (anterior cingulate cortex) descending influences on the autonomic nervous system outflows (see Chapter 4, in this volume). The hypothalamus is also involved in the secretion of vasopressin associated with nausea, but which may also have a role in the cardiovascular changes described above (see Chapters 4 and 6, in this volume). Other changes such as salivation are argued to protect the buccal cavity and esophagus against the gastric contents that may be vomited, while the motility changes in the gut itself (gastric relaxation and RGC) are argued to be part of the toxin defense mechanism and also serve to place the upper gut contents in the location from where they can be most effectively forcefully ejected by the action of the abdominal muscles and diaphragm. These autonomic nervous system–mediated changes in gut motility and secretion as well as the phrenic and abdominal motor neuron outputs are coordinated in the brain stem and do not need regulation from "higher" brain regions (see Chapter 4, in this volume).

A problem is that while recordings of the EGG have the best temporal resolution and may be an indication of autonomic efferent changes, the vast majority of studies in humans have investigated vection-induced nausea, and in addition we have only a patchy picture in humans of other changes in gut function (e.g., blood flow; motility; exocrine, endocrine, and paracrine secretions) that could be detected by the visceral afferents. A related issue is that there are few examples where measurements have been made simultaneously from several physiological systems in humans to investigate the temporal relationship, for example, between events in the gut and the cardiovascular system. The study by Morrow, Angel, and DuBeshter (1992) in patients undergoing chemotherapy shows the potential of studies investigating the relationship among multiple parameters, as it identified what appears to be a clear temporal patterning to the various autonomically mediated cardiovascular changes, with each parameter achieving a maximum value at a different time prior to emesis: temperature > pallor > blood volume pulse > heart rate > blush.

In addition, although changes in the EGG have been variably reported in patients with nausea who are pregnant, undergoing chemotherapy, or have unexplained nausea (Geldof et al., 1986; Koch et al., 1990a; DiBaise et al., 2001; Gianaros et al., 2001; also see Chapter 7, in this volume), the relationship between the onset of nausea and any EGG changes is not as clear as in the vection studies. Long-duration recordings of the EGG are needed to investigate the relationship between the occurrence and intensity of episodes ("waves") of nausea and the pattern of EGG activity, and to correlate these with other parameters such as heart rate and blood pressure. The major outstanding issue regarding the EGG changes is still whether they are simply a biomarker for the presence of nausea and are caused by the changes in autonomic outflow mediated by the brain (e.g., hypothalamus), with the sensation of nausea appearing to arise from the abdomen by "referral," or whether the EGG changes (or their motor correlates), however caused, are detected by the abdominal visceral afferents (probably vagus) and provide a unique signal to the brain that is interpreted as nausea. The central pathways are discussed in Chapter 4 (in this volume), but at present there are insufficient data to decide between the "cause" vs. "effect" options regarding the EGG. Although nausea can be induced in subjects with gastrectomy, this only indicates that there are additional mechanisms and does not exclude the possibility that in intact individuals detected changes in the EGG are not responsible for the sensation. Vection studies indicate that EGG changes precede the onset of the sensation of nausea and increase in magnitude as the time of maximal reported nausea approaches (Koch et al., 1990c; Hasler et al., 1995a), favoring the "cause" rather than "effect" hypothesis, but additional studies are required using nauseogenic stimuli other than vection to test whether the hypothesis can be generalized.

In contrast, studies in animals (particularly dog and cat) have provided a very detailed description of the gastrointestinal and other autonomically mediated changes occurring prior to the onset of vomiting, but it is only an assumption that the animals are experiencing a sensation akin to nausea (see Chapter 8, in this volume). In addition, the published recordings usually only cover the immediate periemetic period lasting a few minutes either side of the retching and vomiting with the most marked gastrointestinal motor events (RGC) beginning about 20–60 s before retching and vomiting (Lang et al., 1986). While it is not possible to comment on the relationship between nausea and the autonomically mediated gastrointestinal tract motor changes in animals, reports of prodromal behaviors raise some interesting questions.

Several authors have noted that following the administration of an emetic agent, animals may become relatively quiescent but that immediately prior to the onset of vomiting they become aroused and adopt a typical posture, as is also the case in humans. For example Hatcher (1924) commented, "If the animal [dog-author] lies down after the injection [apomorphine-author], it gets up at the onset of nausea." Abrahamsson (1973), again in the dog injected subcutaneously with apomorphine, recorded gastric relaxation began 3 min after administration and 2 min later the dog postured as if to vomit. These observations could be used to argue that a signal from the gut provides the animal with an arousing stimulus that makes it aware that vomiting is imminent (i.e., nausea). However, other studies in the dog (Lang et al., 1986) showed that it was possible to uncouple the GI motor events (e.g., RGC) from the occurrence of the prodromal signs of vomiting (yawning, salivation, licking the nose, standing with the head lowered) suggesting that GI motor events may not provide the signal that vomiting is imminent. The recording methods may have constrained the behavioral repertoire of the animals and to assess fully the relationship between GI events and behaviors, studies using telemetry in freely moving animals are required. Examples of such studies in the ferret and *Suncus murinus* can be found in Percie du Sert et al., 2009 and 2010a respectively.

The physiological systems regulated by the autonomic nervous system reflect the central nervous system changes that accompany the onset of nausea and, because they are amenable to measurement using either non- or minimally invasive techniques, they provide an opportunity to obtain a high-temporal-resolution description of CNS activity in the periemetic period. Techniques with high temporal resolution and sensitivity are available to study the cardiovascular system, and wireless telemetric techniques using ingested capsules should facilitate the simultaneous study of the GI tract changes in humans. However, such studies rely on recruitment of volunteers and some of the barriers to recruitment were reviewed in Chapter 4 (in this volume), as these studies also apply to the study of the central nervous system in nausea.

Chapter 6

The Endocrine System and Nausea

Chance observation during previous clinical studies suggested to us
that nausea (N) and /or vomiting (V) from any cause is a potent stimulus
for vasopressin (VP) release.
—(Shelton, Kinney & Robertson, 1977)

INTRODUCTION AND ISSUES

The aim of this chapter is to examine the relationships between the sensation of nausea, and to a lesser extent the induction of vomiting, and the presence of substances detected in the blood. Sensu stricto only the secretory products of the endocrine system (ductless glands) are hormones (derived from the Greek word *hormao*—"I excite or arouse" and introduced by Starling in 1905). But for the purposes of this chapter, we will take a broader definition to include any endogenous substance present in the blood. Early studies recognized the ability of adrenaline (epinephrine) to induce vomiting (Hatcher & Weiss, 1923), and Caspari (1923; cited by Lewis & Crossland, 1970) proposed the existence of a hypothetical emetic substance that he termed a "necrohormone"; however, this idea does not appear to have been pursued.

Interest in substances present in the blood when nausea is reported arises largely from attempts to understand the pathogenesis of nausea and also from the possibility that measurement of a systemic agent may provide a diagnostic marker for the presence and magnitude of nausea (including in laboratory animals, babies, and children) that is not reliant on either self-reporting or observation of behaviors in animal studies (see Chapter 8, in this volume). Some of the obstacles to achieving these aims are outlined below to provide a background against which studies of specific substances can be discussed.

Correlations

If it is assumed that a particular substance has its level altered (either increased or decreased) in a subject reporting nausea, then the issue arises of the relationship between the presence and magnitude of the nausea and the plasma concentration of the substance with respect to time. Irrespective of whether the substance is causing the nausea or is changing as a consequence of the nausea, there should be some degree of correlation between the plasma concentration and the nausea, although not necessarily a linear one. Arguably the relationship would be expected to be stronger if the substance was causally rather than consequentially related because of a more direct mechanistic link. In principle, two types of change could be seen and for simplicity we will assume that changes are increases (but see section below on cortisol):

1. *A threshold-type effect* where an increase above a certain level is associated with the presence of nausea, but the level does not relate to the magnitude of nausea. This pattern could occur with either a substance present normally in the plasma with a physiological regulatory role but which at a higher concentration is somehow involved in nausea (e.g., sensitizing one of the pathways) or with a substance whose only role is an involvement in nausea.

2. *A concentration related effect* where the level of the substance relates directly to the intensity of the nausea. In the case of a substance with a normal regulatory role the relationship would only occur when the concentration exceeded that required for its normal regulatory function; whereas, for a substance with an involvement solely in nausea, in principle any change would be related the presence and intensity of nausea. This is analogous to the situation with encoding pain where there are "high threshold" and "wide-dynamic range" nociceptors (Cervero & Janig, 1992).

In principle, it should be relatively simple to look for correlations between the plasma level of substance and the intensity of nausea, but practical considerations such as the number of times a blood sample can be taken and simultaneously a questionnaire completed or VAS (visual analogue scale) taken in a subject with nausea, make obtaining data difficult. This problem can be overcome to some extent by sampling multiple individuals exposed to the same stimulus, but such an approach assumes that the slope of the relationship between the intensity of nausea and blood concentration is similar across individuals. The best that it may be possible to achieve is to deduce a probability that a given individual is experiencing nausea based on the concentration of a particular substance in the blood. Nausea is often described as occurring in waves, and frequent sampling of blood through one of the cycles would provide an ideal insight, but this "wavelike" nature of nausea has not been studied. The majority of studies have not attempted to relate blood levels to the intensity of nausea but have usually taken blood samples at regular intervals after administration of a subemetic dose of an emetic agent (e.g., apomorphine) or stimulus (vection) and compared blood levels at the same time points in subjects with and without nausea. This approach has proven successful in identification of changes in the level of substances in experimental settings where the stimulus is discrete, but is harder to apply to clinical settings where controlling for the effects of multiple therapeutic drugs may be impossible.

Ideally, experimental stimuli should be used that induce only nausea in order to avoid the possible confounding effect of vomiting following nausea. It is conceivable that an exogenous emetic stimulus could release an endocrine agent that causes both nausea and vomiting with the different effects being mediated by differing blood concentrations (nausea < vomiting) or actions at separate sites. Elevation of blood levels with nausea alone would not necessarily exclude a driving or priming role in vomiting, and this would need to be investigated specifically.

A further factor to consider when looking at plasma levels is that some hormones exist in different molecular forms that may not have the same activity profiles (e.g., acylated and desacylated ghrelin) or in bound and unbound forms (e.g. thyroid hormones) in the blood, and hence both need to be measured as the "signal" may be a change in the ratio.

Cause and Effect Relationships

Even when a substance has been shown to have its blood levels highly correlated with the presence and intensity of nausea, the problem remains of whether it is involved in the genesis of the sensation (i.e., a nauseogenic agent) or is changed as a component of the adaptive response to the presence of nausea (e.g., a response to a stressor). The case for various individual substances is reviewed below, but as a prelude it is possible to identify some criteria by which substances can be categorized.

Temporal Relationships

For a substance to be potentially causal of nausea ideally its level should have a high degree of temporal correlation with the presence and intensity of nausea and should change in the blood *prior to the first report of nausea*. If the agent is directly responsible for the induction of nausea, for example by an action on the area postrema, the change in the blood level may occur shortly before the onset on nausea; whereas, if the substance is indirectly involved, for example by disrupting gastric emptying, then there may be a longer delay between the blood change and the reporting of nausea. For an agent thought to change as a result of the presence of nausea, its level should not change prior to the first report of nausea but should change either coincidentally or immediately after. It is recognized that this is an idealistic and simplistic view and is totally dependent on the report of the awareness and categorization of a sensation as nausea, the ability to take frequent blood samples around this time point, and to have an assay with sufficient sensitivity for the suspected substance. Substances with short plasma half-lives and present in low concentrations would be particularly elusive. If it becomes possible to identify a physiological variable that is diagnostic of the presence of nausea, it may become possible to make more precise measurements of temporal correlations. But all studies performed to date lack sufficient temporal resolution and rely on circumstantial evidence to place them in "cause" or "effect" categories. Vomiting usually follows a period of nausea, and it is possible that a substance could have a clear temporal relationship to nausea but without being implicated in its genesis if, for example, it was involved in other defensive strategies short of vomiting (e.g., a reduction in intestinal blood flow to reduce toxin absorption) or in preparation for the act of vomiting itself.

Induction of Nausea

An endogenous substance implicated in the genesis of nausea should, when given exogenously at a similar concentration to that measured in the blood when nausea is present, induce nausea. If nausea is induced then this provides support for an involvement in the genesis of nausea; but if nausea is not induced then, while suggestive of a lack of involvement, the result must be treated with caution. The reasons are two-fold. First, while it is conceivable that a change in a single substance in the blood may induce nausea, it is also equally likely that a combination ("cocktail") of substances is required so administration of a single agent may not mimic the in vivo situation. Second, even if a single substance is implicated, the brain or other organ (e.g., stomach, vagal afferents) may also need to be primed or made receptive to the substance by other stimuli so again simple administration alone may not mimic the natural situation. Such dual and "gate" mechanisms may be important in preventing the genesis of nausea "accidentally," which could in turn lead to the induction of inappropriate aversive responses for example to the main constituent of the diet.

Selective Antagonists

Selective blockade of the receptor(s) on which a candidate "nauseogenic" substance acts (see cautions in section "Induction of Nausea" above) or prevention of the change in blood levels should block the induction of nausea; whereas, if the substance changes as a consequence of the presence of nausea, the blockade should be without effect on the intensity of nausea. This is a potentially useful criterion but unfortunately selective receptor antagonists are not available for use in humans for all the receptor subtypes of most of the substances of interest (see below), and brain penetration remains a potential issue as many of the antagonists are not small molecules.

Where Would Hormones Act?

If an agent(s) in the blood is somehow involved in the genesis of the sensation of nausea, then where could such a substance(s) act to have such an effect? In principle there are two main mechanisms—direct and indirect. By direct we mean a direct effect on one of the pathways leading to activation of the neural pathways leading to the genesis of the sensation of nausea (see Chapter 4, in this volume), and by indirect we mean an action upon another system or intermediate cell that eventually leads to activation of the pathway leading to the genesis of nausea. These inputs are the same as those leading to induction of vomiting; namely, the vestibular system, the area postrema, the visceral (vagal) afferents, and specific regions of the brain itself. Some of the issues relating to the direct and indirect actions at each site will be discussed, but the discussion is confined to general principles with pathways implicated for specific substances being discussed later.

Vestibular System

While the primary vestibular afferents have receptors for a variety of neurotransmitters, the vestibular system is relatively isolated from the circulation so it is unlikely to be readily accessed by peptides but may be accessed by small molecules, although penetration is likely to be slow. Overall it appears an unlikely site at which endogenous systemic agents act to induce nausea, but we must be cautious as this has not been formally studied and there is at least one study in which the emetic response to an exogenous agent in the dog was affected by labyrinthectomy (Money & Cheung, 1983).

Area Postrema and Other Circumventricular Organs

The area postrema and other circumventricular organs (CVOs) (e.g., subfornical organ, OVLT) are ideal potential sites by which substances in the circulation could access brain pathways leading to the induction of nausea, as the blood-brain barrier (BBB) is relatively permeable in these regions (see Figure 6.1). There is good evidence that hormones from the gut have effects on food intake (Chaudhri, Small & Bloom, 2006) by an action at least in part on the CVOs and hence would provide an ideal mechanism by which disordered gut function could induce nausea in addition to any effects on gastrointestinal afferents (see below). Of particular interest would be a comparison of the dose-sensitivity of peripheral afferent and area postrema pathways to the same substances. Additionally a careful study of the relationship between the dose of an agent required to induce reduced food intake/satiety and that required to induce CTA/pica (see Chapter 8, in this volume) in a rodent would be of interest as many hormones (e.g., CCK, PYY, GLP-1) have a potential to induce both. Penetration of the BBB may be less of a problem in lower vertebrates (e.g., fish), where there is evidence that the BBB is in general more permeable than in mammals, although it must be noted that the area postrema is present in fish, but the microanatomy differs from mammals (Leslie, 1986). While the vast majority of evidence implicates the area postrema in the genesis of nausea and vomiting induced by particular stimuli, it would be unwise to exclude the other CVOs, especially as they are located around the third ventricle in close proximity to the hypothalamic-pituitary axis, which is implicated in a number of the endocrine changes associated with nausea (see below).

In the region of the area postrema the cerebrospinal fluid–brain barrier is also relatively permeable (Leslie, 1986) and could provide a route by which endogenous substances present in the CSF could induce nausea. Finally, dendrites from NTS neurons project into the area postrema (Morest, 1960) and could be the target site for substances either in the blood or the CSF.

Visceral Afferents

The peripheral axon terminals of these afferents, and in particular the abdominal vagal afferents, can readily be accessed by a range of substances in the

Panel A

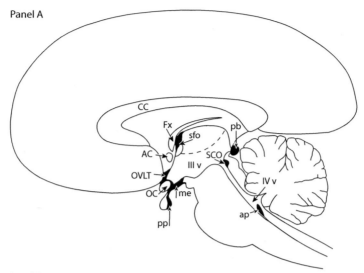

Panel B

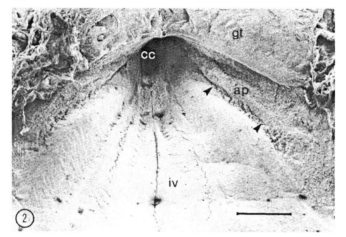

Panel C

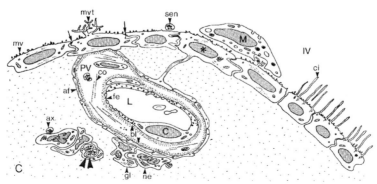

Figure 6.1 **Panel A**. Midsagittal section showing circumventricular organs of the human brain. These specialized brain structures are depicted in black and represent highly vascularized brain regions primarily surrounding the third ventricle or, in the case of the area postrema, the fourth ventricle.AC-anterior commissure; ap-area postrema; CC-corpus callosum; Fx-fornix; me-median eminence; OC-optic chiasm; pb-pineal body; pp-posterior pituitary; sco-subcommissural organ; sfo-subfornical organ; IIIv-third ventricle. Reproduced with permission from Landas et al., 1985. **Panel B**. Scanning electron micrograph of the caudal floor of the fourth ventricle in a human. The tela choroidea has been removed to reveal the ependymal lining of the floor (iv). Along the lateral edges of the floor can be seen the different texture of cells overlying the two lobes of the area postrema (ap); the abrupt transition between the two cell types is indicated on the left lobe by arrowheads. gt-gracile tubercle; cc-entrance to the central canal; bar = 1 mm. Reproduced with permission from Leslie, 1986. **Panel C**. Diagrammatic representation of the AP as seen in section. The abrupt transition between normal ciliated ependyma (*ci*) and nonciliated but microvillous (*mv*) ependyma overlying the AP is indicated. Elaborate microvillous tufts (*mvt*) often occur on apical surfaces of the AP ependymal cells and these have been seen enveloped by the macrophages (*M*) in some preparations. Occasionally supraependymal cell profiles resembling axons in section (*sen*) are seen. *Arrows* indicate the sites of poorly defined tight junction-like apical ependymal membrane specializations that have been shown to be leaky to large tracer molecules. One ependymal cell (=) extends a basal process to form part of the wall of a much-distended perivascular space (*PV*) that encloses a fenestrated (*fe*) capillary (*C*). This basal process forms one of the astrocyte-like endfeet (*af*) delimiting the wall of the perivascular space. The capillary is associated with a dorsally positioned pericyte that is enclosed within the continuous basal lamina (*bl*) of the endothelium. A second continuous basal lamina lines the wall of the perivascular space. The space itself contains abundant collagen fibers (*co*) as well as fibroblasts and profiles of vesiculated axonal varicosities. Several small neuronal somata (*ne*) are represented within the parenchyma of the *Ap* and these are closely associated with astrocyte-like glial elements (*gl*). Several axosomatic synapses are illustrated here (*ax*) although more commonly axodendritic synapses (*double arrowheads*) are seen. Reproduced with permission from Davis et al., 1986.

circulation, including some peptides. Provided the receptors are present, they could be activated directly to induce nausea. In addition, the afferents could be activated indirectly either by an effect of a systemic agent on an adjacent cell, which in turn releases the neuroactive substance, the gut being particularly rich in enteroendocrine cells with evidence for afferents terminating in close proximity, or by the substance producing a change in a function, such as gastric motility, that is itself detected by the afferents (e.g., mechanoreceptors). An additional site for direct activation of afferents would be the cell bodies located in the nodose ganglion (abdominal vagal afferents) and the dorsal root ganglia (DRG, splanchnic afferents), and for indirect activation would be the release of neuroactive substances from macrophages or the induction of ischemia by local changes in gut blood flow. As the nodose and DRG are the sites at which the afferent receptors and neuropeptides are synthesized, there is potential for substances acting on these ganglia to have a long-term impact on afferent sensitivity and hence the threshold for induction of nausea by other substances. Evidence to support this possibility comes from studies of rat nodose ganglion showing inhibition of CB_1 receptor expression by CCK and CART by ghrelin (Burdyga et al., 2004; de Lartigue et al., 2007). Although this section has focused on abdominal visceral afferents, the principles of activation could apply to other afferents capable of inducing nausea (e.g., the trigeminal nerve implicated in migraine). The afferents may also be a site for endogenous substances that reduce the sensitivity of the afferents. For example ghrelin reduces the sensitivity of subpopulations of vagal afferent mechanoreceptors (Page et al., 2007) and, while this may have implications for its role in food intake, such an effect could also reduce a nauseogenic signal from the stomach.

Brain

Substances in the blood could act directly on tissue in the brain if either they penetrated the BBB, were carried across the BBB by transporter mechanisms, or if they initiated a mechanism at the BBB interface that communicated a signal across the barrier (see Figure 6.2). In pathological conditions where capillary permeability is increased (e.g., inflammation, sepsis, trauma),

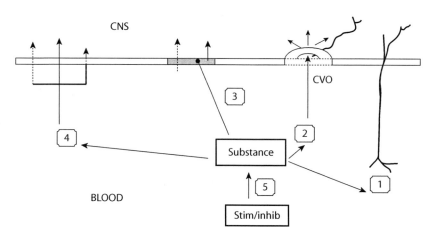

Figure 6.2 Major categories by which blood-borne substances can affect CNS function. Category 1 represents afferent nerve conduction. Category 2 represents CVO-dependent pathways with neural connections and secretions indicated. Category 3 represents alterations in the BBB which can include secretions, disruption, or altered rates of transporters. Category 4 represents direct transport across the BBB by transmembrane diffusion, saturable transport, or the extracellular pathways. Category 5 represents situations in which the administered substance acts by increasing or decreasing the blood level of a substance, which in turn acts through one of the other categories. Reproduced with permission from Banks, 2006.

substances that are normally excluded could gain access. In addition to the classically recognized areas of the CVOs where the BBB is relatively permeable, there is evidence from capillary microstructure that the vascular permeability in some regions of the brain may be higher than in others. Of particular relevance are studies indicating the nucleus tractus solitarius has fenestrated capillaries (Gross et al., 1990) and could in theory be influenced directly by larger molecules in the circulation (see Chapter 4, in this volume). The brain could also be influenced by substances in the cerebrospinal fluid, provided they can cross the cerebrospinal fluid–brain barrier. It is also conceivable that a hormone could affect cranial or brain blood flow, leading to alterations in CNS activity manifest as nausea (cf., migraine).

One Hormone or Many?

Potentially there are hundreds of chemicals that could have their levels changed in the blood in subjects reporting nausea. Conceptually we can classify any substances that change in a person (or animal) with nausea into two groups—those involved in the causation of nausea and those that change either directly or indirectly as a consequence of having nausea. Substances have been identified that appear to fall into both categories (see below), but the levels of only a few substances have been studied, and arguably only one (vasopressin/antidiuretic hormone) has been investigated in any systematic way and in several species. The latter point is worth highlighting, for if an endogenous systemic agent is capable of inducing nausea then it is valid to ask questions such as: Did the substance evolve solely for that function or does it have other additional roles? Is the function conserved across species? Is the induction of nausea a consequence of the evolution of receptor expression and distribution in different tissues?

Ideally, a study is needed that simultaneously measures changes in the profile of as many substances as possible in a way akin to microarrays used to study gene expression. Such a study may be partially possible using proteomics. It is conceivable that it may be possible to identify a unique profile of changes in the blood in subjects experiencing nausea. In addition, current studies focus on "known" substances but it is conceivable that there is an as yet unidentified hormone that is uniquely implicated in nausea—Caspari's "necrohormone." New hormones with major control functions are still the subject of relatively recent discoveries (e.g., ghrelin, oxyntomodulin) and *in silico* studies of the human and other genomes have identified a number of novel 7TM receptors and proteins for study.

SUBSTANCES DETECTED IN THE BLOOD
DURING NAUSEA AND VOMITING

The sections below review studies from both human volunteers and patients as well as laboratory animals.

Vasopressin (AVP) and Oxytocin (OT)

Early scattered reports implicated vasopressin in the physiology of emesis by highlighting that antidiuresis accompanied induction of emesis by a range of stimuli (e.g., Andersson & Larsson, 1954; Taylor, Hunter & Johnson 1957). In the full report of the abstract from which the quotation at the beginning of this chapter is taken, Rowe et al. (1979) drew attention to the complication of clinical studies of AVP secretion by nausea and vomiting and drew particular attention to studies involving ingestion of water loads, infusion of alcohol and hypotensive agents, and cigarette smoking, as well as commenting on the presence of these symptoms in association with inappropriate antidiuresis. From this starting point, the posterior pituitary hormone vasopressin (AVP; antidiuretic hormone, ADH) is the peptide most extensively studied for its potential involvement in nausea, with evidence coming from a number of healthy volunteer and patient studies as well as from experimental animals. As many of the vasopressin studies also investigated oxytocin, this will also be reviewed in this section and, for simplicity, studies in humans will be reviewed separately from those in animals.

Humans—Healthy Volunteers

Apomorphine   In healthy volunteers administration of the dopamine receptor agonist apomorphine, presumed to act on the area postrema, increased the plasma concentration of vasopressin (Rowe et al., 1979; Grant et al., 1986; Feldman, Samson & O'Dorisio, 1988; Nussey et al., 1988) in subjects who reported nausea. These studies merit further discussion as each illustrates particular points.

Rowe et al. (1979) used an apomorphine dose of 16 µg/kg s.c. and showed an increase in the mean plasma concentration from a baseline of 3.8 ± 1.4 pg/ml to 232.0 ± 55.0 pg/ml after 15 minutes. Figure 6.3 plots the results from this study and shows that the major rise occurred between 6 and 15 min after apomorphine.

The paper does not mention how nausea was assessed, but the authors comment on "a dramatic rise in AVP coincident with or *slightly after* [our italics] the onset of symptoms." Although there was a 61× increase in concentration between the mean baseline and the mean peak (15 min), the peak concentration in individual patients occurred at different times after apomorphine, and individual increases ranged from 15.5× to 462× (mean 164.4 ± 44.66×) and values at peak from 93–555 pg/ml. The peak value occurred at either 9 or 15 min in seven out of ten subjects, and in all subjects values had not returned to baseline by 45 min after apomorphine administration. In subjects experiencing both nausea and vomiting the mean plasma levels were similar to those in the nausea-only subjects, although a peak value of 885 pg/ml was measured in one subject at 9 min after apomorphine. Although there was only a small number of subjects with both nausea and vomiting, the duration of the vasopressin response appeared to be curtailed in contrast to the

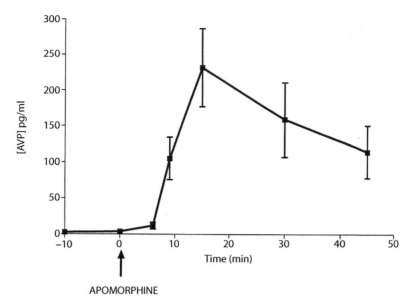

Figure 6.3 The temporal pattern of plasma AVP response to subcutaneous apomorphine (16 µg/kg) in healthy human volunteers. Data plotted as mean ± SEM (N = 9–10 for each time point) from original data in Table 1, Rowe et al., 1979.

nausea-alone group. It is worth noting that in one subject with both nausea and vomiting, a late onset (30 min) insignificant rise in vasopressin was observed (basal 2.8 pg/ml to 3.6 pg/ml). Studies were undertaken that enabled the authors to argue that the effects on AVP were independent of hemodynamic or plasma osmolarity effects.

In patients with hydrocephalus, Sorensen and Hammer (1985) showed a very similar pattern and magnitude (20–50×) of changes in plasma AVP using an apomorphine dose of 16 µg/kg s.c., and simultaneously demonstrated no change in cerebrospinal fluid AVP levels.

Using a similar dose of apomorphine (14 µg/kg s.c.), Grant et al. (1986) also found a rise in plasma vasopressin reaching a peak at 20 min after administration (a time at which nausea was said to be at its peak although no measurements of nausea were presented) and declining by 40 min but not to baseline levels. The median AVP values increased from 0.5 pg/ml (range 12.5–280) to 76 pg/ml (range 12.5–280). The magnitude of this increase (152×) is comparable to the Rowe et al. (1979) study, although the levels of AVP are at the lower end of the range. (Note that different assays were used for AVP in the two studies.) In subjects without nausea given the same dose of apomorphine there was no change in AVP.

Nussey et al. (1988) used a higher dose of apomorphine (50 µg/kg s.c.) which induced both nausea and vomiting in seven out of subjects with the nausea having a latency of 9.5 ± 0.9 min and lasting 5–30 min (mode 15 min) in contrast to the vomiting, which lasted 5–15 min (mode 10 min). AVP levels rose rapidly with the onset of nausea reaching a peak of ~200 – 250× basal 10–15 min after apomorphine but failing to reach basal levels by 30 min. Small but significant increases in oxytocin were reported at 5 and 15 min. A significant additional aspect of this study was an examination of 4 patients with idiopathic diabetes insipidus (IDI). Although these subjects all experienced nausea and three vomited, with a latency comparable to the healthy volunteers, none had an increase in either AVP or oxytocin.

In contrast to the above studies, Feldman, Samson, and O'Dorisio (1988) used an intravenous infusion of apomorphine, which allowed identification of a threshold dose required for induction of nausea. Using two different rates of infusion, it was shown that the dose required to induce nausea was between 5.1 and 8.2 µg/kg (mean 6.4 µg/kg) but with the "high" infusion rate the onset of nausea was 2 min whereas with the "low" rate it was 8–11 min. Vomiting was induced when the total dose reached between 7.8 and 20.5 µg/kg. This study provides clear evidence to support the proposal that nausea can be induced by "low" intensity stimulation of the same pathways in which more intense stimulation also evokes vomiting. In both protocols plasma AVP rose coincidentally with the onset of the reported nausea whenever it occurred, and in the case of subjects who vomited it immediately preceded the onset of emesis. In the subjects who only experienced nausea there was a 5 – 49× increase in AVP, whereas in those who vomited this range was 46 – 75×. There was no significant rise in oxytocin (see Figure 6.4).

Overall, these studies are consistent in demonstrating that nausea induced by apomorphine is accompanied by a marked rise in AVP without a comparable change in OXY, although the magnitude of the AVP rise varies considerably with the range being between 5× and 500× and some evidence of higher levels being seen in subjects who vomited. No studies measured the magnitude of the nausea so it is not possible to comment on any relationship between the magnitude of the AVP change and intensity of nausea. All the studies indicate a close temporal coupling between the onset of nausea and the rise in vasopressin with the increase occurring coincident with the onset of symptom report or immediately after. If the rise in AVP occurs *prior* to the onset of nausea it does not do so by more than a few minutes. Otherwise it would probably have been detected in the Rowe et al. (1979) study.

The Nussey et al. (1988) study is important as it established by studying patients with IDI that nausea (and vomiting) can occur in the absence of a rise in AVP, an observation similar to the finding in the Rowe et al. (1979) study, in which one subject experienced nausea and vomiting induced by apomorphine but unaccompanied by a rise in AVP.

Ipecacuanha   Oral ipecacuanha syrup (30 ml) induced nausea in all subjects with a latency of 16.9 ± 3.2 min and vomiting in five of seven subjects, but there was no significant rise in either AVP or OXT over an hour (Nussey et al., 1988).

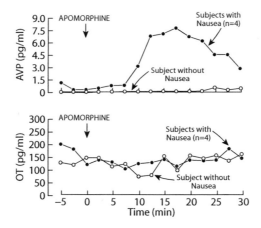

Figure 6.4 Effect of apomorphine infusion, begun at 0 min (*arrows*), on mean plasma vasopressin (AVP) concentrations (*top*) and on mean plasma oxytocin (OT) concentrations (*bottom*) in part 2. Subjects with nausea and 1 subject without nausea are shown separately. Reproduced with permission from Feldman, Samson, and O'Dorisio, 1988.

Because ipecacuanha is considered to have both peripheral (vagal) and central (area postrema) effects, a subsequent study investigated the possibility that the lack of effect on AVP was because blood samples were not taken during the time when a central effect of ipecacuanha might be present (Page et al., 1990). The AVP responses were highly variable during both the "early" (latency 16 ± 2 min) and "late" (latency 130 ± 10.4 min) phases of nausea. In three symptomatic subjects there was no significant change in AVP during either phase, but taking the results overall there was a significant increase in AVP during both the early and late phases with the change being more marked in the former (early basal 0.78 ± 0.12 pmol/l vs. 21.7 ± 9.4 pmol/l, n = 9, 28x rise; late basal 1.1 ± 0.3 pmol/l vs. 5.68 ± 2.55 pmol/l, n = 6, 5x rise). Using a VAS nausea scale, a correlation ($r = 0.64$) was found between the nausea score and the peak incremental AVP level. These two studies indicate that while ipecacuanha is a reliable stimulus for induction of nausea and vomiting, the accompanying AVP response is very variable and, as with apomorphine, nausea can occur in the absence of an AVP response.

Cholecystokinin   Administration of CCK evoked a dose-related increase in plasma AVP with the nausea score being positively correlated with the AVP level; although in some subjects, despite a high nausea score, there was no change in plasma AVP (Miaskiewicz, Stricker & Verbalis, 1989). However, it must be noted that the nausea score used in this study included items such as stomach queasy, weight or pressure in the abdomen, and abdominal cramps as well as nausea itself, which was not graded. Thus the plasma AVP levels rose as the overall symptom score increased, but those reporting nausea on average had a higher AVP secretion than those who did not. AVP secretion is therefore not specifically related to the onset of the sensation of nausea, although the higher the level the more likely it is that the subject is experiencing nausea. As with other stimuli, the magnitude of the increase in AVP was very variable, with the average being ~10× and there was no significant change in OT, although with higher doses of CCK there was some indication that OT was affected. As with apomorphine it was possible to evoke vomiting by using a higher dose for CCK than was required to evoke nausea and other gastrointestinal symptoms. This study also showed that meal-induced gastric distension to a degree evoking nausea was not accompanied by a rise in AVP.

Motion   This is the most extensively investigated stimulus and probably the one that provides the best insights into the temporal relationship between onset of symptoms and AVP levels. In addition, antidiuresis was first proposed as a measure of motion sickness in 1957 (Taylor, Hunter & Johnson, 1957). This topic has been the subject of extensive reviews (e.g. Kohl, 1990; Miller, 1991), and hence only selected papers will be reviewed here to exemplify the relationship between nausea and AVP. One of the earliest studies of Coriolis effect–induced motion sickness included AVP as one of the hormones measured as an index of the effect of this stressful stimulus on the hypothalamic-pituitary-adrenal axis (Eversmann et al., 1978). The group results revealed that the maximal level of AVP secretion almost always occurred after rotation stopped with the levels increasing from 2.2 ± 6.5 pg/ml to 53.7 ± 4.6 pg/ml, a 24.4× increase. A study in eight subjects using more sampling times revealed that plasma AVP rose coincident with the development of motion sickness symptoms (including pallor, sweating, increased salivation) and *before* the onset of vomiting. In addition, subjects with typical motion sickness symptoms prior to emesis had higher levels of AVP than subjects with only emesis.

Increases in plasma AVP but not OT have been reported in numerous studies of nausea induced by illusory self-motion (vection). Using 15 min vection Koch et al. (1990b) showed an elevation from 2.55 ± 0.36 pg/ml prior to vection to 38.4 ± 28.9 pg/ml within 1 minute of the end of vection (15× increase), but there was no correlation between the AVP level and the intensity of nausea, and there was considerable individual variation in the magnitude of the AVP response. Extremely high levels of AVP (183 pg/ml) were measured in one subject who retched 1 minute after the end of vection, suggesting that emesis itself may be associated with higher levels of AVP than occur in association with nausea (e.g., Eversmann et al., 1978; Feldman, Samson & O'Dorisio, 1988). Using a similar vection protocol but taking blood samples during vection rather than after, Xu et al. (1993) showed in healthy Chinese subjects an increase in AVP within the first 5 minutes of vection rising to a peak of 71× basal values (basal 1.73 ± 1.01 pg/ml, peak value of 123.1 ± 29.5 pg/ml) at 6–10 min and declining between 11 and 15 min, although not to baseline, but nausea symptoms resolved in 11 of 12 subjects when AVP levels decreased by 56% (74% if an outlier was excluded) (see Figure 6.5). There was a weak positive correlation ($r = 0.573$) between maximum nausea score and AVP levels, and in

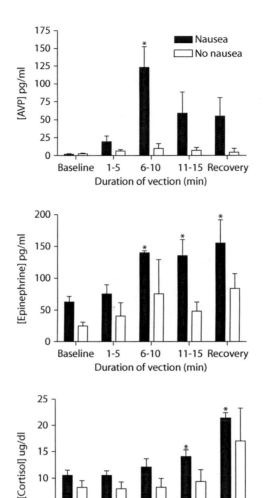

Figure 6.5 Plasma AVP, epinephrine, and cortisol concentrations measured simultaneously in healthy Chinese subjects exposed to vection. Values (mean ± S.E.M) for subjects reporting nausea (N = 12) and those not reporting nausea (N = 3) are plotted separately. Note that the magnitude of the endocrine responses differs between subject with and without nausea and that in subjects reporting nausea the patterns of secretion differs between AVP, which declines during recovery, and epinephrine and cortisol, both of which show sustained responses. Data plotted from values in Table 1, Xu et al., 1993. Significance levels during vection are relative to baseline values (* = p < 0.05).

two subjects it was possible to correlate the onset of the sensation of nausea with a rise in AVP. More modest rises in AVP associated with vection-induced nausea were reported by Kim et al. (1997), who measured a rise from 4.5 ± 1.5 pg/ml to 8.4 ± 2.5 pg/ml (~1.8×) in subjects sensitive to motion sickness; but in those resistant there was no increase in plasma vasopressin, nor did they show the same increase in tachygastria (measured as % of total signal power) as the motion sensitive group.

The temporal relationship between the rise in plasma AVP and the onset of symptoms remains a problem, and although Reichardt et al. (1997; 1998) reported that they used a continuous blood sampling technique to investigate this problem and stated that peak level of AVP followed the maximal nausea ratings in subjects during parabolic flight (see also Kohl, 1987) and a rotating chair model, the results appear to have been published only in abstract form so are difficult to assess fully.

Although the above studies of motion are consistent in demonstrating a release of AVP and some relationship to nausea score in response to vection, a different vection model producing mild nausea has been reported in which the nausea is not associated with a significant rise in AVP, although the AVP levels did correlate with the anxiety score (Kiernan et al., 1997). In this model there were no EGG changes in contrast to the conventional vection model (see Chapter 7, in this volume). These results again provide further evidence that AVP (and EGG) changes are not *essential* for the genesis of the sensation of nausea per se but the differences in intensity of nausea in the Kiernan et al. (1997) study in contrast to the other vection studies suggests that AVP (and EGG changes) may be involved in either signaling or reflecting the intensity of nausea (see below).

Humans—Patients

AVP has been measured in patients undergoing anticancer chemotherapy that is associated with nausea and vomiting. In the first study (Fisher et al., 1982) an increase in AVP occurred in patients with nausea or vomiting, whereas no change was observed in those without nausea or vomiting. AVP levels began to rise (0–40 min) before the onset of emesis and reached a peak (basal 5.53 pg/ml-peak 33.83 pg/ml, 6×) between 28 and 115 minutes (mean 66 min) after emesis. No significant changes in either blood pressure or osmolarity were found that could account for the changes in AVP. A similar study was under-taken by Edwards et al. (1989) in a group of patients the majority of whom were receiving cisplatin, which is associated with a high incidence of nausea and vomiting. In all but one case vomiting was associated with a large rise in AVP with 16-fold being the median increase, although the maximum individual change reported was 129×. As blood samples were only taken at 1, 3, and 5 hours after chemotherapy the temporal resolution is poor, but in two patients a large rise in AVP was apparent prior to the onset of vomiting. This study also quantified nausea (VAS) and found that in patients reporting moderate/severe nausea the AVP increased between 1.3× and 129× (median AVP

7.2 pmol/l, range 0.4–52 pmol/l), values significantly greater than those with mild or no nausea (median 0.65 pmol/l, range 0.3–5.6 pmol/l, 0–5× increase). One patient experienced both vomiting and moderate/severe nausea without a rise in AVP.

In a group of patients undergoing adjuvant chemotherapy for breast cancer and given the antiemetic 5-HT$_3$ receptor antagonist ondansetron, a progressive rise in AVP was measured in patients experiencing nausea and/or vomiting beginning four hours after chemotherapy and peaking at 10 hours (basal 6.3 ± 0.9 ng/l, peak 15.1 ± 3.3 ng/l, 2.4× increase) (Barreca et al., 1996). No change was seen in AVP in patients who did not experience nausea or vomiting. This study also showed that ondansetron had no effect on basal secretion of AVP.

The syndrome of "inappropriate antidiuresis" (SIADH) provides some support for involvement of AVP in nausea and emesis as it is associated with dilutional hyponatremia, which in its mild form has nausea, headache, and anorexia as symptoms, and vomiting as a symptom in moderate disease (Baylis, 1983). Other clinical situations in which AVP is elevated and nausea and vomiting are symptoms include water intoxication, raised intracranial pressure, acute hypertension, and metabolic alkalosis (Rowe et al., 1979; Sorensen, Hammer & Gjerris, 1982; Nussey &Whitehead, 2001).

Experimental Animals

Because of the problem measuring nausea in animals (see Chapter 8, in this volume) and hence making correlations with any plasma changes in AVP, this section will review selected papers that help to illustrate some of the general principles and to make comparisons where possible with the stimuli studied in humans.

Apomorphine-induced emesis has been known for some time to be followed by pronounced and long-lasting inhibition of water diuresis in dogs (Andersson & Larsson, 1954) suggesting a pronounced release of AVP. Administration of apomorphine increases LVP in the pig (Parrott & Forsling, 1994) and AVP in the ferret (Hawthorn, Ostler & Andrews, 1988), with the latter study being conducted under general anesthesia and providing some evidence that the response is not caused by the conscious perception of the stressful nature of the experience. The latter study also showed that abdominal vagal afferent stimulation was also a potent stimulus for AVP but not OT secretion in the ferret (see Figure 6.6). Morphine has also been shown to increase plasma AVP in the ferret (Wilkens & Yates, 2005) and, as was the case in humans (Koch et al., 1996a), there was a trend for ondansetron to blunt the endocrine response to morphine. An inhibition of water diuresis has also been reported following emesis induced by brain-stem stimulation in the goat (Andersson & Persson, 1958).

Cholecystokinin, at doses that induced behavioral changes arguably indicative of nausea but not vomiting, produced a dose-related increase in AVP in the ferret with a ~17× increase at the highest dose (Billig, Yates & Rinaman, 2001) (see Figure 6.7). In monkeys CCK also increased AVP within 5–10 min

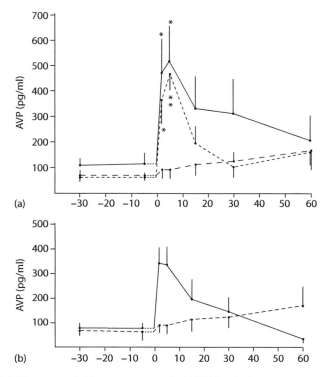

Figure 6.6 Upper panel. Plasma vasopressin (AVP) levels in response to stimulation of the abdominal vagus in the ferret. ●——●, 30-Hz stimulation; ●- - -●, 3-Hz stimulation; ●· - · · -●, control. The stimulus was applied at time zero. Values are mean ± S.E.M. *P < 0.05 **P < 0.01. Lower panel. Plasma vasopressin in response to a bolus i.v. injection of apomorphine (100 μg/kg).●——●, apomorphine, ●- - -●, control. Apomorphine was given at time zero. Results are mean ± S.E.M. *P < 0.05. Reproduced with permission from Hawthorn et al., 1988.

of administration (Verbalis, Richardson & Stricker, 1987), and the authors noted that the peak levels of AVP were higher in the animals that vomited in comparison to those that did not (112.3 ± 21.8 pg/ml vs. 59.8 ± 11.5 pg/ml), and although this difference was not significant it is reminiscent of some of the observations in humans described above. CCK also increased the plasma level of LVP in the pig (Parrott & Forsling, 1992) and AVP in the sheep (Ebenezer, Thornton & Parrot, 1989).

Both lithium chloride (i.v.), which is frequently used in rodent CTA studies, and intragastric copper sulfate, used to induce emesis, evoked a marked rise in AVP in the monkey (Verbalis, Richardson & Stricker, 1987)) with the magnitude of the increase ranging from 4 to 28× basal with a mean of 20 ± 3× (see Figure 6.7).

A single study of the anticancer agent cisplatin in the dog revealed a 25 – 150× increase in AVP at three hours after cisplatin, a time at which emesis was established (Cubeddu et al., 1990). Plasma angiotensin converting enzyme and angiotensin II levels were also measured, and neither changed.

An increase in plasma AVP of up to 27× was found in cats that vomited in response to motion sickness, but there was no change in CSF AVP levels (Fox et al., 1987). Although *Suncus murinus* (house musk shrew) has become established as a model for the study of motion-induced emesis there are no studies of AVP during motion exposure (probably because of technical

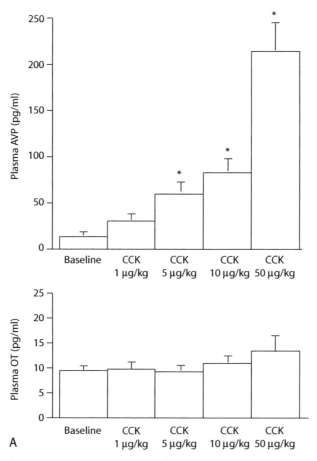

Figure 6.7A Plasma levels of arginine vasopressin (AVP; *top*) and oxytocin (OT; *bottom*) in ferrets just before (baseline) and 8–10 min after intravenous infusion of CCK (1, 5, 10, or 50 μg/kg in 2.0 ml of 0.15 M NaCl). The number of blood samples extracted and assayed for AVP and OT are as follows: baseline, $n = 15$; 1 μg/kg, $n = 5$; 5 μg/kg CCK, $n = 3$; 10 μg/kg CCK, $n = 4$; 50 μg/kg CCK, $n = 3$. Note the 10-fold lower y-axis scale for plasma OT levels compared with plasma AVP levels. *Plasma AVP levels significantly greater than baseline ($P < 0.05$). Reproduced with permission from Billig, Yates, and Rinaman, 2001.

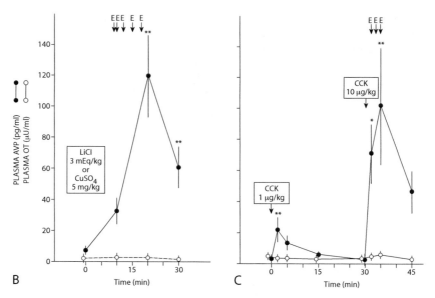

B Time (min)

C Time (min)

Figure 6.7 B, C Plasma levels of arginine vasopressin (AVP) and oxytocin (OT) after intravenous injection of LiCl or intragastric CuSO₄ (*B*) and intravenous cholecystokinin octapeptide (CCK; *C*) to monkeys. Each *point* represents mean ± SE of plasma levels at indicated time points after injection (LiCl + CuSO₄, *n* = 7; CCK 1 μg/kg, *n* = 5; CCK 10 μg/kg, *n* = 4). "E" indicates onset of emesis in individual animals. Significance levels are shown for each stimulated time point relative to basal plasma levels (0 min, except for 10 μg/kg CCK dose, in which case +30 min value was used as basal level; *$P < 0.05$, **$P < 0.01$). Reproduced with permission from Verbalis, Richardson, and Stricker, 1987.

problems in obtaining blood samples), but baseline levels of AVP in this species seem to be high in comparison to other species, with a value of 106.1 ± 27.4 pg/ml reported (Ikegaya & Matsuki, 2002).

All the above studies were performed in species with an emetic reflex, but comparable studies in the rat, which lacks an emetic reflex, have failed to show a significant increase in AVP except at very high doses to the following stimuli: apomorphine, lithium chloride, copper sulfate, cholecystokinin, and motion (Rowe et al., 1979; Renaud et al., 1987; Stricker et al., 1988; Li et al., 2005). However, all the stimuli with the exception of motion have been shown to produce dose-related increases in OT (e.g., see Figure 6.8) in the rat, while the same stimuli failed to produce significant increase in OT in species with an emetic reflex. The issue of whether OT substitutes for AVP in the rat is discussed below.

Vasopressin Receptor Antagonists

The use of selective vasopressin receptor antagonists should provide a clear method for investigating the exact role of vasopressin in the genesis of nausea

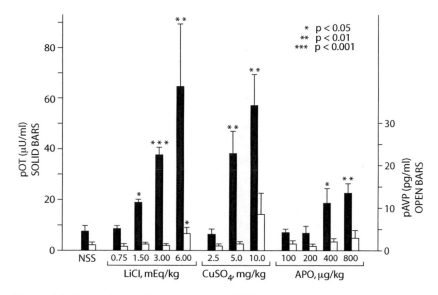

Figure 6.8 Plasma levels of oxytocin (OT; solid bars) and arginine vasopressin (AVP; open bars) after i.p. administration of varying doses of LiCl, CuSO$_4$, and apomorphine (APO). Each bar represents the mean ± standard error of 3–6 rats. Significance levels are shown relative to relative to animals given equivalent injections of 0.15 m NaCl (NSS). Reproduced with permission from Verbalis et al., 1986b.

and vomiting, but progress in this area has been slow because of the lack of availability of nonpeptide brain-penetrant selective antagonists for use in humans. Limited studies of motion sickness in the squirrel monkey reported that emesis was blocked and prodromal symptoms were markedly reduced by selective V$_1$ receptor antagonists but not V$_2$ receptor antagonists or mixed V$_1$/V$_2$ receptor antagonists (Cheung et al., 1994). Despite this encouraging result, data on humans is lacking, although Golding (2006) commented on personal unpublished results that V$_{1a}$ antagonists were ineffective in humans.

In the piglet a nonpeptide V$_{1a}$ receptor antagonist (Relecoptan) given either i.v. or i.c.v. was without effect on either the acute or delayed phase of cisplatin-induced emesis (Grelot et al., 2001).

In the absence of human data it is difficult to draw any firm conclusions based on these results, but developments in this area will be essential for a full understanding of the role of AVP in nausea and emesis, as blockade of an effect is one of the major criteria for implicating an endogenous substance in particular response. Small-molecule selective antagonists for V$_{1a}$, V$_{1b}$, and V$_2$ receptors are becoming available (Serradeil-Le Gal et al., 2002; Ali et al., 2007; Alexander, Mathie & Peters, 2008) and should enable the precise involvement of AVP in nausea to be defined.

Cortisol and Adrenocorticotrophic Hormone (ACTH)

In volunteers measures of cortisol are consistent in showing a significant rise occurring towards the end of the exposure to a motion stimulus and continue to rise in the recovery period (e.g., Eversmann et al., 1978; Koch et al., 1990b; Xu et al., 1993) reaching a level ~2× baseline when symptoms had resolved. Koch (1993) has drawn attention to the similarity of this pattern of cortisol (and adrenaline) secretion to that induced by strenuous exercise in untrained but healthy individuals. In a study using Coriolis effect–induced motion sickness, cortisol peaked 30 min after the end of rotation (Eversmann et al., 1978). In contrast to both AVP and adrenaline measured in the same vection study, cortisol levels did not correlate with the nausea score. These studies measured plasma cortisol, but similar results to the Eversmann et al. (1978) study have been obtained using salivary cortisol (Golding, personal communication). An increase in cortisol has also been reported in subjects experiencing nausea during a parabolic flight (Drummer et al., 1990).

The main stimulus for adrenal cortisol secretion is by ACTH secreted from the anterior lobe of the pituitary in response to corticotrophin releasing hormone (CRH) produced by neurosecretory neurons located mainly in the hypothalamic paraventricular nucleus and carried to the pituitary via the hypophyseal portal capillaries. Of particular note is the finding that AVP secreted from parvocellular neurosecretory cells in the hypothalamic and paraventricular nuclei into the portal capillaries (cf., magnocellular posterior pituitary secretion into the systemic circulation) stimulates ACTH release and potentiates the action of CRH on the ACTH-producing cells (Gillies, Linton & Lowry, 1982; Wotjak et al., 1996). Increases in plasma ACTH have been reported in both terrestrial motion studies and parabolic flights, and when continuous blood sampling was used it showed that the peak level occurred after the maximal nausea score although higher ACTH levels were found in subjects who had experienced severe as opposed to mild nausea (Reichardt et al., 1998; Otto et al., 2006).

Cortisol has been studied in patients undergoing chemotherapy in part to understand the antiemetic action of the synthetic corticosteroid dexamethasone. In patients given either cisplatin or carboplatin for ovarian cancer, a significant reduction in plasma cortisol was found over a 6-hour period following drug infusion and was present during two consecutive cycles of treatment (Morrow et al., 2002a). This effect was attributed to a direct effect of cisplatin and was argued to be involved in the mechanisms by which cisplatin induced nausea for several reasons including the finding of a negative correlation between prechemotherapy nocturnal cortisol and the severity of chemotherapy-induced nausea and vomiting (Hursti et al., 1993) and that nausea/vomiting are clinical symptoms of cortisol deficiency, for example in Addison's syndrome.

ACTH has been investigated following ingestion of ipecacuanha (Page et al., 1990) in healthy volunteers with significant increases of ~5–6× during both the early (mean 16 min) and late (mean 106 min) phases of nausea and vomiting and the elevation of ACTH outlasting that of AVP. A positive correlation ($r = 0.62$) was found between the nausea score and ACTH levels, as was also the case with the AVP levels.

Prolactin, Growth Hormone, and Thyroid Hormones

Although the anterior pituitary hormone prolactin is best known for its effects on lactation, it has been noted that it has been implicated in more than 300 functions, a greater number than the total for all the other pituitary hormones (Nussey & Whitehead, 2001). One of these additional effects is in reduction of fluid and sodium ion loss by the kidney and gut (cf., AVP), and this may provide a rationale for the doubling of its plasma levels evoked by motion sickness (Eversmann et al., 1978). However prolactin and growth hormone are considered to be "stress hormones" and consistent with this is a motion sickness–induced 14× rise in growth hormone levels (Eversmann et al., 1978), with the peak level occurring after that of prolactin. Both prolactin and growth hormone have been shown to increase following parabolic flights (Drummer et al., 1990). The gastrointestinal hormone ghrelin is involved in the regulation of pituitary growth hormone secretion, but no increase in ghrelin levels was detected in a study of vection-induced nausea, although there was a ~2× increase in ACTH and a 50× increase in AVP (Otto et al., 2006).

Using rotation and the Coriolis effect to induce motion sickness, Habermann et al. (1978) reported an increase in urinary output of both thyroxine (T4) and triiodothyronine (T3) together with a decrease in the plasma level of thyroid stimulating hormone (TSH). More extensive studies of the possible involvement of the thyroid hormones in emesis have been undertaken during pregnancy. Elevated levels of T4 and decrease in TSH were found during early pregnancy in women experiencing "morning sickness," with the levels correlated with the severity of symptoms and returning to the normal range as symptoms resolved (Mori et al., 1988). Levels of hCG also increased and were correlated with symptoms as well as with levels of T4 and inversely with levels of TSH. This basic finding has been confirmed in several studies, which have provided additional information by showing an increase in T3 and including subjects experiencing hyperemesis gravidarum (Kimura et al., 1993).

Gastrointestinal Hormones

There are scattered reports of measurements of a number of gastrointestinal hormones following a number of emetic stimuli but, perhaps surprisingly, there appears to have been no systematic investigations comparable to those for AVP.

In response to apomorphine in humans a rapid onset (~10min) marked (~7–16×) rise in pancreatic polypeptide (PP) was found in subjects reporting nausea, while there was no concomitant change in either vasoactive intestinal polypeptide or substance P (see Figure 6.9). PP levels are used as an index of the vagal efferent drive to the pancreas, as secretion of PP is under vagal control. This observation is important, as it emphasizes that it is unwise to make generalizations about activity in the parasympathetic nervous system during nausea based on either heart rate variability (Chapter 5, in this volume) or the electrogastrogram (Chapter 7, in this volume), both of which have led to proposals of decrease in vagal efferent activity in subjects with nausea. Apomorphine produced a prompt rise (~4×) in plasma gastrin in the dog, reaching a peak within 5 min of i.v. administration (Goiny & Uvnäs-Moberg, 1987). Elevation of gastrin has also been reported in decerebrate dogs, in which retching was induced by vagal afferent stimulation with the secretion of gastrin being dependent on an intact ventral vagal trunk (Qu, Furukawa & Fukuda, 1995).

A study in patients undergoing chemotherapy showed a significant increase in plasma insulin lasting three days after chemotherapy administration, and a nonsignificant increase in gastrin on day one, although there was a significant relationship between the prechemotherapy levels of gastrin and the presence of delayed emesis following chemotherapy. No changes were seen in

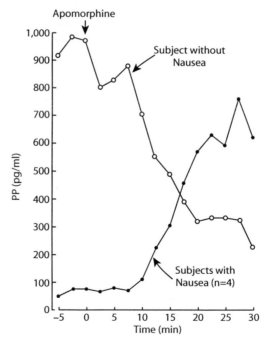

Figure 6.9 Effect of apomorphine infusion, begun at 0 min (*arrow*), on mean plasma pancreatic polypeptide (PP) concentrations in part 2. Subjects with nausea and 1 subject without nausea are shown separately. Reproduced with permission from Feldman, Samson, and O'Dorisio, 1988.

cholecystokinin (CCK) levels, but a significant decrease in motilin concentration occurred on day one and recovered on day two (Hursti et al., 2005). In the dog the pattern of emesis induced by the chemotherapeutic agent cisplatin was closely matched by an increase in the plasma level peptide YY (PYY) with a strong correlation ($r = 0.99$) between PYY concentration and emesis (Perry, Rhee & Smith, 1994). The rise in plasma levels of PYY was significantly reduced by the 5-HT$_3$ receptor antagonists ondansetron and granisetron. The latter observation is consistent with the observation by Talley et al. (1989) that ondansetron reduced the PYY response to a meal in healthy volunteers.

Indirect evidence for an involvement of CCK comes from studies showing that instillation of lipid into the duodenum (a potent stimulus for CCK release) can give rise to the sensation of nausea when accompanied by distension of the proximal stomach in healthy volunteers (Feinle & Read, 1996) and that the nausea score can be reduced by both a 5-HT$_3$ receptor antagonist and a CCK-A receptor antagonist. These results raise an important point because of the synergism between the stimuli of gastric distension and duodenal lipids in determining the resulting sensation. In the presence of duodenal lipid, gastric distension induced a sensation more akin to that experienced following a meal and, more significantly, altered the end point of distension from pain to nausea. Overall these results argue that under some conditions nausea may not arise from an effect at a single site but an effect at a given site may sensitize or prime the system to an effect at a different site. In this case the presence of lipids in the duodenum releases 5-HT and CCK to act on vagal afferents projecting to the nucleus tractus solitarius, where, if there is an appropriate concomitant level of gastric distension activating vagal afferent mechano-receptors, then a signal indicative of nausea will be projected rostrally from the NTS (see Chapter 5, in this volume). Note that this does not exclude an involvement of a duodenal hormone also acting on the area postrema, which in turn modulates NTS activity.

Adrenaline, Noradrenaline, and Dopamine

The level of plasma catecholamines provides an indicator of sympathetic nervous system activity with adrenaline indicating sympathetic drive to the adrenal medulla while noradrenaline reflects release from sympathetic nerve terminals.

Significant elevation in both adrenaline and noradrenaline has been reported in response to motion (Coriolis- or vection-induced) (Kohl, 1985; Koch et al., 1990b, Xu et al., 1993). The most detailed studies have used vection and showed that both adrenaline and noradrenaline were elevated in subjects reporting symptoms but dopamine levels were unaffected in either group (Koch et al., 1990b). Significant elevation of adrenaline occurred within 6–10 min of the start of vection and noradrenaline within 11–15 min and although declining had not returned to basal values by 15–20 min after the end of vection (Xu et al., 1993), the magnitude of the change in adrenaline ($\sim$2–3×) is larger than that for noradrenaline ($\sim$1.10–1.3×). Nausea score had a weak but positive correlation with adrenaline ($r = 0.566$) level, but it is important to note that in contrast to the AVP response the adrenaline levels were sustained during symptom resolution. An interesting observation is that there was a significantly higher basal level of adrenaline but not noradrenaline in the group that was susceptible to vection. 3× increase in plasma adrenaline concentration has been reported in healthy volunteers reporting nausea in response to apomorphine (Grant et al., 1986). Dopamine, adrenaline, and noradrenaline may all be produced in excess by pheochromocytomas, but nausea and vomiting are not the predominant symptoms. They are also not major symptoms in dopamine β-hydroxylation deficiency, where there is an increase in plasma dopamine. In Riley-Day syndrome (familial dysautonomia) there is a relationship between the periodic episodes of vomiting and dopamine levels (Axelrod, 1999).

Prostaglandins

Although prostaglandins have been implicated in nausea and vomiting induced by ionizing radiation (Dubois et al., 1987), malignancy and chemotherapy (Curry et al., 1981), Sato syndrome (Sato et al., 1988), ethanol ingestion (Kaivola et al., 1983), and infection (Jett et al., 1990), and nausea can be a side effect of prostanoid-based medications (e.g., the chloride channel activator Lubiprostone; Lacy & Levy, 2007), there is a paucity of studies of plasma levels of prostaglandins in emesis. In patients receiving cisplatin Curry et al. (1981) failed to see a significant rise in either $PGF_{2\alpha}$ or 6-keto-$PGF_{1\alpha}$ but did detect a decrease in PGE_2. In the monkey no increase in plasma 6-keto-$PGF_{1\alpha}$ and PGE_2 was detected 2 hours after exposure to ionizing radiation at a time when emesis was present, but a significant increase in both was found in samples of gastric juice (Dubois et al., 1987).

In patients undergoing anticancer chemotherapy Hursti et al. (2005) noted a significant increase in plasma $PGF_{2\alpha}$ sustained for three days following treatment. Although prostaglandins would perhaps be expected to have local effects and hence not to be elevated in the plasma, the experience with prostanoid-based medication suggests that this remains a possibility although perhaps an unlikely one.

β-Endorphin

Plasma levels of β-endorphin have been shown to increase (~2.4×) following a cross-coupled motion stimulus with no correlation between susceptibility and plasma level (Kohl, 1987). Koch et al. (1990b) showed an increase in β-endorphin levels following the vection stimulus with the levels continuing to increase throughout the 20-min recovery period. Baseline β-endorphin (and cortisol) levels were higher in subjects in whom vection induced symptoms as opposed to those in which it did not.

Endorphins have been implicated as potentially protective "antiemetic" factors, as naloxone (an opiate receptor antagonist) increased the sensitivity to motion stimuli in the cat (Crampton & Daunton, 1983). In humans it had a similar effect and furthermore appeared to have a prolonged effect, with recurrent nausea lasting 3 days following motion exposure.

Further studies of β-endorphin are needed to examine whether it could be responsible for the "high" or immediate sensation of relief reported by some subjects immediately following vomiting, which could function to ensure that vomiting (in contrast to nausea) does not induce an aversion as it may be maladaptive to discourage an activity that leads directly to toxin expulsion from the gut and enhances survival.

5-Hydroxytryptamine (5-HT) and Substance P (SP)

5-HT and the metabolite 5-hydroxyindoleacetic acid (5-HIAA) have been studied exclusively in chemotherapy-induced emesis because of the considerable body of data implicating 5-HT release from enterochromaffin cells in the mechanism and because of the efficacy of 5-HT$_3$ receptor antagonists in the treatment of this form of emesis (Cubeddu & Hoffmann, 1993; du Bois et al., 1997; Janes et al., 1998; Castejon et al., 1999; Hesketh et al., 2003b; Higa et al., 2006; Roila, Hesketh & Herrstedt, 2006; Hesketh, 2008). However, the evidence that blood levels of 5-HT itself increase following chemotherapy (as opposed to during vomiting itself) is sparse (for review and references see Rudd & Andrews, 2005). The current view is that during the acute phase of chemotherapy-induced emesis the 5-HT released from the gut enterochromaffin cells acts locally on 5-HT$_3$ receptors located on the abdominal vagal afferent terminals (Rudd & Andrews, 2005; Hesketh, 2008). An increase in the urinary level of the 5-HT metabolite 5-HIAA and the plasma level of the secretory vesicle protein chromogranin A (Cubeddu et al., 1995) have provided support for the "5-HT hypothesis" together with numerous preclinical studies (for reviews see Sanger & Andrews 2006; Darmani et al., 2009), the most recent of which showed that a selective reduction in gut 5-HT levels by a tryptophan hydroxylase inhibitor decreased the emetic response to cisplatin in the ferret (Liu et al., 2008). It must be noted that the predominant evidence for an involvement of 5-HT and 5-HT$_3$ receptors in chemotherapy-induced emesis is for the acute phase. However, there are some unexplained observations such as the lack of rise in 5-HIAA and chromogranin A in patients treated with cyclophosphamide-based therapies despite its sensitivity to 5-HT$_3$ receptor antagonists (Cubeddu et al., 1995). The consistency of the 5-HIAA response even to cisplatin has also been questioned (Higa et al., 2006). This may indicate an effect of chemotherapeutic agents on 5-HT release/turnover from sources other than enteroendocrine cells (e.g., neurons), which would not be associated with an increase in plasma chromogranin A or a large rise in urinary 5-HIAA (Cubeddu et al., 1995). Central neurochemical changes (e.g., 5-HT, SP turnover) induced by chemotherapeutic agents have been reported by Darmani et al. (2009) and may provide additional mechanisms by which such treatments induce emesis. The efficacy of 5-HT$_3$ receptor antagonists in postoperative nausea and vomiting (see Chapter 13, in this volume) indirectly implicated 5-HT in its genesis, but extensive studies of plasma 5-HT and 5-HIAA and urinary chromogranin A levels have not been undertaken. In addition it is unclear whether the 5-HT_3 receptors involved are central (e.g., brainstem) and/or peripheral (e.g., vagal afferents).

The peptide substance P has been implicated in emesis partly because of the efficacy of tachykinin NK_1 receptor antagonist in chemotherapy-induced emesis, especially in the delayed phase of cisplatin-based therapies (see Chapter 14, in this volume; Hesketh et al., 2003b; Andrews & Rudd, 2004, for review of preclinical evidence). Changes in plasma levels of substance P in patients during chemotherapy have not been the subject of extensive study, but two studies of cisplatin-based therapy have shown increases in the delayed phase with some evidence that the magnitude is dose-related (Matsumoto et al., 1999; Higa et al., 2006). Although this provides some support for a central site (e.g., area postrema) of action for substance P the majority of evidence favors a neuronal source of substance P and a related neuronal location (e.g., brain stem) for the site of action of NK_1 receptor antagonists (see Andrews & Rudd, 2004; Darmani et al., 2009, for reviews). However, additional studies are needed before a role for circulating substance P can be excluded.

EFFECT OF SYSTEMICALLY ADMINISTERED EXOGENOUS AGENTS IN HUMANS AND ANIMALS AND THEIR POTENTIAL SITE(S) OF ACTION

Although demonstration of a rise in the plasma level of an endogenous substance in response to an emetic challenge is indicative of an involvement in nausea (either directly or indirectly as an element of a more generalized stress response), the demonstration that administration of the endogenous substance can itself evoke nausea adds considerable weight to the case. While this would appear to be a relatively straightforward criterion to investigate, matching the secretory pattern and plasma concentration of a given substance may be difficult, and negative effects should be treated with caution as the substance may have a synergistic effect with another input or an as yet unidentified cofactor. In addition, for substances capable of inducing nausea the potential site(s) of action are discussed.

Vasopressin

Effect of Administration

Vasopressin has been shown to have the potential to induce vomiting in the dog (Carpenter, Briggs & Strominger, 1984; Wu et al., 1985; Chen et al., 2003; Tatewaki et al., 2005), *Suncus* (Ikegaya & Matsuki, 2002), and humans (Thomford & Sirinek, 1975) when given systemically, so arguably at lower doses has the potential to induce nausea. In the ferret, intravenous AVP did not evoke emesis (Knox et al., 1993). The emetic response to intravenous AVP in the dog was markedly reduced (~80%) by vagal blockade using cooling

(Tatewaki et al., 2005) implicating a peripheral, vagal afferent, site of action
for the major component of the emetic response to AVP. If the systemic AVP
was having a central action (e.g., area postrema) then vagal blockade would
not be expected to interfere with the ability of AVP to induce retching and
vomiting, as the vagus is not required for these motor acts, an observation
supported by the minimal effect of abdominal vagotomy on the emetic response
to apomorphine. A similar study used surgical truncal vagotomy and obtained
a similar result and in addition showed a marked reduction in the effect of
AVP on gastric dysrhythmias and behavioral changes "suggestive of nausea"
(Chen et al., 2003). These results could be argued to indicate that AVP has a
peripheral (gastric) effect that is signaled to the CNS in the vagal afferents;
but also that the induction of gastric dysrhythmias by AVP is either peripheral,
but requires a permissive action of the vagal efferents, and/or is central and
is mediated via the vagal efferents. These pathways will be considered further
in attempting to explain the relative roles of the vagus, AVP, and EGG disturbances in the genesis of nausea.

Studies in humans have demonstrated a dose-related induction of nausea
by intravenously administered AVP (see Figure 6.10). Kim et al. (1997)
and Caras et al. (1997) both reported that AVP induced nausea but not retching or vomiting at a plasma concentration of 322.1 ± 10.3 pg/ml and 420 ± 99
pg/ml to 687 ± 89 pg/ml respectively. It should be noted that in addition
to reporting nausea, subjects in the Caras et al. (1997) study also reported

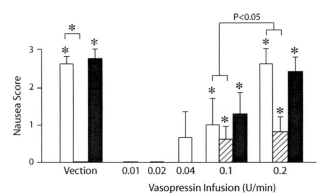

Figure 6.10 Effects of vasopressin infusion on nausea in the absence (open bars) and
presence (hatched bars) of atropine administration and indomethacin pretreatment
(solid bars) are compared with circular vection results. Vasopressin evoked a dose-
dependent induction of nausea, which was significant at doses at and above 0.1 U/min
($P < 0.05$ compared with basal). Magnitude of symptoms at 0.2 U/min was similar to
that achieved during circular vection. Atropine blunted the symptomatic effects of
vasopressin ($P < 0.05$, analysis of variance [ANOVA]), although a small but significant
level of nausea persisted ($P < 0.05$ compared with basal). In contrast, indomethacin did
not affect vasopressin-induced nausea ($P < 0.05$ compared with basal). All results are
means ± SE, $n = 14$, *$P < 0.05$. Reproduced with permission from Kim et al., 1997.

abdominal cramp and bloating as symptoms at both plasma levels. Together with nausea, these are all typical symptoms of dyspepsia. Both cramping and nausea were significantly more intense at the higher plasma AVP level with nausea beginning within 5 min of the start of the infusion and symptoms resolving over 15–30 min during the washout period.

The above studies demonstrate that AVP has the potential to induce nausea provided that the plasma concentration reaches a sufficiently high level. It should be noted that the plasma levels reached in the infusion studies are in general higher than those seen in the experimental studies described above; for example in the Kim et al. (1997) study a plasma AVP concentration of 322.1 ± 10.3 pg/ml was required to induce a similar nausea score to that induced by circular vection when the plasma AVP concentration was only 8.4 ± 2.5 pg/ml. However, even the high plasma values achieved in the infusion studies do overlap with values seen in some individual subjects experiencing nausea induced by stimuli other than motion (see above).

Site(s) of Action

The function of the large rise in vasopressin associated with nausea and vomiting has been the subject of considerable discussion (e.g., Kucharczyk, 1991; Yates, Miller & Lucot, 1998) with proposals including: the signal for nausea (direct or indirect), antidiuresis in anticipation of fluid and ionic loss including renal and intestinal sites of action, mesenteric vasoconstriction to reduce intestinal absorption of ingested toxins and also indirectly via ischemia to reduce motility, reduced gastric blood flow and hence acid secretion in anticipation of vomiting, gastrointestinal motility changes (including EGG) to delay absorption of ingested toxins, and cutaneous vasoconstriction to protect against the pressure changes associated with vomiting.

The plasma levels that can be reached during nausea in humans are in the main above those normally considered to induce substantial antidiuresis (via V_2 receptors) such as after 24–48 hours dehydration when the levels go from 2–4 pg/ml to ~10 pg/ml. During hemorrhage when vasoconstriction (via V_{1A} receptors) occurs, levels are 100–500 pg/ml (Robertson, 1977) with the magnitude of change being similar to that reported during nausea, and the concentration being within the "nausea range." Thus during nausea AVP levels are sufficiently elevated for it to exert its normal physiological functions of water conservation and widespread vasoconstriction (except brain, heart, and lungs) both of which can be argued to be potentially beneficial. Vasopressin causes a marked decrease in splanchnic blood flow (Jodal & Lundgren, 1989), and this will not only reduce perfusion of the gastrointestinal mucosa leading to reduced gastric acid secretion and intestinal absorption but will also lead to a reduction in muscle blood flow and consequently reduced motility (e.g., Liberski et al., 1990). In vascular smooth muscle, AVP potentiates the constrictor effect of catecholamines enhancing the effects of sympathetic activation occurring during stress and nausea (see Chapter 5, in this volume).

Considerable attention has focused on potential effects of AVP on gastrointestinal motility, which in turn could provide the signal for nausea via activation of abdominal visceral afferents, but there is surprisingly little data on the dose-response sensitivity of the gastrointestinal tract to AVP. mRNA for V_{1A}, V_{1B}/V_3, and V_2 receptors have all been found in full thickness biopsies from human gastrointestinal tract including the stomach (Monstein et al., 2008), although the cellular location of the receptors is not known. In vitro studies of the effects of AVP in animal tissue have demonstrated a potential for it to induce contraction of gastric and intestinal muscle, but these effects are only apparent at higher concentrations in contrast to the effects on blood vessels (threshold 10^{-12} to 10^{-13} M) (Percie du Sert, Rudd & Andrews, 2008). In the ferret, AVP was without effect on the stomach and duodenum at 10^{-12} M, the baseline AVP concentration in this species, and was also without effect when applied at 10^{-9} M, the concentration measured in the plasma of ferrets exposed to an emetic stimulus (Billig, Yates & Rinaman, 2001). Using a higher concentration of AVP, 10^{-7} M, contractile responses were evoked (Percie du Sert, Rudd & Andrews, 2008). In the cat gastric corpus, vasopressin evoked dose-related contractile responses over the range 1.5×10^{-9} to 2.1×10^{-7} M (Mircic, Jankovic & Beleslin, 1998). These studies indicate that in vitro upper gastrointestinal tract tissue is relatively insensitive to the effects of AVP; and that if AVP is involved in the pathogenesis of nausea by an effect on the stomach, then either the effect is more subtle than revealed by in vitro studies of tension or other factors are required (e.g., extrinsic autonomic nerves; see below) that render the tissue more sensitive. Direct effects of high concentrations of AVP on the gut could explain the abdominal cramping reported in some infusion studies (e.g., Caras et al., 1997); and in the monkey, giant contractions in the colon have been reported in response to vasopressin (Zhu et al., 1992).

Studies in vivo in both dogs and humans have investigated the effects of AVP on gastric motility primarily by recording the EGG. The relationship between EGG changes and nausea are reviewed in Chapter 7 (in this volume), but in essence dysrhythmic changes in the EGG induced by vection preceded the onset of nausea and the plasma elevation of AVP (Koch et al., 1990b; Xu et al., 1993). In a study of healthy Chinese subjects, gastric dysrhythmias began 3.4 ± 0.8 min after the onset of vection; whereas the first report of nausea symptoms was at 6.8 ± 1.1 min and AVP levels increased significantly in the 6–10 min measurement period. Although this indicates that AVP is not the originator of the dysrhythmic changes, it could be involved in sustaining the response and facilitating the response to other factors such as the autonomic efferents. In addition, vection may not be generally representative of all situations where nausea occurs, so a potential role for AVP in the genesis of gastric dysrhythmias remains an issue. In humans, AVP infusion producing plasma levels of 300–700 pg/ml evoked dysrhythmias, with both bradygastric and tachygastric changes being reported (Kim et al., 1997; Caras et al., 1997;

Lien et al., 2003). Caras et al. (1997) argued from their results that symptoms of nausea induced by the AVP infusion preceded the EGG disturbances.

Extensive studies in the dog have shown that AVP infusion induces gastric and small intestinal dysrhythmias with an onset of a few minutes and a delay in gastric emptying probably due to antral hypomotility (Chen et al., 2003; Xing, Qian & Chen, 2006; Xu, Brining & Chen, 2005). Chen et al. (2003) also showed that vagotomy reduced the degree of EGG disruption induced by AVP, implicating either a central role for AVP in EGG disruption via the vagus or a peripheral action of AVP to potentiate the effect of the vagus.

Several pieces of evidence suggest that the area postrema provides a credible target for a central effect of systemic AVP: it is outside the BBB and hence accessible to small peptides, it has V_1 receptors (Tribollet et al., 1988),   50% of neurons tested in the dog AP were activated by AVP microinjection (Carpenter, Briggs & Strominger, 1983), in the rat circulating AVP influences the AP with both increases and decreases in firing being recorded (Smith, Lowes & Ferguson, 1994), circulating AVP can increase the sensitivity of the baroreceptor reflex via a central action (Harris & Loewy, 1990), and a similar effect on the gastrointestinal vagal reflexes or central processing of vagal afferent signals from the gut could contribute to the vagally dependent gastric effects of AVP (see above) as well as the genesis of the rostrally projected signal for nausea.

Does Oxytocin Substitute for Vasopressin in the Rat?

The striking differences in the secretion of vasopressin and oxytocin between the rat and species with an emetic reflex such as humans, monkey, dog, and ferret should provide an insight into the function of these endocrine changes. There are really two questions to consider: first, why doesn't vasopressin increase in the rat as this appears to be the more usual mammalian pattern, and second, does the rise in oxytocin in the rat fulfill the same role(s) as vasopressin in other species? In the rat vasopressin plays a key role in regulation of fluid excretion with levels being modulated by dehydration, hemorrhage, hyperosmolar stimuli, and baroreceptor activation, as is the case in other mammals. The lack of a rise in vasopressin in the rat in response to potentially emetic stimuli could be used to argue that because the rat does not vomit there is no expectation of a loss of fluid by this route and hence no requirement to anticipate this loss by a large elevation of vasopressin secretion. Such a conclusion could also be used to argue that the large elevation in vasopressin secretion is more a marker of the likelihood of impending vomiting that of the sensation of nausea, although the two are of course related. Although oxytocin does have some activity at the renal V_2 receptor, hyperosmolar stimuli in rats evoke oxytocin and vasopressin secretion (Verbalis et al., 1986).

The absence of a rise in vasopressin in the rat could simply be explained by a difference in the relative connectivity of the nucleus tractus solitarius, where the area postrema and abdominal vagal afferents project with the supraoptic and paraventricular nuclei, but this appears not to have been studied in detail. This does not appear likely as carotid sinus baroreceptors terminating in the nucleus tractus solitarius modulate the magnocellular cells of the supraoptic nucleus in the rat, as occurs in dogs and cats (Harris & Loewy, 1990), and the NTS has been shown to provide an input to these nuclei although it is not major projection (Day & Sibbald, 1988). Indirect projections from the nucleus tractus solitarius could also reach the supraoptic nuclei via the median preoptic nucleus. Also, the bed nucleus of the stria terminalis and an ascending noradrenergic projection (A1/C1 cell groups) from the ventrolateral brain stem to the magnocellular hypothalamic neurons is the major ascending pathway by which cardiovascular information influences vasopressin secretion (Harris & Loewy, 1990). Thus on gross anatomical grounds there is no reason that rats could not increase vasopressin secretion if required, but further comparative studies are required specifically investigating the pathways activated by emetic stimuli. For example, Billig, Yates, and Rinaman (2001) reported that in response to emetic stimuli in the ferret, hypothalamic neurons showing an increase in c-Fos were CRF-, AVP-, and OT-positive; while in the rat there was little or no activation of AVP-positive neurons but clear activation of CRH- and OT-positive neurons.

If AVP secretion is somehow essentially involved in nausea then, as there is no rise in the rat, it can be argued that rats do not have nausea or a functionally equivalent sensation (see Chapter 8, in this volume, for discussion). This does not appear to be the case, as rats develop conditioned taste/food aversion/avoidance to stimuli known to evoke nausea in humans and behavioral changes such as emesis in other species. However, although there is a large secretion of oxytocin by stimuli capable of inducing CTAs (e.g., CCK, apomorphine, copper sulfate, lithium chloride) in the rat, systemic administration of oxytocin itself does not induce CTA (Verbalis et al., 1986b) and immunoneutralization of circulating oxytocin did not prevent the development of CTA to other stimuli (Verbalis et al., 1986a). In addition, although there is an inverse relationship between plasma levels of oxytocin and the reduction in food intake induced by lithium chloride and CCK and an associated decrease in gastric emptying rate, exogenous oxytocin does not inhibit food intake or gastric emptying in rats (McCann, Verbalis & Stricker, 1989). In this respect oxytocin appears to differ from vasopressin in species with an emetic reflex, as exogenous vasopressin is capable of inducing a sensation of nausea and even vomiting, and induces gastric dysrhythmias and a delay in gastric emptying (see above). While there may be debate about the equivalence of effects of endogenous and exogenous hormones, it does argue that oxytocin and vasopressin are not interchangeable.

In the rat oxytocin is recognized as a "stress" hormone, and plasma levels increase in response to a range of stressful stimuli including tail hanging, foot shock, immobilization, and swimming. However, these levels are substantially lower than the levels evoked by emetic stimuli, although as with the latter stimuli no significant secretion of vasopressin was observed (Lang et al., 1983; Verbalis et al., 1986a). It can be argued that the stressful nature of visceral illness accounts for a proportion of the oxytocin secretion but not for the majority, and the same argument can be made for vasopressin secretion in emetic species.

If the systemically released oxytocin is not involved in either the genesis of CTA, delay in gastric emptying, or reduction of food intake associated with administration of emetic agents, then what is its role? It is impossible to answer this question; but it is likely that, at the concentrations reported, effects on vascular smooth muscle occur. As has been proposed for vasopressin, such constrictor effects are argued to reduce absorption of the presumed ingested causal toxin. Although this is plausible, it has not been formally investigated. In addition one should ask why a hormone rather than the sympathetic nervous system would be used to achieve this effect. Also, as vasopressin is a more potent vasoconstrictor than oxytocin, is there some explanation why a large rise in vasopressin would be maladaptive in response to an emetic in the rat whereas it is not in other species? Whatever the function, plasma oxytocin appears to provide a marker for visceral illness in the rat with the level being able to differentiate between the increase associated with normal feeding, and with a range of stressful stimuli, and that evoked by emetic stimuli (Verbalis et al., 1986a; Renaud et al., 1987). Understanding the different patterns of secretion of vasopressin and oxytocin between emetic and nonemetic species may provide the best insight into the function(s) of the high levels of vasopressin secreted in response to emetic stimuli in species with this reflex.

Adrenaline, Noradrenaline, and Dopamine

Direct central application (i.c.v.) of adrenaline has been shown to evoke emesis in cats and dogs (Hatcher & Weiss, 1923; Feldberg & Sherwood, 1954; Borison, 1959), as has intravenous (i.v.) and intraperitoneal (i.p.) administration of adrenaline, noradrenaline, and dopamine (Peng, 1963; Cahen, 1972), with the emetic effect of noradrenaline being potentiated by pretreatment with a monoamine oxidase inhibitor. The latency for the emetic effect of i.p. or i.v. catecholamines was ~ 1.5 min. These studies reveal the potential that these catecholamines have for induction of vomiting, but shed little light on the potential that circulating endogenous catecholamines have for induction of nausea; although by analogy with the effect of subemetic doses of apomorphine in humans, it is likely that they are all capable of inducing nausea. The induction of nausea and vomiting in patients given L-DOPA without co-administration of carbidopa supports a potential role for systemic dopamine in induction of nausea and vomiting (Markham, Diamond & Treciokas, 1974). The most likely target site is the dopamine receptors (primarily D_2 but also D_3) in the area postrema, which is also the likely anatomical site for the action of adrenaline and noradrenaline; although with all three catecholamines, peripheral effects—for example on gastrointestinal motility and blood flow—cannot be excluded.

Gastrointestinal Hormones

A cholecystokinin-1 receptor (previously called CCK_A receptor) agonist and pentagastrin are both capable of inducing nausea and vomiting in humans (Castillo et al., 2004; Hursti et al., 2005) and vomiting at higher doses in the monkey within a few minutes of i.v. administration (Verbalis, Richardson & Stricker, 1987). Emesis was not evoked by CCK in the dog or ferret, although in the ferret a dose-related increase in licking and salivation indicative of sub-emetic activation of emetic pathways was reported (Billig, Yates & Rinaman, 2001). Area postrema recording in the dog failed to identify any neurons that responded to CCK, although neurons were identified that responded to gastrin (Carpenter, Briggs & Strominger, 1983), and CCK_A receptors (now called CCK 1R) have been identified in the AP (Hill et al., 1990). There is considerable evidence that CCK_A receptors (now called CCK 1R) are present on abdominal vagal afferent terminals (Richards et al., 1996; Sternini et al., 1999), and this would appear a likely site for the nausea and emesis effects of CCK and perhaps gastrin reported above. The vagal afferents activated by CCK would in turn project to the NTS/AP, which subsequently in addition to activation of emetic pathways leads to the large elevation of AVP associated with CCK administration. In addition, systemic CCK is also likely to act via the AP to activate the NTS and its outputs. An endogenous agonist at the CCK_A receptor (now called CCK 1R) may be involved in the central pathway by which vasopressin secretion is regulated as the antagonist devazepide antagonized the vasopressin response to the dopamine receptor agonist apomorphine in the pig (Parrott & Forsling, 1994).

In the dog an investigation of the potential emetic activity of porcine intestinal extracts revealed that peptide YY was a potent emetogen when given intravenously, that the related peptide NPY was less emetic, and pancreatic polypeptide was not emetic (Harding & McDonald, 1989). PYY was also emetic in the ferret (Tuor, Kondysar & Harding, 1988; Perry, Rhee & Smith, 1994). The proposed site of action is the area postrema as it has PYY binding sites in the dog, and area postrema ablations abolished the emetic response to PYY (Harding & McDonald, 1989; Leslie, McDonald & Robertson, 1988). Despite this evidence and the subsequent observation that plasma PYY levels increase in the dog following treatment with cisplatin, and that the pattern parallels emesis (Perry, Rhee & Smith, 1994), the potential role of systemic PYY in nausea and emesis has not been pursued.

It is notable that both CCK and PYY have been implicated in the physiological regulation of food intake in humans and rodents, both leading to a reduction, and in view of this it is not unreasonable to propose that at higher plasma concentration both could be involved in nausea and perhaps emesis, as arguably satiety and nausea are part of a continuum of sensations associated with the stomach (Sanger & Andrews, 2006). Teleologically it is also arguable that a hormone from the gut with the potential to induce nausea independent of an action on the vagal afferents would have survival value. Conversely, there is also a growing list of gut endocrine factors, which can stimulate food intake and stimulate gastric emptying and which have the potential to be antiemetic, with ghrelin being a good example (Malik et al., 2008; Rudd et al., 2006).

Although insulin and glucagon have not been the subject of systematic study, it is worth recalling that nausea and vomiting can be induced by the administration of either; for example, in the glucagon test ~ 30% of subjects report nausea and ~ 10% vomiting (Rao & Spathis, 1987). While the effect is likely to be secondary to the hypoglycemia, although the mechanism is unclear, it should be noted that insulin is emetic in the dog and induces activation of area postrema neurons when applied directly (Carpenter & Briggs, 1986).

Prostaglandins and Cytokines

Although there is a paucity of data on the plasma levels of systemic prostaglandins following administration of emetic agents, there is a considerable body of data to show that exogenously administered prostaglandins or their analogues are capable of inducing nausea and vomiting as well as diarrhea in humans (e.g., PGE_2 and $PGF_{2\alpha}$; see Kan, Rudd & Wai, 2006 for refs.). In addition, in animal models such as the ferret and *Suncus*, evidence has been produced to implicate DP, EP, and TP prostanoid receptor types in emesis (Kan, Rudd & Wai, 2006). Agonists of all the aforementioned PG receptors depolarize the ferret vagus (Kan et al., 2004), providing a possible substrate for their nausea and emesis effects, but prostaglandins also have central effects on the brainstem neurons including the area postrema (Avanzino, Bradley & Wolstencroft, 1966; Briggs & Carpenter, 1986).

Prostaglandin synthesis can be stimulated by cytokines; and although cytokines (IL-1, IL-6, TNFα) are implicated in the induction of "sickness behavior" following bacterial or viral infection, there is almost no work on the role of cytokines in nausea and vomiting despite the area postrema and vagal afferents being implicated in the pathogenesis of several aspects of sickness behavior (Konsman, Parnet & Dantzer, 2002; Dantzer & Kelley, 2007). In the cat recombinant IL-2 given i.m. induced vomiting, and the effect was not abolished by area postrema ablation (Gonsalves et al., 1991). In humans nausea was an early symptom in subjects who received the anti-CD28 antibody TGN1412 (Suntharalingam et al., 2006), which triggered a "cytokine storm."

ENDOCRINE CODING OF NAUSEA? AN ATTEMPT AT A SYNTHESIS

The above review has provided evidence that a number of endogenous substances when administered in an experimental setting can induce the sensation of nausea and evoke vomiting and in some cases produce gastric dysrhythmias. Some distinction needs to be made between the substances. For example, adrenaline is likely to be secreted in nausea as a component of the general autonomic arousal because of the "stressful" nature of nausea. CCK is involved in regulation of food intake and has the potential to induce nausea possibly by intense activation of the vagal and CVO "satiety" pathways, perhaps as part of a continuum of sensations from hunger to satiety to nausea. Vasopressin is involved in the regulation of fluid homeostasis and blood pressure, but at higher concentrations can induce nausea and is secreted in response to emetic stimuli. The evidence supports the concept that a hormone *could* be involved in the genesis of the sensation of nausea either by a direct effect on brain or indirectly via disruption of gastric motility. However, because an injected substance can induce nausea does not mean that it does so when released endogenously. Note that for both endogenous and exogenous causes, evidence that nausea is blocked by prior administration of selective receptor antagonists is lacking, making any conclusions tentative until such data are available. While the area postrema is a likely site at which a hormone could act because of its involvement in vomiting and CTA (see Chapter 8, in this volume), the other circumventricular organs (OVLT, subfornical organ, median eminence) should not be overlooked as they have been implicated in drinking and feeding, which are regulated in part by hormones (e.g., angiotensin II, ghrelin) and are associated with the sensations of thirst and hunger/satiety, which are themselves associated with peripheral structures, namely the tongue/pharynx and stomach. The OVLT has also been implicated in cytokine-induced sickness behavior, which has some features, such as decreased appetite and lethargy, in common with nausea. In principle there is nothing unusual in the genesis of a sensation such as nausea with a relationship to an organ such as the stomach being induced by a hormone acting on the brain. But is this what happens and if so which hormone(s) is involved?

The consistency of the evidence relating to the secretion of vasopressin in relatively high concentrations in several emetic species, by a range of stimuli with emetic potential and with a time course similar to the occurrence of nausea (in humans) is consistent with the conclusion that vasopressin can be secreted in response to activation of pathways capable of inducing vomiting. As the pathways for vomiting converge in the brain stem (see Chapter 4, in this volume), this demonstrates the rostral projection of information to the hypothalamus. For plasma vasopressin to be the cause of the sensation of nausea, the paraventricular nucleus of the hypothalamus should be activated at levels of stimulation below those evoking vomiting. This could be investigated using fMRI, as the temporal resolution should be sufficient to allow correlation with reported sensations, which is a limitation with plasma measurements of vasopressin. Correlation with the onset of EGG changes should be possible. It appears unlikely that vasopressin would be secreted in such concentrations solely for the purpose of evoking the sensation of nausea, irrespective of whether this is direct (e.g., via the CVOs) or indirect (via the EGG and the vagus), especially as the midbrain already "knows" about the originating stimulus, and it is likely that projections to the forebrain are already active and could more easily give rise to the sensation of nausea. The secretion of a hormone by the brain to produce a motility change in the stomach (EGG), which is then detected by the visceral afferents to transmit the signal for the genesis of nausea to the brain appears a rather circuitous mechanism. However, this does not exclude an involvement of vasopressin (or other hormones) in the GI motility changes either via an action of the area postrema–NTS and vagal efferents (see Chapters 4 and 5, in this volume) or directly on the stomach. Although the vasopressin secreted has several functions (fluid retention, cutaneous vasoconstriction) should vomiting ensue, we should ask if vasopressin would be secreted in such quantity solely in the anticipation that vomiting will ensue shortly? The concentrations reported in some studies are disproportionate if this is indeed the sole function of the vasopressin secretion, and in view of this, other roles for vasopressin need to be considered including effects on the gastrointestinal tract such as reduction of blood flow. The sensations (if any) associated with markedly reduced gut blood flow have not been investigated, but nausea is a symptom of ischemic mesenteric syndrome (Liberski et al., 1990). Circulating vasopressin will act wherever there are receptors and where it gains access. There is considerable evidence that vasopressin acts as a neurotransmitter at multiple points in the brain and that it is involved in pathways mediating the response to stress and aggression with both the hypothalamus and the amygdala implicated (Pittman & Spencer, 2005). The latter has been shown to be critical for induction of CTA (see Chapter 4, in this volume). It is conceivable that systemic vasopressin could act on the vasopressin receptors in the brain, especially in regions where the blood-brain barrier is relatively permeable, to have behavioral effects, but this requires direct investigation. An increase in plasma vasopressin is not an absolute requirement for the induction of nausea, as the study by Kiernan et al. (1997) demonstrated, but the intensity of nausea was low in their study in contrast to others. Nevertheless this illustrates that, as perhaps would be expected, other mechanisms exist; but it may also indicate that vasopressin is secreted only when the nausea is relatively intense and hence there is a higher probability of vomiting ensuing.

In conclusion, although endogenous circulating substances have the potential to cause nausea, it appears unlikely that this is the main mechanism by which the brain pathways leading to the genesis of a conscious sensation are activated (see Chapter 4, in this volume). The existence of a hormone with a specific function of signaling nausea, "nauseaphorin," is unlikely. With regard to vasopressin it provides a potentially useful biomarker (in humans and species with an emetic reflex) that the emetic pathways have been activated at a level not necessarily sufficient to evoke vomiting, but further work is needed to establish the levels that are likely to be associated with the presence of nausea in humans and behavioral changes in animals.

Chapter 7

Gastric Dysrhythmias and Nausea

Gastric dysrhythmias are abnormal electrical rhythms emanating from the corpus and antrum of the stomach. In humans, the normal gastric pacesetter potentials range from 2.5 to 3.6 cycles per minute (cpm). Gastric dysrhythmias, on the other hand, are categorized as tachygastrias, which range from 3.6 to 10 cpm, and bradygastrias, which range from 1 to 2.5 cpm. The possibility of gastric dysrhythmias was suggested soon after the first normal EGG was recorded by Walter Alvarez (Alvarez, 1922). He hypothesized that abnormal electrical activity may exist in patients with a variety of symptoms related to the stomach.

Gastric dysrhythmias can be measured by several different methods. Improvements in amplifiers and analysis techniques, such as running spectral analysis, led to improved recordings of gastric electrical signal in animals and humans (Koch & Stern, 2004). There has always been some confusion with the terminology and understanding of the stomach electrical activity because the signal recorded from the serosa of the stomach has a different wave configuration than the electrogastrogram (EGG) signal recorded from the skin with EKG-type electrodes placed on the epigastrium (see Koch & Stern, 2004). The relationships between gastric dysrhythmia and upper GI symptoms such as nausea are described in this chapter.

LABORATORY STUDIES

In the 1960s and 1970s there was considerable interest in gastric dysrhythmias in France and other European countries. A number of studies showed that gastric dysrhythmias were present in patients with gastroparesis, postoperative ileus, and with Billroth II procedures. In the United States, You et al. (1981) reported antral tachygastria in patients with chronic, unexplained nausea and vomiting. Several of these patients underwent antrectomy to extirpate the source of the dysrhythmias and reduce their symptoms. However, this radical surgical approach to the treatment of gastric dysrhythmias was abandoned.

The correlation of nausea and the onset of gastric dysrhythmia was documented in a number of papers. The normal 3 cpm gastric rhythm can be disrupted by medications. Abell and Malagelada (1985) showed that the administration of glucagon resulted in gastric dysrhythmias and nausea.

Hasler et al. (1995b) showed that estrogen and progesterone induced gastric dysrhythmias and nausea of pregnancy. Koch et al. (1996b) showed that morphine infusions induced gastric dysrhythmias and increased vasopressin levels, and evoked nausea in healthy individuals. Hasler et al. (1995b) also showed that intravenous infusions of glucose that produced levels over 200 mg/dl induced gastric dysrhythmias and upper GI symptoms. Recent studies by Coleski and Hasler (2009) used mucosal electrodes and showed that hyperglycemia-induced tachygastrias in healthy subjects developed in the distal antrum. Studies such as these supported the concept that the normal 3 cpm gastric electrical rhythm was not fixed and that it could be shifted into gastric dysrhythmias. Furthermore, the shift to these dysrhythmic frequencies, either tachygastria or bradygastria, was associated with nausea.

Stern et al. (1985) published the results of the first of a series of studies that used a rotating optokinetic drum, as shown in Figure 7.1, to induce nausea and other symptoms of motion sickness in healthy subjects. EGGs and other

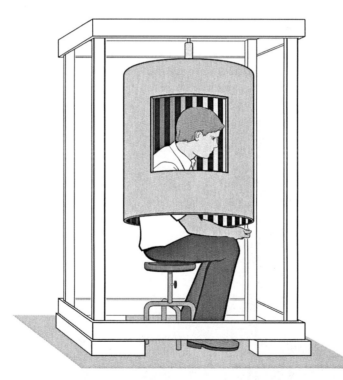

Figure 7.1 Illusory self-motion (vection) is produced by rotating a drum around a seated subject. The inner surface of the drum is painted with black and white stripes. The drum is rotated at a speed of ten revolutions per minute to induce the illusion of self-motion. The subject's chin is on a chin rest to provide stability for the head. Nausea and motion sickness symptoms are induced in susceptible subjects.

physiological measures were recorded during optokinetic stimulation. Stern et al. recorded EGGs from 21 healthy human subjects who were seated within the optokinetic drum, the rotation of which produced vection (illusory self-motion). Fourteen subjects developed symptoms of motion sickness during vection, and in each, the EGG frequency shifted from the normal 3 cpm to tachygastrias. In six of seven asymptomatic subjects, the 3 cpm EGG pattern was unchanged during vection. It was concluded that the sensory mismatch created by the illusory self-motion evoked tachygastria and nausea and other symptoms of motion sickness in susceptible subjects. In a follow-up study (Stern et al., 1987a), 15 healthy subjects were exposed to the rotation of the same drum. Similarly, approximately two-thirds (ten subjects) showed a shift of the 3 cpm EGG signal to tachygastria during drum rotation and reported nausea and other symptoms of motion sickness. In these studies running spectral analysis of the EGGs and symptom reports revealed a close correspondence over time between the onset of tachygastria and the development of nausea and other symptoms of motion sickness (see Figure 7.2).

The strong temporal correspondence between the development of tachygastria and nausea and other symptoms of motion sickness can be seen. In subjects exposed to the rotating drum turning at different speeds, there was a very strong correspondence between reports of nausea and other symptoms of motion sickness and tachygastria (Hu et al., 1989). Gastric dysrhythmias preceded the onset of nausea by approximately one minute and plasma vasopressin increased shortly thereafter (Koch et al., 1990c), suggesting the perturbation of rhythm in the stomach occurs before symptoms and before the release of vasopressin from the pituitary. Thus, the shift to gastric dysrhythmias may alter ongoing gastric vagal afferent activity, which then modulates neuronal activity in the tractus solitarius and hypothalamus, and ultimately results in vasopressin secretion from the posterior pituitary (see Chapter 6, in this volume).

Koch et al. (1990b) reported that vasopressin levels in the blood of symptomatic subjects increased along with reports of nausea, and decreased as nausea subsided. In contrast, levels of stress hormones such as epinephrine increased with reports of nausea, but did not decrease until long after nausea subsided. Asymptomatic subjects developed neither gastric dysrhythmias nor increased vasopressin release during drum rotation. For a review of possible neurohumoral mechanisms involved in the generation of gastric dysrhythmias see Owyang and Hasler (2002).

It is important to note that during tachygastria, antral motility decreases or even completely shuts down (e.g., Koch & Stern, 2004). Many years ago, Wolf (1943) showed that nauseogenic stimuli, i.e., putting cold water in one ear or swinging on a swing while rotating the head, inhibited gastric contractile activity *and* provoked nausea. To quote from Wolf, "These experiments show that the same bodily changes were induced by swinging as by caloric stimulation. Decreased gastric motility was a constant occurrence, but further gastric changes and the more widespread autonomic effects occurred only when

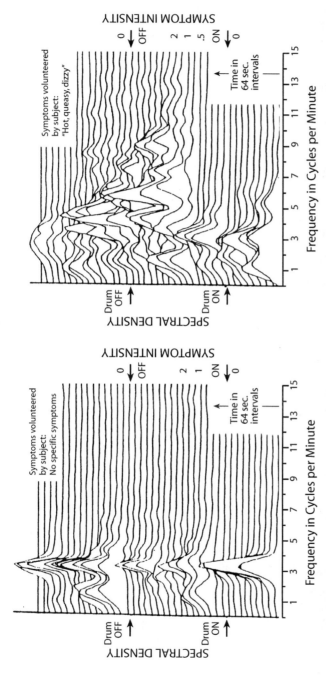

Figure 7.2 The panel on the left shows a running spectral analysis of the EGG signal recorded from a subject who did not develop motion sickness during illusory self-motion. The EGG frequencies in cycles per minute (cpm) from 1 to 15 cpm are shown on the X-axis. The Y-axis indicates times when the drum was turned on and off. Total drum rotation time was 15 minutes. The Z-axis shows power, and the peaks indicate the EGG frequencies present in the EGG signal. Note peaks at the normal 3 cpm rhythm at baseline (before the drum is turned on), during the period of illusory self-motion, and also the 3 cpm peaks after the drum is turned off. This subject maintained the normal EGG rhythm and did not report nausea. The panel on the right, on the other hand, shows the running spectral analysis of the EGG recorded from a different subject who developed nausea and queasiness, symptoms of motion sickness, during the drum rotation period. The subject developed a variety of peaks at faster frequencies of 4, 6, and 9 cpm, all consistent with tachygastria during illusory self-motion and nausea. When the drum was turned off, these dysrhythmias disappeared, and small 3 cpm peaks are noted in the late recovery period. Thus, the development of gastric dysrhythmias during illusory self-motion was associated with development of nausea and motion-sickness symptoms. Reproduced with permission from Stern et al. 1987a.

nausea or discomfort was induced" (p. 880). Motion sickness induced by drum rotation and the illusion of motion was associated with decreased oral-cecal transit time and loss of 3 cpm EGG patterns (Muth, Stern & Koch, 1996). Patients with tachygastria have poorer gastric emptying rates when compared with patients with bradygastria or normal 3 cpm EGG signals (Koch, Xu & Hong, 2000). Thus, the onset or presence of tachygastria is associated with decreased antral contractions and delayed gastric emptying, or gastroparesis.

Wolf's subjects had a balloon positioned in their stomach to record gastric pressure changes. Wolf grappled with a problem inherent in all studies that relate some bodily change to a perceived sensation, in this case the relationship of decreased gastric contraction activity and the sensation of nausea. To what extent is the altered stomach physiology (decreased antral contraction or tachygastria) essential to the occurrence of the sensation (nausea)? In a series of ingenious experiments, unfortunately with only three subjects, Wolf gave his subjects a combination of two drugs, prostigmine and atropine, and he reported that this combination prevented the inhibition of gastric contractile activity. He then exposed the subjects to the stress situations that had previously provoked nausea, and found that no nausea was reported. Wolf (1943) concluded as follows: "The fact that nausea may be prevented, despite strong nauseating stimuli, by controlling with drugs the pattern of gastric motility indicates that gastric relaxation and hypomotility are essential to the occurrence of nausea" (p. 882). In this respect, researchers today continue to look for drugs that will prevent or treat antral hypomotility and gastric dysrhythmias.

NAUSEA OCCURRING IN CLINICAL CONDITIONS

The nausea and vomiting of pregnancy (NVP) is another type of nausea that like motion sickness occurs "naturally." NVP affects about 80% of women (see Chapter 12, in this volume). Koch et al. (1990a) recorded EGGs in 32 women during the first trimester. On the day of the study, 26 of the women reported nausea and 65% had tachygastria, 29% had bradygastria, and 6% had arrhythmias (flatline pattern). Six women did not have nausea and each had a normal 3 cpm EGG rhythm. These observations indicated that morning sickness was associated with the presence of the gastric dysrhythmia, and a normal 3 cpm EGG was not. Moreover, these gastric dysrhythmias appear to be temporary, as the 6 subjects who had EGGs recorded after delivery showed normal 3 cpm signals. Jednak et al. (1999) reported that a high protein meal decreased dysrhythmic EGG activity and nausea significantly better than a high carbohydrate or high fat meal in patients with NVP. Levine et al. (2004) followed this study with a motion sickness study and demonstrated that a high protein meal consumed prior to exposure to a rotating drum decreased tachygastria and the symptoms of motion sickness. Thus, control of tachygastria by ingestion of food was a unique treatment modality for nausea of pregnancy and motion sickness. These results are concordant with Wolf's concept that control of the gastric dysfunction, in these later cases the gastric dysrhythmias, would decrease or eliminate the nausea.

DETECTION OF GASTRIC DYSRHYTHMIAS

Gastric dysrhythmias may be recorded from electrodes attached to the mucosa or serosa of the stomach or with EKG-type electrodes positioned on the surface of the skin in the epigastric region (Figure 7.3). Recordings from the skin using EKG-type electrodes are termed electrogastrograms or EGGs, a term similar to that used for electrical recordings from the heart that are obtained with electrodes placed over the surface of the chest (electrocardiograms or EKGs). Electrical recordings from the serosa of the stomach or the mucosa of the stomach should be termed mucosal or serosal gastric myoelectrical recordings.

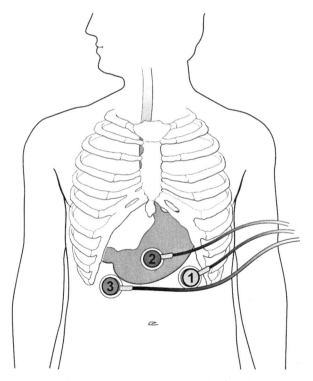

Figure 7.3 Standard EKG-type electrodes are positioned on the abdominal skin in order to record electrogastrograms (EGGs). Electrode one (1) is located in the mid-clavicular line three fingerbreadths below the lower rib margin. Electrode two (2) is located midway between the xiphoid and umbilicus. Electrode three (3) is the reference electrode.

Mucosal Recordings

Recordings of electrical activity from the stomach using electrodes attached to the mucosa (gastric pacesetter potentials or slow waves) have been accomplished in humans (Abell & Malagelada, 1985; Hamilton et al., 1986). This technique requires an endoscopy procedure to pass electrodes into the stomach and fix them to the mucosa with suction electrodes or with clips. The electrode wires are then brought out through the mouth and connected to the amplifier and recorder. Using this type of electrode, reliable recordings of gastric pacesetter potentials can be obtained for minutes to hours. However, peristaltic waves tend to dislodge suction electrodes resulting in their being stable for only hours to days. Electrodes may be attached to the mucosa with clips that are applied to the electrodes during placement at endoscopy. These electrodes exit from the mouth, and may provide reliable mucosal electrical recordings for 3–5 days (Coleski & Hasler, 2004).

Serosal Recordings

Serosal electrodes may be placed on the corpus or antrum at the time of laparoscopic surgery to record gastric electrical activity. High quality gastric electrical rhythms have been obtained during animal and human studies (Mintchev, Kingma & Bowes, 1993; Mintchev & Bowes, 1994; Lin et al., 2000). Recordings from the mucosa or the serosa all indicate that the normal gastric myoelectrical rhythm in healthy people ranges from 2.5 to 3.6 cpm, a range that encompasses the mean of approximately 3.0 cpm, plus or minus 2 standard deviations. Serosal electrodes can be placed temporarily and then removed by pulling the wires out after 7–10 days without any adverse events. Serosal electrodes may remain in place for years when they are used as stimulating electrodes for gastric electrical stimulation (Abell et al., 2003). However, a small incidence of adverse events can occur with prolonged implantation as the electrode wires may fracture. Recently gastric electrodes were inserted transmurally by endoscopic methods in dogs for gastric electrical stimulation (Xu, Pasricha & Chen, 2007).

Cutaneous Electrodes

Cutaneous electrodes (EKG-type electrodes) are used to record EGGs from the abdominal surface of the epigastrium. Electrodes are placed in a standard bipolar configuration to detect the maximum amplitude of the gastric pacesetter potential as it migrates from the pacemaker area of the greater curvature of the stomach to the pylorus (Koch & Stern, 2004). Typically a 3 cpm sinusoidal wave is recorded using these techniques. The normal 3 cpm rhythm, as well as tachygastria and bradygastrias, can be reliably recorded using EGG methodologies (Mintchev, Kingma & Bowes, 1993; Hamilton et al., 1986; Lin et al., 2000). Commercial EGG recording devices are available, and additional information concerning recording and analysis of EGG can be found in the *Handbook of Electrogastrography* (Koch & Stern, 2004).

VISUAL AND COMPUTER ANALYSIS OF GASTRIC DYSRHYTHMIAS

A high quality EGG signal is required before computer analysis of the signal is performed; that is, the EGG signal should be artifact-free and interpretable by visual inspection. A sinusoidal 3 cpm wave should be apparent in healthy people, although baseline EGG recording may show instability of the signal. In the postprandial period, the EGG signal reflects the gastric electrical and contractile activity of postprandial mixing and emptying of the specific meal. Thus, different EGG signal patterns are produced by different meals.

The EGG analog signal is digitized and subsequently analyzed by a variety of methods (Koch & Stern, 2004). Electrical signals from the mucosa or serosa may also be analyzed by computer methods. A common method is the running spectral analysis. In the running spectral analysis, the EGG signal is digitized and a fast Fourier transform is produced. Typically, a 4-minute period of EGG signal is digitized and subjected to Fourier transform. The EGG data are overlapped 75% as one new minute of data is added to the previous three to analyze the 4-minute time period of any given experiment. This method allows detection of gastric dysrhythmias with approximate duration of 1 minute (Koch & Stern, 2004). The digitized data can be quantified further by calculating the percentage of EGG power in a given amount of time in four relevant frequencies: 1–2.5 cpm (bradygastria), 2.5–3.6 cpm (eugastria), 3.6–10 cpm (tachygastria), and 10–15 cpm (duodenal-respiratory range). The data can also be expressed as power ratios from postprandial to baseline. Figures 7.4, 7.5, 7.6, and 7.7 show a normal 3 cpm EGG, a 4 cpm tachygastria, a 1–2 cpm bradygastria, and a mixed gastric dysrhythmia, respectively.

PROVOCATIVE TESTING AND EGG RECORDINGS

Baseline or "at rest" EGG recordings are sometimes made either for their inherent value or to compare with the results of provocative testing. Many investigators use provocative testing to stimulate electrical and contractile activity of the stomach. Various meals increase the amplitude of the 3 cpm EGG signal and thus the ratio of postprandial to preprandial EGG power (Koch, Hong & Xu, 2000; Lin et al., 2000). Of interest, "disgusting meals" actually decrease the 3 cpm activity (Stern et al., 2001a). Caloric and noncaloric meals have been used to stimulate the stomach by eliciting gastric neuromuscular work in the postprandial period. For example, during "satiety testing" patients are asked to consume nutrient drinks until the point of maximum satiety tolerated to assess the volume of liquid calories they can ingest (Boeckxstaens et al., 2001). EGGs recorded in healthy subjects during the time of maximum tolerated satiety showed increased tachygastria and decreased 3 cpm activity compared to baseline EGG patterns (Talley et al., 2006). Furthermore, the majority of subjects reported nausea and three vomited the meal. These studies indicate that maximum satiety is closely related to nausea and tachygastria, presumably via stretch on the gastric wall and metabolic changes (e.g., hyperglycemia).

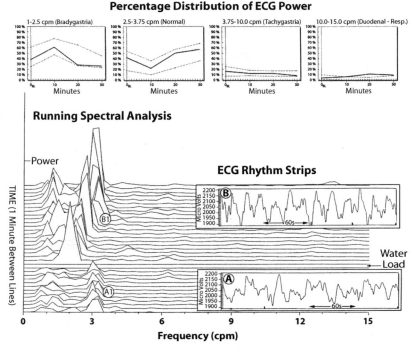

Figure 7.4 Normal electrogastrogram and running spectral analysis after the water load test. EGG rhythm strips, before and after a water load is consumed, are shown. The baseline fasting rhythm strip (A) shows normal 3 cpm EGG waves, and after the water is ingested (B) stronger 3 cpm EGG signals are seen. The water load test involves drinking water until full over a 5-minute period. The running spectral analysis shows peaks in the 3 cpm range at baseline before the water load (A1). After the water load, there is a decrease to 2 cpm for several minutes and then a series of 3 cpm peaks develops as shown at B1. The four panels above the running spectral analysis show the distribution of EGG power as percentages of all of the power from 1 to 15 cpm. Note the gradual increase in the percentage of 3 cpm power after the water load test and the absence of tachygastria or bradygastria (the abnormal EGG rhythms from 1.0 to 2.5 cpm and 3.5 to 10 cpm, respectively). Reproduced from Koch and Stern, 2004.

During the water load test, water is consumed over a 5-minute period until the subject is full. The distention of the stomach with the noncaloric physical load of water elicits reproducible EGG responses in normal subjects that differ when compared with patients with unexplained nausea, dyspepsia, and gastroparesis. The water load frequently elicits nausea and bloating, and concurrent gastric dysrhythmias compared with healthy subjects. Furthermore, patients with functional dyspepsia ingest significantly less volume of water compared with normal subjects. Thus, the water load test is a convenient provocative test of the capacity of the stomach and of gastric electrical activity (Koch, Hong & Xu, 2000). The stretch of the water volume on the

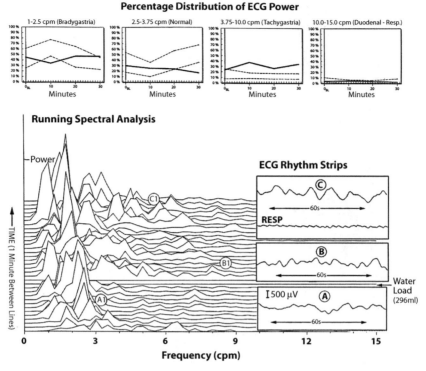

Figure 7.5 Tachygastria in the EGG rhythm strip and running spectral analysis. EGGs in this figure show a nonspecific baseline rhythm (A) and after the water load test volume of 296 ml was ingested, a low amplitude tachygastria is seen at approximately 8 cpm. The tachygastria is also shown in B1 in the running spectral analysis as a series of peaks at 8 cpm. Another run of tachygastria is seen in the EGG (C) with a frequency of approximately 5 cpm. This 5 cpm tachygastria is also shown in the running spectral analysis at C1. The four panels above the running spectral analysis show the distribution of power from 1 to 15 cpm in the four relevant EGG frequency ranges. The black line shows increased tachygastria, whereas the normal 3 cpm percentage is diminished. Overall this is a pattern of tachygastria in response to a water load test. Reproduced from Koch and Stern, 2004.

wall of the antrum and corpus is the presumed mechanism that elicits gastric dysrhythmias, but the precise mechanism has not been elucidated.

Drugs may also be used to stimulate the stomach neuromuscular activity. For example, the contrasting effects of erythromycin and morphine on EGG activity have been documented. In a study by Gonlachanvit et al. (2003b), erythromycin accelerated and morphine delayed solid- and liquid-phase gastric emptying compared to placebo ($p < 0.05$). Morphine infusions increase tachygastria and induce nausea in healthy subjects (Koch et al, 1993).

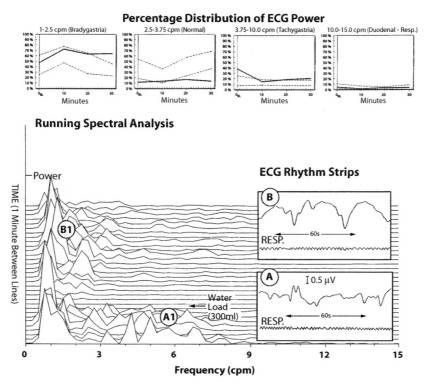

Figure 7.6 Bradygastrias in the EGG rhythm strips and running spectral analysis. The EGG rhythm strips at baseline show a nonspecific rhythm and after the water load test (B), large 1–2 cpm EGG waves, consistent with bradygastria, are seen. The running spectral analysis shows a variety of peaks at baseline (A1) and after ingestion of the 300 ml water load, peaks in the 1–2 cpm range, consistent with bradygastria are seen. The four panels above the running spectral analysis also show that the percentage of power in the bradygastria range is increased at 20 and 30 minutes after ingestion of water, whereas there is no increase in the normal 3 cpm response in this patient. Reproduced from Koch and Stern, 2004.

GASTRIC DYSRHYTHMIAS IN GASTROINTESTINAL NEUROMUSCULAR DISORDERS

Gastric dysrhythmias have been recorded in patients in whom nausea or dyspepsia are the predominant symptoms. Tachygastrias, bradygastrias, and mixed gastric dysrhythmias have been described in patients with functional dyspepsia, gastroparesis, GERD, and IBS plus dyspepsia (Koch & Stern, 2004). In a minority of patients (10%) with unexplained nausea and vomiting, the normal 3 cpm EGG signal has been recorded. In patients with normal 3 cpm EGG signals and gastroparesis, a noncongruent finding, the underlying cause of the symptoms was found to be mechanical obstruction of the stomach due to pyloric stenosis secondary to peptic ulcer disease. This pattern of normal

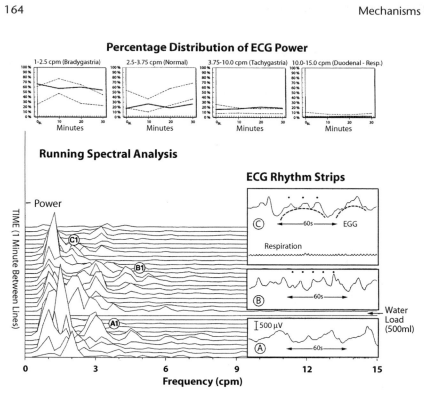

Figure 7.7 Mixed gastric dysrhythmia with normal water load test. The electrogastrogram (EGG) rhythm strips show normal 3 cpm baseline rhythm (A). In the post–water load phase, as shown in rhythm strip B, there is a tachygastria with 5 cpm pattern, but in rhythm strip C a 1–2 cpm wave is noted which is a bradygastria. The running spectral analysis also shows some 3 cpm peaks at baseline, but after ingestion of water, peaks appear in tachygastria ranges (B1) and bradygastria ranges (C1). This is a mixed gastric dysrhythmia. Similarly the four graphs above the running spectral analysis show a slight increase in the percentage of tachygastria power at minutes 20 and 30 and an increase in percentage of bradygastria power at minute 30, all of which are consistent with a mixed gastric dysrhythmia. Reproduced from Koch and Stern, 2004.

3 cpm EGG rhythm and gastroparesis is discordant and strongly suggests gastric obstruction (Brzana, Koch & Bingaman, 1998). Obstruction may also occur in the postbulbar duodenal area or further distal in the small bowel. Thus, examination of the various electrical patterns that are recorded from patients with nausea, vomiting, or dyspepsia symptoms is helpful in detecting the cause of the symptoms when standard diagnostic tests such as upper endoscopy or abdominal CT scans are normal.

Functional Dyspepsia

Functional dyspepsia is a common syndrome in which postprandial nausea, vomiting, early satiety, and fullness are the chief symptoms (Tack et al., 2006). In approximately 60% of these patients, gastric dysrhythmias such as tachygastria or bradygastria are present. In patients with tachygastria there is an increased incidence of gastroparesis compared to bradygastria (Koch, Xu & Hong, 2000). Thus, tachygastria appears to be a more disruptive rhythm and more relevant to gastroparesis compared with bradygastria. Several studies have shown that eradication of gastric dysrhythmias using domperidone, metoclopromide, or cisapride resulted in restoration of the normal 3 cpm electrical rhythmicity and decrease in nausea and dyspepsia symptoms as shown in Figure 7.8. (Koch et al., 1989; Cucchiara et al., 1992; Bersherdas et al., 1998).

Diabetic Gastroparesis

Koch et al. (1989) reported that in patients with diabetic gastroparesis and gastric dysrhythmias, domperidone treatment for six months resulted in decreased symptoms of dyspepsia, decreased gastric dysrhythmias, and improvement in 3 cpm activity. On the other hand, gastric emptying did not

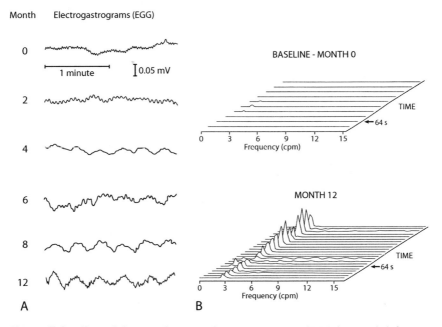

Figure 7.8 Effect of domperidone on electrogastrograms (EGGs) recorded from a patient with nausea and diabetic gastroparesis are shown from Month 0 (before domp-eridone) to Month 12 in A. At Month 0 a low amplitude 1-2 cycle per min (cpm) bra-dygastria is seen. By Month 4 a normal 3 cpm EGG rhythm is noted and remains present at Month 12. The patient's nausea symptoms improved and disappeared during this time. At B, the top and bottom figures are running spectral analyses of the EGG record-ings obtained at Month 0 and at Month 12. Note at Baseline (Month 0) the lines are flat and only two tiny peaks at 1-2 cpm are present; in contrast, at Month 12 of domperi-done treatment, a series of peaks at 3 cpm are present, reflecting the improved 3 cpm EGG signal. This patient had sustained relief from nausea and a stable 3 cpm EGG pattern. Reproduced with permission from Koch et al., 1989.

improve significantly, suggesting the gastric dysrhythmias (not the delay in food emptying) were more relevant to nausea.

Patients with Type 1 and Type 2 diabetes often have gastric dysrhythmias and almost 50% have gastroparesis (Intagliata & Koch, 2007; Hasler, 2007). Almost 75% of patients with poorly controlled Type 2 diabetes have gastric dysrhythmias (see Chapter 11, in this volume).

Idiopathic Gastroparesis

In idiopathic gastroparesis, a variety of gastric dysrhythmias have been reported (Brzana, Koch & Bingaman, 1998). Gastric dysrhythmias may also be present in patients who have gastroparesis on the basis of hypothyroidism or hyperthyroidism. Optimal regulation of the thyroid replacement therapy results in decreased dysrhythmia and decreased nausea.

Ischemic Gastroparesis

Gastric dysrhythmias have also been recorded in patients with ischemic gastroparesis (Liberski et al., 1990). In the patients who underwent mesenteric artery bypass operations, the gastric dysrhythmias resolved and normal 3 cpm activity was restored. These data suggest that chronic ischemia is a mechanism that may underlie some gastric dysrhythmias, since the dysrhythmia resolved with restoration of normal blood flow. Delays in gastric emptying also improved after revascularization.

Gastroparesis and GERD

Patients with gastroparesis and gastroesophageal reflux disease frequently have a mixed gastric dysrhythmia in which both tachygastria and bradygastria are prominent in the period after the standard water load test (Koch, Xu & Noar, 2001). Of interest, by eradicating gastroesophageal reflux in patients with GERD and gastroparesis with radiofrequency treatment of the lower esophageal sphincter area, gastric dysrhythmias improved and the rate of gastric emptying increased (Noar & Koch, 2003; Noar & Noar, 2008). Radiofrequency therapy presents a novel approach to the related entities of gastroparesis and gastroesophageal reflux disease.

MECHANISMS OF GASTRIC DYSRHYTHMIA

Unfortunately, the mechanisms that underlie tachygastria, bradygastria, and mixed gastric dysrhythmias are very poorly understood. This lack of understanding has limited the design of drugs to eradicate gastric dysrhythmias and restore normal 3 cpm activity. Normal gastric rhythmicity is maintained by a delicate balance of activity from interstitial cells of Cajal activity, smooth muscle, the enteric nervous system, the sympathetic and parasympathetic nervous system activity, and ambient hormonal levels (Koch & Stern, 2004; Kim, Azpiroz & Malagelada, 1986; Kim et al., 2002). For example, gastric dysrhythmias are common in the first trimester of pregnancy, but subjects who displayed tachygastria during the first trimester and reported nausea showed normal gastric activity and no nausea following delivery of the baby (Koch et al., 1990a). Thus, fluxes in estrogen and progesterone (or medications) may be one mechanism of gastric dysrhythmias (see Chapter 12, in this volume).

Hyperglycemia induces gastric dysrhythmias, and nonsteroidal anti-inflammatory agents block this effect of hypoglycemia (Hasler et al., 1995). These data suggest that hyperglycemia-induced prostaglandin synthesis may produce gastric dysrhythmias in some circumstances. Infusion of prostaglandin E increases the pacesetter potential frequency in the rabbit ileum and in the human stomach. Several reports show that nonsteroidal anti-inflammatory agents eradicate gastric dysrhythmias and restore normal electrical rhythm (Sanders, 1984; Hasler et al., 1995b)

Morphine induces nausea and gastric dysrhythmias and suggests mu-pathways are involved in the mechanisms underlying gastric dysrhythmias (Koch et al., 1993). On the other hand, epinephrine infusions and glucagon infusions also elicit dysrhythmias temporarily, indicating other neural or smooth muscle pathways can elicit gastric dysrhythmias (Kim et al., 1989; Abell & Malagelada, 1985).

Finally, vagotomy results in temporary gastric dysrhythmias, suggesting that vagal cholinergic influences may also play a role in stabilizing the normal gastric electrical rhythm (Stoddard et al., 1975; Hinder & Kelly, 1977). More subtle reduction of vagal inhibitory activity can result in "sympathetic dominance," and gastric dysrhythmias originating in the antrum may then develop spontaneously.

To summarize, drugs or foods that increase the normal 3 cpm EGG activity and/or decrease tachygastria appear to decrease nausea. Examples of this relationship include eating a breakfast meal before being exposed to vection (Uijtdehaage, Stern & Koch, 1992), deep breathing (Jokerst et al., 1999), gastric electrical stimulation (Hu, Stern & Koch, 1992), and drugs (Weinstein & Stern, 1997). On the other hand, unappetizing food, certain drugs and hormones, motion sickness, and other stimuli that decrease normal 3 cpm EGG activity and increase tachygastria or bradygastria are associated with sensations of nausea. This relationship is consistent with an evolutionary explanation, which would suggest that if one's stomach is not functioning normally (presence of gastric dysrhythmia or antral hypomotility), then one should not eat—the primary message delivered by the sensation of nausea.

Gastric dysrhythmias represent an exciting pathophysiological signal because there is much to discover in terms of the basic science of gastric dysrhythmias, the pathophysiology of dysrhythmias in human nausea syndromes, and improved treatments with drugs and devices.

Section III: Measurement of Nausea

Chapter 8

The Functions, Identification, and Measurement of Nausea and Related Behaviors in Animals

For each kind of investigation we shall be careful to point out the proper choice of animals. This is so important that the solution to a physiological or pathological problem often depends solely on the appropriate choice of the animal for the experiment so as to make the result clear and searching.
—(Claude Bernard, 1949/1865, p. 226)

At this point, it should be realized that almost every writer who has discussed nausea in an experimental animal, and who has written in his protocols the words, "Nausea exists," has reached these conclusions because he has seen the animal salivating, because he has seen a look of dejection about the animal, and he has realised that when these phenomena are present in man, man then experiences the sensation of nausea.
—(Keeton, 1925, p. 696)

SOME LESSONS FROM THE STUDY OF HUMANS

Can you tell by observation only what sensations a human being is experiencing? The answer is, "No," and the same answer applies to animals. When one observes the best actors playing a role in which their character is feeling sick or is in pain, the portrayal is by adopting the posture (e.g., limping, head bowed, hunched); appearance (e.g., pallor, florid, staring eyes); actions (e.g., writhing, holding the head, clutching the stomach); and demeanor (e.g., drawn facial expression, withdrawn) associated with these sensations. The actor conveys what their character would be feeling in that situation by adopting the behaviors that would be familiar to the audience when they have been in a similar situation. A range of sensations and emotions are conveyed to the audience by the actor's behavior and especially facial expressions: tears and down-turned mouth for sadness; wide eyes, open mouth, and a scream for fear; or snarling flushed appearance for anger. In his book *The Expression of the Emotions in Man and Animals*, Darwin (1872) described a range of facial expressions in humans that he believed were universal and that he argued were signs of underlying emotions. In each of the above human examples a naive observer would be challenged to say whether they were observing someone actually experiencing the relevant sensation or emotion or an actor portraying someone having it. Studies in over 20 literate cultures using photographs of the faces of subjects exhibiting fear, anger, sadness, disgust, happiness, and surprise have shown a very high level of agreement in linking the expression to an emotion. A similar study was undertaken with natives of the Papua New Guinea Highlands, and similar results were obtained (Ekman, 1999; Ekman also discusses the controversial nature of the proposal of the universality of facial expressions).

In the specific contexts of nausea and pain a naive observer would not be able to tell if the subject was actually experiencing the sensation and even if they thought they were, they would have no idea what they were experiencing except by reference to their own experience or perhaps a clinical definition based on consensus. Outside the theater, humans are probably quite good at assessing other humans by nonverbal communication as this has clear survival advantage whether it is assessing a potential rival or deciding whether to order the same menu item as the person on the adjacent table who has gone pale, clutched their stomach, and put a hand to their mouth. In the transcultural studies of facial expression outlined above, Americans had no problem in identifying the facial expression of disgust in a Papua New Guinea Highlander who was asked to mimic how he would look if he saw a dead pig that had been lying there for some time. Interestingly, there is growing evidence that rodents communicate information to each other about health status including by "inadvertent social information" (see Stamp Dawkins, 2003; Kavaliers et al., 2006).

As first discussed in Chapter 1 in this volume, if one is able to ask subjects about their experience then, assuming that they are being truthful and can accurately describe their sensations, their appearance becomes largely irrelevant. However, if the observer is a cynical clinician who demands independent evidence before believing what a patient is reporting, then what can be studied? In the earlier chapters we have seen that changes in the autonomic nervous system (Chapter 5), an elevated plasma level of antidiuretic hormone (Chapter 6), and changes in the frequency of the electrogastrogram (EGG; Chapter 7) are all associated with the sensation of nausea in humans. Appropriate changes in these parameters would increase the probability that the patient was indeed experiencing nausea although neither would necessarily indicate the degree.

From the above paragraph it can be seen that there are three broad approaches to determine if a human is experiencing nausea (or in principle any sensation):

- Ask them to describe what they are experiencing
- Look at them and examine their behavior
- Measure physiological variables (biomarkers)

The first approach only applies to humans once they are capable of speech and can understand the meaning of the word nausea in relation to their own experience and that of others. In neonatology and pediatrics, nausea (and pain) is diagnosed mainly using the second approach with the mother being an important source of behavioral data. However, we do not have any real insight into the qualitative sensory experience of nausea in a neonate as opposed to an adult. The third approach has been used in both adults and neonates, but is usually used to refine or refute a diagnosis or as a research tool. Ideally measurements using either the second or third approaches should be equivalent to asking the subject if they are experiencing nausea in terms of categorizing the sensation and its magnitude. In attempting to study nausea in animals (in this chapter the word "animals" will be taken to exclude humans), we are confined to using the second and third approaches but are unable to validate the measurements because the first approach is not possible (currently!).

It is impossible for us to get "inside the mind" of an animal so we are sure we know exactly what it is experiencing, and to some extent this is also true as far as knowing what other humans are experiencing. What we can consider is how a species responds to a stimulus within its own behavioral repertoire and under a particular set of environmental conditions which in a human we would expect to evoke a sensation described as nausea and which may also trigger retching and vomiting (probably at a higher intensity or dose). The interpretation we place on the behavioral responses is then a matter for scientific debate. To some extent the issues that surround nausea are similar to the issues involved in the study of pain in animals (e.g., the sensory experience vs. the motor response) (Morton & Griffiths, 1985; Blackburn-Munro, 2004; Mogil, 2009).

Above, three approaches were mentioned for the identification and measurement of nausea in humans. For obvious reasons approaches two and three are the ones that have been applied to nonhuman animals (cf., neonates) and although we are unable to "ask" animals directly about the sensory experience resulting from a particular stimulus, we can "ask" indirectly by observing whether they categorize the stimulus as having positive or negative hedonic properties. While it may not be possible to observe an immediate behavioral response associated with a sensation of either nausea or an equivalent in an animal, it is possible to identify if the animal perceived the stimulus as unpleasant by investigating whether it avoids or becomes averted to it on a future exposure or to another stimulus (e.g., a novel food) with which it was paired. This is perhaps the nearest insight we can obtain into the nature of the sensory experience in a nonhuman animal.

Related to this is the question of how developed a central nervous system is required to be for the perception of a conscious sensation akin to nausea in humans, and also what is the evolutionary advantage of a conscious sensation resulting from a stimulus as opposed to the genesis of a reflex or learned response not involving consciousness? (See Chapter 4, in this volume.) It is probably reasonable to assume that the more advanced nonhuman primates and some cetaceans (i.e., dolphins and whales) with a similar cortical architecture (Dunbar & Shultz, 2007; Marino, 2007) do experience a sensation of nausea comparable to that experienced by humans, but the sensory experiences of other mammals, "lower" vertebrates, and invertebrates can only be imagined.

In humans, it is possible to obtain an insight into the temporal pattern of nausea induced by a particular stimulus or disease by questionnaires, but the most widely accepted (although not necessarily valid) techniques used in animals lack temporal resolution (e.g., pica, conditioned taste aversion). The "wave" like nature of nausea is a commonly reported feature in humans (although there are no quantitative data on this phenomenon), but we have no evidence for this from animal studies. In animals such as marmosets, dogs, ferrets, and shrews, all of which have the ability to vomit, it could be argued that based on observations in humans that nausea frequently (but not always) occurs prior to the onset of retching and vomiting. Hence, characterization of behavior and physiological parameters in the time between administration of a stimulus and onset of vomiting would give insights into the prevomiting sensory experience of an animal. Novel behaviors occurring close to the time of vomiting or behaviors that increased in frequency from stimulus onset to the time of vomiting would arguably be most relevant. However, laboratory species such as rats and mice are unable to vomit, so what is the equivalent relevant time period to look for indices of nausea? The absence of vomiting in these species raises the issue of whether they even experience nausea.

Despite the considerable technical and interpretational difficulties, a range of techniques that have been used to identify and quantify "nausea" in nonhuman animals are critically reviewed below. But first we will outline the reasons why such studies are of importance and some of the theoretical considerations relating to the measurement of nausea in animals.

WHY ATTEMPT TO STUDY NAUSEA IN ANIMALS?

Since the 1980s there have been substantial advances in our understanding of the neuropharmacology of vomiting and in the identification of novel drugs (e.g., 5-Hydroxytryptamine$_3$ receptor antagonists, tachykinin neurokinin$_1$ receptor antagonists) to treat vomiting. These advances have had an especially beneficial impact on the treatment of chemotherapy- and radiotherapy-induced emesis (see Chapter 14, in this volume) and the emesis following anesthesia and surgery (see Chapter 13, in this volume). However, in general nausea is treated less effectively than vomiting (e.g., Foubert & Vaessen, 2005; Hesketh, 2008). There are at least two reasons for this and they are interdependent. First, until relatively recently there was a relative paucity of studies in humans focusing on the mechanism(s) of nausea. These studies are discussed elsewhere in this book, but it is worth noting that the vast majority of studies have investigated motion sickness (including vection) and not nausea in clinical settings. Especially notable is the paucity of brain imaging studies of subjects experiencing nausea in either experimental or clinical settings (see Chapter 4, in this volume). The lack of such studies in humans makes it difficult to look for similar changes or pathways activated in animals and hence to provide some validity to any animal model that may be developed. Second, there is no widely accepted animal model for the study of nausea that could be used to identify agents to treat nausea in humans with a reasonable expectation of success. Apart from the philosophical problems of assessing conscious sensations in animals outlined above, the lack of critical pieces of information in humans (e.g., brain regions active in nausea, plasma biomarker) further limits the validity of any animal model. Despite these limitations there is a growing body of evidence reviewed below to indicate that if we are unable to measure nausea directly, we are able to identify surrogate markers which although requiring careful interpretation nevertheless have a degree of predictive value. In addition to identification of drugs to treat nausea in humans, there is also a need to identify drugs targeted against a variety of diseases but which have nausea (and or vomiting) as a dose-limiting toxicity (Holmes et al., 2009). While vomiting may be detected by testing in species such as the dog and ferret, although nausea may be suspected based on animal studies it may not be identified until studied in healthy volunteers or even clinical trials. In one analysis of Phase 1 (first in human) studies, nausea was found to be the second most commonly encountered side effect with headache being the first (see Figure 8.1). Therefore there is a need to identify whether there are animal models of nausea from which the data can be translated to humans with a high degree of sensitivity and specificity. Such models could contribute to reducing the time and hence cost of drug development and reduce the attrition in the later phases of development.

Identification of novel treatments for nausea in humans is the major drive for attempting to study nausea in animals, but improved understanding of how various animal species express unpleasant sensations will potentially improve veterinary diagnosis. In experimental laboratory settings there is often an emphasis on pain as a humane end point (Morton & Griffiths, 1985). While there is no doubt about its importance in welfare terms, this focus probably reflects our lack of understanding about other unpleasant sensations such as nausea and the special significance *humans* attach to pain. Identification of patterns of behavior that may be indicative of nausea rather than of other sensations will help refine some experimental protocols and reduce suffering by the recognition of the signs of nonpainful but perhaps equally unpleasant sensations. Such sensations may be unidentified but significant confounding factors in some experiments.

SOME THEORETICAL CONSIDERATIONS

General Issues of Studying Behavior in Animals

The Nobel prize–winning ethologist Niko Tinbergen posed "Four Questions" (Tinbergen, 1963) that apply to all studies of animal behavior and are useful to

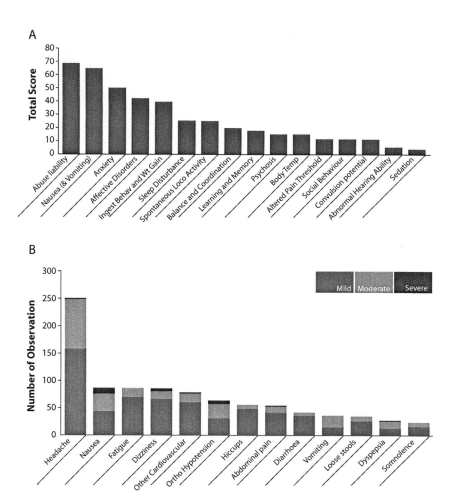

Figure 8.1 The impact of nausea and vomiting on the development of NCEs. (A) An analysis by Pfizer assessing how various side-effects encountered in preclinical safety studies impacted on the development of a medicine for humans. More than 70 novel therapeutics, including antivirals, agents to promote tissue repair, neurology, sex health, allergy and respiratory, cardiovascular, gastrointestinal, and urogenital disease targets were used in this analysis. The targets included were agents with both peripheral and central sites of action and were assessed during the period 1998–2000. The total score represents the number of compounds progressing to clinical development that interact with targets that have known or suspected safety liability based on experimental data or from literature reports. This analysis took into account not only the impact to the patients but also to the drug development program through the need for additional studies to investigate the extent and seriousness of the safety issue and also to support regulatory acceptance by bodies such as the European Medicines Agency and the U.S. Food and Drug Administration. Whereas factors such as sedation, convulsion potential, and changes in body temperature were important, they easily could be examined both clinically and preclinically. In contrast nausea and vomiting were considered

Figure 8.1 (*continued*) second only to abuse liability as having an impact on the development of the drug. (B) A further analysis of side effects encountered in sixteen Phase 1 clinical studies conducted by Pfizer between 2003 and 2005. While the most commonly encountered side effect was headache, with approximately 250 instances, the next most encountered was nausea, which accounted for over 80 instances, nearly half of which were rated as either moderate or severe. There were also a similar number of observations of moderate vomiting. The sixteen trials averaged approximately 35 individuals each. Reproduced with permission from Holmes et al., 2009.

consider when exploring behaviors associated with the administration of emetic agents:

1. *Function*—How does the behavior increase the chances of the animal surviving or reproducing?
2. *Evolution*—How has the behavior changed during the course of evolution?
3. *Causation*—What external and internal factors are responsible for that specific behavior occurring at a particular moment in time?
4. *Development*—How does the behavior develop during the life of an animal and what factors affect this?

Of these questions, "Function" and "Causation" are the ones that will be most relevant to the behaviors outlined below and they will be used to guide the discussion.

It should be noted that these questions do not address what animals are "feeling" (if anything) when initiating or performing a particular behavior, and do not address the question of whether animals can think and reflect on their actions. An introduction to this controversial issue can be found in Manning and Stamp Dawkins (1998), who use a quote known as "Morgan's Canon" from 1894 by the comparative psychologist C. Lloyd Morgan, to caution against invoking anthropomorphic explanations and take a "sensible" approach to the analysis of animal behavior: "In no case may we interpret an action as the outcome of the exercise of a higher psychical faculty, if it can be interpreted as the outcome of one which stands lower in the psychological scale."

In all cases where we attempt to study nausea in animals, we are attempting to identify a specific behavioral change that reflects a sensation or feeling that we are assuming a particular species has at the time when it is exhibiting the behavioral change. This issue is related to the nature of conscious sensations and indeed consciousness in animals, which was discussed in Chapter 4 (in this volume) together with central processing of emetic signals in humans. We will return to some of the arguments at the end of this chapter as they help to determine whether we are actually measuring nausea in animals.

General Characteristics of a Model for Nausea

Basic characteristics of all animal models are face, construct, and predictive validity (Blackburn-Munro, 2004), and these provide sensible criteria against which experimental studies can be judged. *Face validity* requires that the model should be similar to a human experiencing nausea as judged by the presence of a multiplicity of signs and symptoms. In essence an animal thought to be experiencing nausea should "look" in the broadest sense like a human experiencing nausea. We will take this to include not only behaviors but also changes in physiological parameters. *Construct validity* demands that the theoretical basis for the genesis of the condition or disease in the animal model matches that known to occur in humans. This is problematic for the study of nausea as we are lacking some critical information in humans, although data on vomiting mechanisms is considerable in both humans and animals and helps with problems of construct validity. There are two main tools available for investigating the mechanisms by which a particular drug, stimulus (e.g., motion), or disease induces emesis in an animal: pharmacological tools and surgical lesions to pathways (usually neural). We will see several examples of these approaches in this chapter with drugs and lesions that block potential behavioral indices of nausea and/or vomiting. *Predictive validity* in this case requires that the model can be used to identify either drugs or other treatments that will have antinausea activity in humans. This important criterion of course requires that drugs be studied in humans in order to validate the predictive (translational) nature of the model as a tool for the identification of novel agents. Such data are also needed to enable calculation of the sensitivity of a model/assay. It is important to appreciate that for a model to be predictive it does not necessarily have to be a model of nausea itself. It just has to reliably identify treatments that either induce nausea in humans as a side effect or that block nausea in humans. Development of models (including in vitro models) with predictive validity requires more extensive studies in humans to improve knowledge of the neuropharmacology of nausea. Without such knowledge it will be difficult, if not impossible, to refine current animal models and eventually to replace them with nonanimal alternatives. These three criteria will be used to assist in judging whether any of the models described below is an animal model of nausea.

Specific Issues Relating to the Study of Nausea in Animals

If we are to attempt to measure nausea in animals by indirect means, then we need to consider a number of practical issues to optimize the validity of any such measurements.

When Should We Look for Nausea?

In humans nausea usually (but not invariably) precedes the onset of vomiting and hence in attempting to look for any surrogate marker (behavioral or physiological) of nausea in an animal, this should be the period of most interest. This of course can only apply to species with an emetic reflex; in rats and mice lacking an emetic reflex there is no obvious equivalent to a vomit to demarcate a window of interest for the study of nausea-related behaviors. In the case of stimuli where multiple bouts of vomiting occur over an extended time scale, it is likely that similar (but probably not identical) changes in the proposed marker for nausea will occur as the next emetic episode becomes more likely. A potentially confounding problem with attempting to study nausea after the first emetic episode is the observation in humans that emesis can abolish the sensation of nausea (e.g., in migraine; Sacks, 1981). Although infrequently studied, any measurements taken following the administration of an emetic and during the time when emesis is occurring will have added validity if it is shown that they eventually return to preemetic administration levels.

Presence, Pattern, and Dimensions

Ideally two questions need to be answered: first, is the animal experiencing nausea as opposed to another sensation; and second, how much nausea is it experiencing at a given time? In humans both questions are relatively easily answered by some form of questionnaire although definitions of nausea vary (see Chapter 1, in this volume); but in animals, these questions are much more complex. Whatever method we choose in animal studies must, at the most basic level, be able to distinguish reliably between an animal with, and one without, nausea as this would at least permit it to be used for studies of potential antinausea agents. Ideally, we should be able to ascribe some magnitude to the nausea at any given time point so that temporal patterns can be mapped (especially important if we are attempting to make correlations of physiological measures with behavioral changes) and also so that relative efficacy and potency of potential antinausea agents can be studied. In humans, while we can assess the magnitude of nausea, it is important to appreciate that all subjective measures are related to an individual's experience (e.g., VAS scales with the anchor points "no nausea" and "worst nausea I have ever felt"; Del Favero et al., 1990). Even with physiological measurements of plasma vasopressin and EGG in humans, we can only give a probabilistic estimate of whether or not the person is experiencing nausea and the magnitude (see Chapters 6 and 7, in this volume).

Sensory Qualities

Definitions of nausea in humans (see Chapter 1, in this volume) frequently include phrases such as "unpleasant sensation," "awareness of the urge to vomit," (Watcha & White, 1992), and "referred generally to the epigastrium and abdomen" (Sarna, 1989). While we are probably able to detect in some animal species if they are experiencing (or have experienced) an unpleasant sensation, we have little concept of the nature of their sensory experience ("what does it *feel* like?") except by being anthropomorphic. In an animal it may be very difficult, if not impossible, to distinguish between a sensation of nausea and a less specific sensation of "malaise" or "visceral illness," both of which could include nausea as a component (cf., dyspepsia in humans). It is probably not unreasonable to assume that species with brains of similar organization and complexity to the human brain (e.g., chimpanzees) have a similar capacity for sensory experiences to the same stimulus, but we do not actually know this nor can we be certain of what emotional qualities are associated with such experiences. And outside the advanced nonhuman primates (and possibly some cetaceans) we can only speculate on the entire problem.

With regard to the "awareness of the urge to vomit" and "referred generally to the epigastrium and abdomen" it may be possible to gain insights into these aspects indirectly from behavioral studies (e.g., suddenly adopting a characteristic posture) but the problem remains of linkage to a specific conscious sensory experience.

An additional, even more problematic issue relates to whether the sensory experience is similar between species. It is known that dogs and house musk shrews will readily ingest their own vomit (Andrews et al., 2005) something that humans would find very distasteful. Does this mean that nausea and vomiting are of less consequence to dogs as compared to humans?

TECHNIQUES USED IN AN ATTEMPT TO STUDY NAUSEA IN ANIMALS

This extensive section will review the range of techniques brought to bear on the measurement of "nausea" in a variety of animal species. Each measurement will be discussed using a similar format: (1) What is it? (2) Why might it be indicative of nausea? (3) How is it measured? (4) Species in which it has been demonstrated and stimuli for induction, (5) Effects of antiemetics, and (6) Advantages and disadvantages. For some of the measurements where there is a paucity of information in all areas, the various aspects are discussed under a single heading. The possible utility of indices used in humans such as plasma vasopressin (AVP) levels and the electrogastrogram (EGG) are discussed in Chapters 6 and 7 in this volume for ease of direct comparison with the more extensive human data, and the same is true for the brain pathways reviewed in Chapter 4.

Pica

What Is It?

The word "pica" derives from the Latin word for the common magpie (*Pica pica*), presumably reflecting its eclectic foraging habits. Clinically, pica is classified as an eating disorder or perversion of appetite in which a patient has strong cravings for and as a result ingests a range of nonnutritive substances (allotriophagia) (Green, 1925). The term is most often used to refer to ingestion of soil or clay when it may be referred to by the specific term "geophagia" (Stokes, 2006), but a diverse range of other substances may be ingested including (but not limited to) ice (pagophagia), lead (plumbophagia), feces (coprophagia), hair (trichophagia), stones (lithophagia), bones (osteophagia), and raw potatoes (geomelophagia) (Green, 1925; Cooper, 1957). Pica commonly occurs in the first trimester of pregnancy (the time when pregnancy sickness is most common), in children, and in those with psychiatric illnesses. Pica has often been ascribed to specific dietary deficiencies (e.g., iron [rust ingestion], calcium [osteophagia]) in humans and animals; but in humans there is also evidence for cultural determinants particularly for ingestion of soil or clay, and this appears to be a widespread practice (Laufer, 1930). In many parts of the world clays are mixed with food as an extender to stave off hunger in times of food shortage (e.g., Kieselghur-diatomaceous earth), and may even be specially prepared and baked as in the case of "ampo" in Java (Root-Bernstein & Root-Bernstein, 1997). Clays also have a long history of use in detoxification of food when mixed with foods that otherwise would be toxic (e.g., wild potatoes) and have also been used to ameliorate the effect of poisons as exemplified by the case in 1581 C.E. of a prisoner who asked a court if he could take the poison mercuric chloride instead of being hanged. He also requested that he take *terra sigillata* ("sealed earth") following the mercuric chloride. The court agreed and although the prisoner was very ill he survived this lethal dose (Root-Bernstein & Root-Bernstein, 1997). Clays and earth in general have been used since ancient times to relieve nausea and vomiting. This latter observation provides the link with animals, as many animal species in the wild have been reported to ingest clay or earth under similar circumstances and this is discussed more fully in the next section.

Why Might Pica Be Indicative of Nausea in Animals?

If an animal eats clay (or other nonnutritive substance) as a manifestation of pica, we need to examine the *causation* and *function* of this behavior within the context of nausea and vomiting. In the wild, clay or earth consumption in animals is most often associated with some form of gastrointestinal illness. This may be caused by toxic constituents of food, infection, or parasites and may be manifest as vomiting (in species with an intact emetic reflex) or diarrhea, but other manifestations of gastrointestinal malaise (referred pain, jaundice) may be difficult to observe. In the wild, pica, usually involving earth or clay consumption, has been observed in a wide range of species either as a preparatory behavior to eating foods that are known to be toxic or that become toxic in particular seasons and following ingestion of a food that has induced gastrointestinal malaise. This behavior may give some species an evolutionary advantage by allowing them to eat foods that cannot be exploited by other species and by reducing the magnitude of illness or enabling more rapid recovery if a toxin is accidentally ingested. Clay consumption is most commonly (but not exclusively) observed in plant-eating animals, most likely because of the range of toxic secondary metabolites (especially alkaloids) used as defensive agents. Studies in macaws have demonstrated that clay ingestion reduced the plasma level of an ingested alkaloid by 60% (Gilardi et al., 1999). Clay (or soil) consumption linked to ingestion of toxins or gastrointestinal illness has been reported in cattle, chachalacas, chimpanzees, currassows, deer, dogs, forest elephants, macaws, macaque monkeys, mountain gorillas, guans, parrots, peccaries, tapirs, and tigers (Krishnamani & Mahaney, 2000; Attenborough, 2002;

Engel, 2002). Clay is not the only substance eaten by animals to ameliorate the effects of toxins in the diet. Charcoal is also used by some species, as is the case in humans. Charcoal consumption has been documented in red colobus monkeys that eat a diet containing secondary toxic metabolites and is especially high in phenols (Krishnamani & Mahaney, 2000; Engel, 2002). There is evidence that this behavior is learned by imitation, whereas in laboratory rats the ingestion of kaolin following administration of an emetic agent appears to be an innate behavior (see below). Ash eating has also been reported in elephants and chimpanzees and has been proposed to act as an antacid (Engel, 2002).

Before considering laboratory observations of clay consumption, we need to make some comments on the above observations under the headings of *function* and *causation*. The *function* is relatively clear: to minimize the impact of either deliberate or accidental toxin ingestion, which would have a clear survival advantage at several levels (e.g., reduction of mortality prior to reproductive age, reduced vulnerability during the period of illness, reduced impact on growth and hence reproductive fitness). In considering geophagy among nonhuman primates, Krishnamani and Mahaney (2000) conclude that all hypotheses suggest that it has some medicinal value primarily in treating gastrointestinal problems for example by toxin adsorption or an antacid action and as a micronutrient source.

Causation is more of a problem. It can be argued that the animals are ingesting clay either prophylactically to avoid or minimize gastrointestinal illness, which arguably would require them to have previously experienced and remembered some illness that elicited either a behavioral change (e.g., vomiting, diarrhea), conscious sensation (e.g., nausea, pain), or internal state change that could be linked to the food and to have found that ingestion of clay (by trial and error?) alleviated the problem. Based on the experience, the animal may have generalized the response to a range of foods, but the learning process may need to begin again if the animal were forced to switch diets because of a shortage. The causal factor here would be the recognition of a toxic food. It may not be necessary for all individuals of one species in a particular locality to have previous experience of toxic food as the response may have been learned from a parent, or by mimicking the behavior of other members of the same species when eating the same food, or even by observing the behavior of other species. Rats made ill by an ingested toxin do communicate information about the hazard to others in the colony (Stamp Dawkins, 2003), but there is no indication that they "tell" each other about how to deal with the problem except to avoid that food. This of course raises the issue of how species that do not feed in groups or live in social groups learn the response. Recruitment of behaviors is common where the behavior of an individual is noted by others who in turn change their behavior. This can be seen in city pigeons, where one individual alighting on the tiniest piece of food will quickly recruit many others despite the size of the food portion. It also is seen in cleaner fish, who recognize the change in behavior of a shark indicating that it is safe to approach to clean ectoparasites.

Another possibility is that the ingestion of clay may be innate. This is hard to study in the wild, but laboratory studies suggest that it is an innate behavior, and this is mentioned below where we review the extensive laboratory studies of pica that help with the *causation* question. It is a particularly interesting ingestive behavior as, at the same time as there is an increased appetitive drive for a nonnutrient substance such as kaolin, there is usually a reduced appetitive drive for ingestion of food but not usually water (e.g., Malik et al., 2006). It should be noted that provided kaolin is available the desire or urge to ingest it following toxicosis may not require the genesis of a conscious sensation such as nausea or malaise, and hence the ingestion would be a measure of the degree of toxicosis and not nausea per se, although the two may be related.

De Jonghe et al. (2009) studied the effect of kaolin consumption on food intake by rats treated with cisplatin (see below) and showed that the suppression of food intake recovered more rapidly in animals allowed access to kaolin (see Figure 8.2), but this effect was only apparent three days after cisplatin and after peak kaolin consumption (day 1). A similar study (Malik, N. & Andrews, P.L.R., unpublished observations) investigated only the first two days after cisplatin and failed to see any difference between rats allowed access to kaolin in food intake, body weight, locomotor activity, or the weight of gastric contents. These studies indicate that kaolin consumption may be beneficial in the longer term, but for this effect to manifest the animal must survive the initial acute challenge. It was noted above that clay ingestion reduced the plasma level of ingested plant toxins in a bird, supporting the proposal that the clay binds toxins in the gut lumen. However, in the cisplatin studies while the kaolin is in the gut lumen the cisplatin is given intraperitoneally making toxin binding an unlikely explanation for its beneficial effect in this setting. A final issue in relation to clay consumption in a broad biological context relates to which species exhibit it, especially in relation to the presence or absence of vomiting, and this is dealt with below.

How Is It Measured?

In a laboratory setting pica is usually measured using kaolin consumption, although a few studies have used soil (e.g., Mitchell et al., 1976; Mitchell, Krusemark & Hafner, 1977). The kaolin (China clay, hydrated aluminium silicate) is mixed with water and bound with 1% gum arabic. The resulting paste is extruded (using a modified syringe) into relatively uniform pellets that are as similar in size and shape to the pelleted food of the species under study, and the pellets are either dried at room temperature or baked in an oven on a wire mesh tray (e.g., Mitchell, Krusemark & Hafner, 1977; Takeda et al., 1993a; Rudd et al., 2002; Liu et al., 2005). The pellets are usually presented in a divided hopper with food in the other compartment, but it would be interesting to examine the effect if the kaolin pellets were mixed with food pellets. One disadvantage of placing kaolin in a food hopper is if the stimulus reduces the ability of the animal to reach the hopper then not only will a reduction in

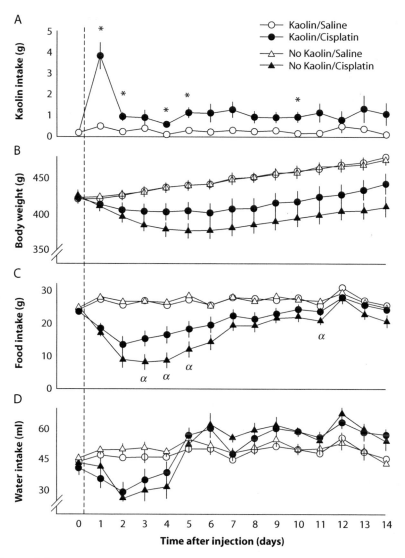

Figure 8.2 Effects of cisplatin, a chemotherapy agent, on kaolin consumption and body weight, food intake, and water intake in rats with or without kaolin access. One day of baseline measures is shown (Day 0) before injection (i.p.) of cisplatin (6 mg/kg) or saline. The dashed vertical line indicates the time of injection. A. Cisplatin increased kaolin consumption in rats with access to kaolin. * = statistically significant mean comparison for saline vs. Cisplatin, Benjamin-Hochberg correction for multiple comparisons. B. Effects of cisplatin on body weight. C. Food intake. D. Water consumption in animals with or without kaolin access "α" = $p < 0.05$, significant two-way ANOVAs injection by kaolin access for food intake at 3, 4, 5, and 11 days after injection. Reproduced with permission from De Jonghe et al., 2009.

food intake be seen (as may be expected) but there may not be an increase in kaolin consumption. Even if kaolin is taken from the hopper, the pattern and magnitude of consumption may be influenced by concurrent illness other than nausea. Rearing to reach into a food hopper requires a degree of coordination and muscular strength, and hence a failure to see an increase in kaolin intake in response to a treatment is not necessarily an indication of the absence of "nausea" but may be due to the treatment inducing fatigue or even dizziness. Careful observation of general behavior should accompany measurements of pica to assess such potentially confounding factors. However, in rats treated with cisplatin where rearing is reduced by ~25% and other indices of locomotion are also reduced (Malik et al., 2006), kaolin consumption is increased.

Kaolin is introduced into the hopper several days before exposure to the test stimulus or substance. One to five days appears to be the range, with three days a commonly used adaptation period (e.g., Mitchell, Krusemark & Hafner, 1977; Takeda et al., 1993a; Rudd et al., 2002; Liu et al., 2005). In general, rats will nibble some kaolin over the adaptation period. Rudd et al. (2002) reported a consumption of 0.7–1.2 g on the first adaptation day and 0.3 to 0.5 g on the following two days. In our experience, spillage of kaolin in the adaptation period is higher than following drug treatment, with consumption most often measured daily and account taken of spillage. In some studies, animals are housed in wire-bottom cages to facilitate collection of spilled food and kaolin; however, such housing may impose additional stress on the animals, and this must be taken into account in the interpretation of the results especially if the experiment has a long duration. In principle, shorter measurement periods could be used to obtain better temporal resolution, but this is not commonly done. In addition there are almost no data on the latency to ingest kaolin following administration of the stimulus. One exception is Mitchell, Laycock, and Stephens (1977), who noted that following rotation kaolin consumption began within a few minutes and subsided over the next 2 to 3 hours. Interestingly, in this study the rats were trained to bar-press to obtain kaolin, a technique that appears not to have been used recently but which deserves consideration as it may give useful insights into motivation.

A modified technique has been used to investigate pica in the mouse. This used kaolin prepared as described above but during preparation it is mixed with the coloring agent carmine (see Yamamoto et al., 2002, for details) which, like kaolin, is not absorbed in the gastrointestinal tract and hence will appear in the feces. Feces are collected over two days and the carmine extracted, measured, and used to calculate the consumption of kaolin after correcting for carmine retained in the gut (the recovery rate in Yamamoto et al., 2002, was 68.8% so this is a major correction factor). This method is particularly applicable to situations where either the species is expected to consume a relatively small amount of kaolin (e.g., mouse), and hence measurement of actual consumption may be problematic, or perhaps where one is looking for very small changes. The temporal resolution of this method is not good because of the time delay between ingestion of kaolin and production of feces, especially when many of the stimuli under study induce delays in gastric emptying. A method utilizing radio-labeled kaolin would enable precise measurement of consumption with a high temporal resolution and if the detection method had sufficient resolution, transit time though various regions of the gut could be measured.

The duration of the period of study is determined by the nature of the stimulus under study and the purpose of the study. For example, after a single exposure to motion, systemic lithium chloride, apomorphine, cholecystokinin, or intragastric copper sulfate, a period of 24 hours appears adequate to assess the impact of these "emetic" stimuli and antiemetic agents (e.g., McCutcheon, Ballard & McCaffrey, 1992; Takeda et al., 1993a; Takeda et al., 1995b). Note that with cytotoxic anticancer agents such as cyclophosphamide and cisplatin, where protracted or delayed emesis is the focus of the study, measurement periods of several days may be necessary to characterize the effect (e.g., Rudd et al., 2002). Mitchell, Krusemark, and Hafner (1977) measured kaolin consumption daily over 20 days in rats in a study of repeated rotational stimulation, and a 5-week period has been used in a cisplatin study (Vera et al., 2006). In studies of kaolin consumption it is essential that food and water intake and body weight be measured simultaneously for welfare reasons and also to examine the relationships among the parameters, which may provide added insights into the significance of kaolin consumption.

In all studies of pica, when the effect of a potential antiemetic agent is to be investigated, it is essential that appropriate control groups receiving exactly the same number of injections as the test animals are included, as there is evidence that the number of injections can influence the pattern of the response to cisplatin and that the 5-HT$_3$ receptor antagonist ondansetron can itself induce pica in rats (Rudd et al., 2002; Malik et al., 2006).

Pica studies usually report the results as mean kaolin consumption in grams ± S.E.M. and do not report whether all animals given an emetic stimulus responded. Some studies mention selecting only animals that exhibit pica in response to a given stimulus (Yamamoto, Takeda & Yamatodani, 2002). Some indication of the variability in the response can be gained from the relatively large standard errors and numbers of animals per group often seen in pica studies (e.g., Takeda et al., 1993a). In our experience individuals that appear not to respond to a stimulus by kaolin consumption do occur, and this may represent a form of neophobia. Across a range of studies the maximum mean consumption of kaolin reported in adult rats is up to 10g/day (Aung et al., 2003).

In studies of pica it is essential that food and water intake be measured simultaneously especially when the effect of pharmacological agents is being investigated. The reason for this is that agents that suppress food intake could also suppress kaolin consumption, perhaps leading to an erroneous conclusion that they had anti-nausea/emetic properties. As most (if not all) experimental agents that induce pica also reduce food intake, candidate antiemetic drugs should reduce kaolin consumption while stimulating food intake (see below).

Laboratory Species in Which Pica Has Been Studied
and Stimuli for Induction

Rat (*Rattus norvegicus*)   The rat has been the main species in which pica has been used as an index of the effects of emetic agents, but studies have been confined to male animals so we do not know if females behave in the same way. An age-related effect of motion sickness on kaolin consumption has been reported, with older rats (20 months) being less susceptible than younger (2 and 11 months) animals (McCaffrey & Graham, 1980).

Pica has been reported in several strains of rat including laboratory bred strains such as Wistar (Takeda et al., 1993a), hooded Long-Evans (Mitchell, Winter & Morisaki, 1977), Sprague-Dawley (McCaffrey & Graham, 1980), and wild rats caught in two different locations around Seattle (Mitchell, Beatty & Cox, 1977). Little attention has been paid to possible strain differences with the exception of the study by Mitchell, Winter, and Morisaki (1977) that showed a difference in the pattern of the response to cyclophosphamide between Wistar and Long-Evans strains, with the former having a larger and more protracted response. In addition a marked difference was observed between the responses in the wild rats caught in different locations. This study also showed differences in the neophobic tendencies between the two groups of wild rat and this could be a reflection of an "anxious" phenotype associated with enhanced activity of the corticotrophin-releasing factor system reported in mice (Contarino & Gold, 2002). It is worth noting that even the same strain of rat from different commercial breeders may have marked phenotypic differences as has been reported for metabolic and hypothalamic pituitary adrenal axis function in Sprague Dawley rats from three suppliers (Pecoraro et al., 2006).

Pica has been reported in the rat in response to stimuli acting via all the main pathways that when activated are known to evoke both nausea and vomiting in humans and vomiting in species capable of emesis: vestibular system (motion: Mitchell, Krusemark & Hafner, 1977; Mitchell, Laycock & Stephens, 1977; McCaffrey, 1985; Takeda et al., 1993a; Takeda et al., 1995a); area postrema (apomorphine: Takeda et al., 1995a; morphine: Aung et al., 2003; buprenorphine: Clark et al., 1997); abdominal visceral afferents (cisplatin: Takeda et al., 1995b; Rudd et al., 2002; Aung et al., 2003; Yamamoto et al., 2004; Liu et al., 2005; radiation: Yamamoto, Takeda & Yamatodani, 2002; cholecystokinin: McCutcheon, Ballard & McCaffrey et al., 1992; copper sulfate: Takeda et al., 1993a). Pica can also be induced by cytoglucopaenia caused by 2-deoxy-D-glucose (Watson et al., 1987), cyclosporine-A (Fujisaki et al., 2001) and by neuropeptide Y (NPY; Woods et al., 1998). In addition Mitchell, Winter, and Morisaki (1977) demonstrated that it was possible to induce

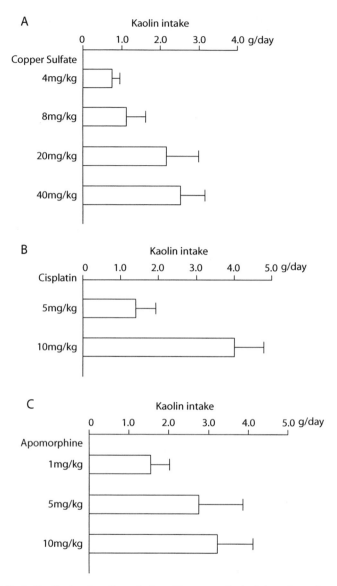

Figure 8.3 A. Kaolin intake of rats induced by peroral administration of copper sulfate. Columns and bars represent mean intakes ± SE of 11 animals for 24 h after treatment. B. Kaolin intake of rats induced by intraperitoneal injection of cisplatin. Columns and bars represent mean intakes ± SE of eight animals for 24 h after the injection. C. Kaolin intake of rats induced by intraperitoneal injection of apomorphine. Columns and bars represent mean intakes ± SE of 13 animals for 24 h after the injection. Reproduced with permission from Takeda et al., 1993.

conditioned pica. In this paradigm the cyclophosphamide or lithium chloride administration was paired with saccharine solution; when animals were exposed subsequently to saccharine, they consumed kaolin.

In all cases where the intensity of the stimulus has been varied, either the amount of kaolin consumed and/or its pattern of consumption has changed in proportion, indicating that pica is a graded phenomenon, as are both nausea and vomiting (see Figures 8.3 and 8.4). Using a range of anticancer drugs, Yamamoto et al. (2007) reported that both the amount and duration of kaolin consumption were related to the clinical emetic potential (high: cisplatin and cyclophosphamide; medium: actinomycin and 5-fluouracil; low: vincristine). Kaolin intake has also been used to study the effects of weekly injection of a "low" dose (1 mg/kg) of cisplatin intended to mimic the cyclical nature of chemotherapy, and it was shown that over 5 weeks each injection induced an increase in consumption for at least 24 hours following injection (Vera et al., 2006).

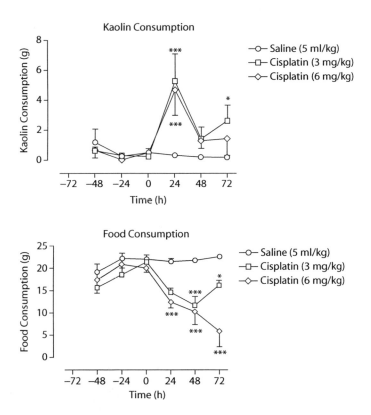

Figure 8.4 Action of cisplatin to modify kaolin and food ingestion in the rat. Cisplatin or vehicle (saline 0.9% w/v, 10 ml/kg, i.p.) was administered at $t = 0$. Data represents the means ± S.E.M. of 5–6 determinations. Data significantly different from the respective vehicle-treated cisplatin animals are indicated as $*P < 0.05$, $**P < 0.01$, $***P < 0.001$ (repeated measures ANOVA with preplanned contrasts of specified means). Reproduced with permission from Rudd et al., 2002.

Mouse (*Mus musculus*)   Surprisingly few studies have attempted to demonstrate pica in the mouse despite the utility that this would have because of the availability of genetically modified animals. Yamamoto et al. (2002) showed an increase in kaolin consumption in mice (ICR strain) by cisplatin (5 mg/kg, i.p.) using indirect measurement by carmine labeling of kaolin. Consumption increased from 0.33 ± 0.08 g to 0.45 ± 0.16 g. However, Liu et al. (2005), using direct measurement of kaolin consumption in one inbred (C57/6J) and one outbred (MF1) strain of mouse, failed to see an increase in kaolin consumption with cisplatin (6 mg/kg, i.p.); although there was a decrease in food intake and an increase in the weight of stomach contents at 48 hours, both effects seen in rats in which pica occurs (see Figure 8.5). A higher dose of cisplatin (20 mg/kg, i.p.) also failed to induce pica. The reason for the difference between the results of the two is unclear but may reflect strain differences or the different methodologies used. Santucci et al. (2000; 2002) using an outbred Swiss-derived CD-1 strain of mice reported an increase in kaolin consumption following exposure to hypergravity. This study considered the three prerotation and five postrotation days as repeated measures using a mixed-model ANOVA. The effects of rotation appeared to be confined to males, and the values reported for consumption are surprisingly high (6.3 ± 1.9 g) when compared to the range reported for rats (<10 g). Using whole body X-radiation, Yamamoto et al. (2005) reported a dose-related increase in kaolin consumption in OCR strain mice, the same strain in which they demonstrated an increase in kaolin consumption in response to cisplatin. The few studies undertaken in the mouse using a combination of different methods, strains, and stimuli do not allow firm conclusions to be drawn about pica in the mouse although a priori one would expect the mouse to exhibit pica. One explanation may be that it is not such a robust response as in the rat and may be highly strain-dependent.

Rabbit (*Oryctolagus cuniculus*)   There are no studies of pica under controlled conditions, although Green (1925) reported what he termed "evanescent" pica following apomorphine injection. The pica was manifest as the animal becoming restless and gnawing anything in reach. This observation has not been pursued but is of interest as the "purposeless chewing" seen in response to some drugs has been argued to be a reflection of nausea rather than dyskinesia (Rupniak, Tye & Iversen, 1990).

House Musk Shrew (*Suncus murinus*)   There has been considerable interest in whether any of the laboratory species with an emetic reflex exhibit pica in response to an emetic challenge. While there are anecdotal reports of dogs eating nonnutritive substances such as soil or grass when ill (Mitchell, Winter & Morisaki, 1977), there have not been any formal studies of this. The house musk shrew, an insectivore, has become an established small-animal model for studies of emesis (Ueno, Matsuki & Saito, 1988). To date it has not been possible to demonstrate pica, as indicated by an increase in kaolin consumption (see Figure 8.5), in *Suncus* in response to cisplatin, nicotine, copper

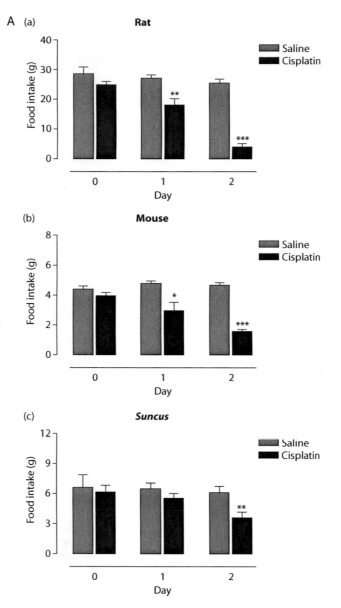

Figure 8.5A Effect of cisplatin on daily food intake in a. rats (6 mg/kg; i.p.), b. mice (6 mg/kg; i.p.), and c. *Suncus* (20 mg/kg; i.p.). Results are mean ± S.E.M; $n = 6$ for rats and mice; $n = 8$–10 for *Suncus* (10 saline-treated and 8 cisplatin-treated with emesis). $*P < 0.05$, $**P < 0.01$, $***P < 0.001$ vs. Saline-treated group.

(*Continued*)

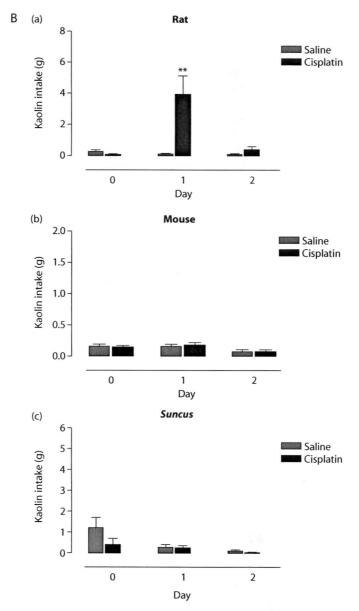

Figure 8.5B Kaolin consumption pre– and post–cisplatin treatment in a. rats (6 mg/kg; i.p.), b. mice (6 mg/kg; i.p.), and c. *Suncus* (20 mg/kg; i.p.). Results are mean ± S.E.M; $n = 6$ for rats and mice; $n = 8$–10 for *Suncus* (10 saline-treated and 8 cisplatin-treated with emesis). $*P < 0.05$, $**P < 0.01$, $***P < 0.001$ vs. Saline-treated group. Reproduced with permission Liu et al., 2005.

sulfate, or lithium chloride (Yamamoto et al., 2004; Liu et al., 2005) given at doses that either induced emesis and/or conditioned food avoidance in *Suncus* (see below).

Pigeon (*Columba livia*)   Although the pigeon has been used extensively for studies of emesis and conditioned food avoidance and several species of birds in the wild (e.g., macaws; Gilardi et al., 1999) exhibit pica, there do not appear to be any laboratory studies of pica in the pigeon.

Effects of Antiemetic Agents and Nerve Lesions

The effects of pathway lesions and pharmacological agents will be discussed separately and will be confined to studies in the rat, as this is the species in which pica has been most extensively studied.

Pathway Lesions   In the rat, Morita et al. (1988a) reported that following bilateral labyrinthectomy (a procedure that abolishes motion-induced emesis; Reason & Brand, 1975) rats exposed to motion failed to have pica. This is consistent with pica being an index of motion sickness, but it fails to enable any distinction to be made between motion-induced nausea and vomiting. In a related study in labyrinthectomized animals in contrast to intact rats, Takeda et al. (1986) found no increase in histamine levels in the hypothalamus. The effect of abdominal vagotomy or area postrema ablation on pica has not been studied extensively. De Jonghe and Horn (2008) demonstrated that section of the common hepatic branch of the abdominal vagus in the rat markedly reduced (61%) cisplatin-induced pica as well as ameliorating the loss in body weight and reduction of food intake also associated with cisplatin administration (see Figure 8.6). Pica induced by apomorphine (presumed to act on the area postrema) was unaffected by vagotomy. These results are consistent with the hypothesis that pica in the rat is induced by activation of the same pathways as are responsible for the induction of emesis by the same stimuli in species with an emetic reflex.

Pharmacological Agents and Other Interventions

For simplicity the section below will discuss each "emetic" challenge in turn and will be confined to studies in the rat.

Apomorphine   In the rat, kaolin consumption induced by apomorphine was markedly reduced (approx. 80%) by the dopamine D_2 receptor antagonist domperidone (Takeda et al., 1993a) and by diphenidol (Takeda et al., 1995a) but was unaffected by either diphenhydramine or the 5-HT$_3$ receptor antagonist ondansetron (Takeda et al., 1995a). Apomorphine is a well-characterized dopamine receptor agonist inducing emesis via the area postrema, and its emetic effect in the ferret can be blocked by domperidone but not by ondansetron (Andrews & Bhandari, 1993). Therefore these pharmacological studies are supportive of the contention that pica induced by a stimulus capable of inducing emesis in other species is a result of activation of pathways that in other species would lead to the induction of nausea and vomiting.

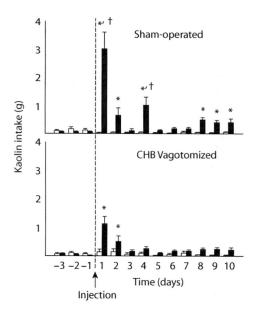

Figure 8.6 The effects of common hepatic branch vagotomy (CHB) on cisplatin-induced pica. Cisplatin (6mg/kg) or saline was injected (ip) after three days of baseline measurements.* = p < 0.05, saline versus cisplatin.† = p < 0.05, sham-operated versus CHB vagotomy cisplatin conditions. Reproduced with permission from De Jonghe and Horn, 2008.

Cisplatin   Cisplatin has been the subject of the most intense investigation, reflecting its clinical significance as an anticancer drug and also the recognition that it is a highly emetogenic agent (Hesketh et al., 1997) so that agents demonstrating efficacy against it are likely also to have efficacy against other, lesser emetogenic stimuli acting via the same pathway. A wide variety of substances including natural products have been tested against cisplatin, with the majority of studies investigating the effects in the first 24 hours and in a few the later effects with the two time points argued to be analogous to the "acute" and "delayed" emetic effects of cisplatin seen in the clinic (Hesketh et al., 2003b) and in emetic species such as the ferret (Rudd et al., 1994).

The acute effects of cisplatin (doses between 6 and 10 mg/kg i.p.) on kaolin consumption was unaffected by diphenydramine (20 mg/kg i.p.) and domperidone (2 mg/kg i.p.) but was reduced (> 50%) by diphenidol (30 mg/kg i.p.) The selective 5-HT$_3$ receptor antagonist ondansetron has been investigated in several studies using cisplatin doses of 6–10 mg/kg i.p. Takeda et al. (1993a; 1995b) reported a dose related (1–2 mg/kg i.p.) decrease in kaolin consumption although it was not abolished. A similar result was obtained by Saeki et al. (2001), who measured kaolin intake over three days and reported that while ondansetron reduced kaolin consumption to control levels on the first day after cisplatin, it was without effect on the subsequent two days (see below). Using twice-daily injections of ondansetron (1 mg/kg i.p.) Malik et al. (2006) failed to demonstrate a significant reduction in kaolin intake over the first 24 hours after cisplatin, although there was significant reduction on day 2. This failure of ondansetron to reduce cisplatin-induced kaolin consumption was also reported by Rudd et al. (2002) using a lower dose of cisplatin (3 mg/kg i.p.) and a higher dose of ondansetron (2 mg/kg i.p. x 2). Rudd et al. (2002) noted that ondansetron increased kaolin consumption in their cisplatin-treated (but not control) animals and Malik et al. (2006) reported that given alone, ondansetron significantly increased kaolin intake in the first 24 hours after administration. Rudd et al. (2002) argued that in their study the additional handling required for the administration of additional ondansetron or saline may have acted as a conditioning stimulus to the cisplatin, inducing non–5-HT_3 sensitive kaolin-intake mechanisms. The stimulation of kaolin consumption by ondansetron but not saline administration in the Malik et al. (2006) study suggests that ondansetron may have a paradoxical emetic-like effect analogous to that reported in the pigeon (Preziosi et al., 1992) and *Suncus murinus* (Torii, Saito & Matsuki, 1991). The discrepancies between these studies indicates that the effects of ondansetron on the acute phase of cisplatin-induced kaolin consumption are not very robust and may be particularly sensitive to the individual experimental conditions (e.g., number of injections, cisplatin dose, period of measurement, rat strain). These observations also indicate the critical importance of including drug-treated control groups in addition to saline treated groups.

The NK_1 receptor antagonists HSP-117 and CP-99,994 when given intraperitoneally caused a dose-related reduction in cisplatin-induced (10 mg/kg i.p.) kaolin consumption over the first 24 hours (Sacki et al., 2001), although in the case of the latter a very high dose was required (60 mg/kg i.p.), reflecting the low affinity of this compound for the rat NK_1 receptor (rat 111 nM, ferret 1.7 nM, human 0.3 nM) and perhaps a nonselective effect (Andrews & Rudd, 2004). Both compounds were also effective when given via the intracerebroventricular route, representing one of the few studies of pica to compare central and peripheral routes of administration of antiemetic agents. However, Malik et al. (2007) using a selective NK_1 receptor antagonist GR205171 with a relatively high affinity for the rat receptor (0.32 nM; see Andrews & Rudd, 2004) failed to show a significant effect on kaolin consumption on day 1, although there was a clear trend to a reduction and it did produce a significant reduction on day 2.

The synthetic corticosteroid dexamethasone has also been investigated in the cisplatin-induced pica model. Using a cisplatin dose of 3 mg/kg i.p., Rudd et al. (2002) showed that dexamethasone (1 mg/kg i.p. ×2) reduced kaolin consumption by 74.3% in the first 24 hours. With a higher dose of cisplatin (6 mg/kg i.p.), Malik et al. (2006) reduced kaolin consumption by 60% in the first 24 hours and by 75% on day 2.

Models of cisplatin-induced pica have been developed in the rat, in which the pattern of kaolin consumption appears to match the acute and delayed phases of emesis characteristic of cisplatin-induced emesis in humans and animals such as the ferret (Rudd, Jordan & Naylor, 1994; Hesketh et al., 2003b). The delayed phase is taken as the consumption of kaolin, which occurs between 48 and 72 hours following administration of cisplatin, with studies using either 10 mg/kg i.p. (Saeki et al., 2001) or 3 mg/kg i.p. (Rudd et al., 2002). In this phase ondansetron was without effect on kaolin consumption (Saeki et al., 2001; Rudd et al., 2002), but dexamethasone reduced consumption by 94% (Rudd et al., 2002).

The cisplatin-induced pica model has also been used to test the "antiemetic" potential of a number of natural products with antioxidant activity. Reductions in kaolin consumption have been reported with extracts of *Scutellaria baicalensis* and American ginseng berry (Aung et al., 2003; Mehendale et al., 2004; 2005).

Radiation   Pica induced by total body irradiation (TBI) in the rat was reduced by ~50% by treatment with ondansetron (Yamamoto et al., 2002), an observation consistent with the effect of ondansetron on emesis induced by TBI in ferrets and humans (Harding, 1995; Spizer, 1995). Ondansetron and dexamethasone reduced X-ray-induced kaolin consumption to 48% and 57% of control values respectively in mice, but this effect was not statistically significant (Yamamoto et al., 2005) although in combination they did produce a significant reduction. The NK_1 receptor antagonist CP-99,994 did not have any effect on kaolin consumption when given alone, although it did appear to enhance the effect of the ondansetron/dexamethasone combination.

Morphine   The opioid analgesic morphine, which has dose-dependent emetic and antiemetic effects in species with an emetic reflex (e.g., ferret, Thompson et al., 1992; dog, Foss et al., 1998), induces kaolin consumption in the rat without affecting food intake. Kaolin consumption was reduced by both ondansetron, a 5-HT$_3$ receptor antagonist, and by methylnaltrexone, a quaternary peripherally acting opioid antagonist (Aung et al., 2004). The latter has been shown to block the emetic effects of morphine in the dog (Foss, Bass & Goldberg, 1993). It should be noted that the emetic effects of morphine are abolished by area postrema ablation (Wang & Glaviano, 1954) and that although quaternized compounds are poorly brain penetrant, the blood-brain barrier in the region of the area postrema is relatively permeable (Leslie, 1986).

Motion   In a double rotation-model (simultaneous rotation in two parallel axes designed to cause otolith-canal conflict) of motion sickness, kaolin consumption was inhibited by administration of α-fluoromethyl histamine (a depleter of neuronal histamine), diphenhydramine (H$_1$ receptor antagonist), methamphetamine (a releaser of neuronal catecholamines), scopolamine (a muscarinic receptor antagonist), and diphenidol (Takeda et al., 1993b; 1995a;

Morita et al., 1988b). Motion-induced kaolin consumption was unaffected by either domperidone or ondansetron (Takeda et al., 1995a). The efficacy of antagonists of the central histaminergic and cholinergic systems are consistent with studies in animals with an emetic reflex in which these neurotransmitter systems have been implicated in motion-induced emesis. The lack of efficacy of both a D_2 and a 5-HT_3 receptor antagonist is also consistent with the view that kaolin consumption is induced via activation of the same central pathways that activate emesis in susceptible species.

Advantages and Disadvantages of Pica—Summary

Advantages: a natural behavior observed in wild animals; noninvasive; simple to measure kaolin consumption; response is dose-related within a particular stimulus; spontaneous "innate" behavior not requiring any preconditioning of the animal (cf., CTA, below) but can be conditioned; not dependent on recent learning and memory; can be used to study dose-related effects of candidate anti-nausea/emetic agents; may be amenable to a pharmacological "intervention" study when a candidate antiemetic is able to stop emesis after it has started; can be combined with other measures of behavior.

Disadvantages: poor temporal resolution, although potentially this could be improved using automated real-time measurement of kaolin consumption (Yamamoto et al., 2010) provided the time point at which consumption increases above baseline can be identified for an individual animal; may be difficult to apply to species where intake may be small (e.g., mouse); unmeasured spillage may be a source of error especially if relatively small quantities are consumed; a species may have the potential to exhibit pica but does not do so because of a dislike for kaolin; can be induced by stimuli that are not necessarily nauseogenic or emetic such as stress, pain, and arthritis (Burchfield, Elich & Woods, 1977), hence caution in assessing predictive validity; may only occur in a restricted range of laboratory species and not be widespread among species with an emetic reflex; agents blocking pica could be acting via induction of satiety rather than anti-emesis/nausea; pathways involved (e.g., vagal afferent, area postrema) poorly investigated; the pattern of kaolin consumption may be influenced by factors such as concurrent illness unrelated to the genesis of nausea/emesis; fine discrimination between candidate anti-nausea/emetic compounds may not be possible as the maximal intake of kaolin in 24 hours in the rat is about 10g with 3–6g being more usual; involvement of forebrain structures not investigated; arguably weak face validity.

Conditioned Taste Aversion (CTA), Conditioned Food Avoidance (CFA), and Related Phenomena

What Are They?

Pavlov was probably the first to recognize the potential of conditioned responses or reflexes as a tool for studying learning (Pavlov, 1927). Our individual experience provides evidence that we have mechanisms by which we learn to avoid foods that caused "illness" on a previous occasion, and such "adaptive selection" of food would clearly be of evolutionary advantage to both humans and other animals. Garcia and colleagues (Garcia, Kimeldorf & Koelling, 1955; Garcia, Ervin & Koelling, 1966; Garcia & Koelling, 1967) were the first to adapt this learned aversion paradigm to the laboratory, although this phenomenon was reported in chickens in 1887 (Poulton, E.B., cited by Garcia & Hankins, 1977). In essence an animal will learn to become averted to a flavor that was associated with toxicosis on a prior occasion. The phenomenon is often referred to as "conditioned taste aversion" (CTA), although it is argued that "conditioned flavor avoidance" (CFA) or aversion may be a more appropriate term (see below and Andrews & Horn, 2006) because the relative roles of gustation, olfaction, and chemaesthesia to the conditioned stimulus is not usually known. In addition, a distinction should also be drawn between conditioned *aversion* and *avoidance* (Parker, 2003). This is because when there has been a pairing between a novel flavor and a toxin, the consequence is that the animal will *avoid* consumption of that flavor on subsequent exposure; whereas, to ensure that the animal has developed an *aversion*, it is necessary to demonstrate that the animal exhibits rejection reactions (e.g., gaping, chin rubbing, paw treading in rats). The latter can be tested using intra-oral infusions of the flavor previously paired with the toxin; this is called the taste reactivity test (Grill & Norgren, 1978a) (see Figure 8.7).

The term "conditioned food avoidance" (CFA) has also been particularly used (Garcia & Hankins, 1977) in studies where toxicosis and a resulting aversion have been induced by a food, or a toxic stimulus was paired with a particular food, which the animal learns to avoid or to which it becomes averted. All the above are considered to be examples of classical "Pavlovian" conditioning. The literature on this topic is vast and complex and has been the subject of books (e.g., Barker, Best & Domjan, 1977) and extensive reviews (Braveman & Bronstein, 1985) with a database on CTA alone containing 2600 papers in 2004 (Riley & Freeman, 2004). Hence, this review will be selective and will focus on studies in the rat as most research has been undertaken in this species.

Why Might They Be Indicative of Nausea in Animals?

The phenomena of CFA/CTA have been demonstrated with varying degrees of rigor in a diverse range of mammals (see Table 8.1) and birds (Gustavson, 1977) and also in some fish (Gerhart, 1991), arguing that this behavior is of *functional* significance in aiding the survival of an animal. In humans, if nausea is produced following ingestion of a food then a dislike develops, although other consequences of ingestion such as diarrhea, rashes, and respiratory distress can have similar but less potent effects (Pelchat & Rozin, 1982). Taste aversion has been induced in humans using apomorphine, radiation, and chemotherapy (Bernstein, 1978; Cannon et al., 1983; Carrell et al., 1986). A face value comparison of the animal and human studies would suggest that CFA/CTA are indeed indices of nausea (or an analogous sensation) because

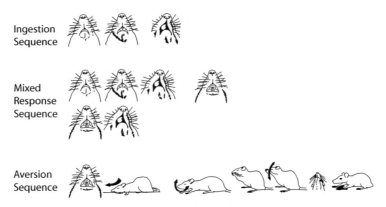

Figure 8.7 Taste reactivity for unpaired and paired stimuli. (Either novel or familiar sucrose, NaCl, and HCl stimuli when presented intraorally elicit an ingestive sequence [top] composed of rhythmic movements of mandible and tongue followed by non-rhythmic lateral tongue protrusion. After a single pairing of familiar NaCl or HCl with LiCl injection, a mixed response pattern [middle] is evoked. The mixed pattern generally adds the gaping component to the ingestion sequence. This mixed pattern is also characteristic of the response elicited by novel 3 X 10^{-15} M quinine HCl. After two pairings of sucrose, NaCl, or HCl with LiCl injection, an aversive sequence is elicited. This sequence [bottom] is generally composed of some set of the following response components: gaping, chin rubbing, head shaking, face washing, forelimb flailing, and paw pushing. This same aversive sequence is elicited by novel quinine HCl in concentrations 3 X 10^{-4} M or greater.) Reproduced with permission from Berridge, Grill, and Norgren, 1981.

their genesis appears in humans to rely heavily on induction of the sensation of nausea. However, this relies on the animal experiencing a sensation analogous to nausea and with the same adaptive significance. These aversive phenomena are of particular interest because in the wild they rely on the animal associating the ingestion of a particular food with an unpleasant consequence, which the animal recalls on a future occasion when that food is presented again. The term "bait shyness" is often used to express the potential protective nature of this learned response (Borison, 1989). A pivotal issue is whether the consequence needs to be an unpleasant conscious sensation (i.e., nausea) or whether the association can be made at a "subconscious" level. It is conceivable that the latter may represent a "primitive" form of the response such as the aversive responses reported in *Drosophila melanogaster* larvae (Wu, Zhao & Shen, 2005), the nematode *C. elegans* (Zhang, Lu & Bargmann, 2005), the gastropod mollusc *Lymnaea stagnalis* (Elliott & Susswein, 2002), and perhaps fish (especially when the development of the cerebral hemispheres is taken into account), whereas in mammals, the subconscious learning may be reinforced and the memory refined by the accompanying conscious sensation. Studies in the sea anemone (*Aiptasia pallida*) showed that while it was capable of regurgitating toxic food it appeared incapable of forming a learned aversion (Lindquist & Hay, 1995).

There is evidence from lesion studies that rats require the cerebral hemispheres (see Chapter 4, in this volume) and in particular the amygdala in order to form a learned taste aversion (Grill & Norgren, 1978b; Nachman & Ashe, 1974), but there is also evidence that the unconditioned stimulus is also effective at producing CTA if it is presented while the animal is under general anesthesia (Grill, 1985).

An additional factor is whether nausea/malaise (especially gastrointestinal) is the only sensation(s) that can lead to the development of a learned avoidance. Although in the wild it is likely that this is the case, in the laboratory it has been possible to design experiments in rats that indicate that "nausea is neither necessary nor sufficient for the establishment of conditioned taste avoidance" (Parker, 2006). For example, taste avoidance can be induced by conditioned fear (Parker, 2003), and by drugs such as amphetamine and cocaine, which have "rewarding" rather than emetic properties. And while the development of conditioned flavor avoidance was unaffected by an antiemetic (5-HT$_3$ receptor antagonist), the learned flavor aversion was blocked by the same treatment (Rudd, Ngan & Wai, 1998; Limebeer & Parker, 2000). However, this may not apply to species with an emetic reflex such as *Suncus murinus* (see below and Parker, 2006). Finally, pairing a novel flavor with a painful cutaneous stimulus failed to induce CTA in the rat, and this observation has been used to argue that for the unconditioned stimulus to induce CTA it must induce an "internally" generated sensation (Garcia et al., 1985). It would be of interest to know if pairing of the novel flavor with a stimulus inducing visceral pain would lead to CTA.

How Are They Measured?

There are a large number of different experimental designs used to induce learned aversions, and only the basic designs used in mammals will be described to illustrate the principles involved. In the simplest form, paradigms involve some baseline period in which the animal becomes adapted to a palatable but novel food or liquid. In the case of the latter, saccharine or sucrose solution is often used and drinking confined to a specific time and duration each day. This novel taste stimulus is the conditioned stimulus (CS). It is important that the CS does not itself induce any behavioral change as it is the avoidance of this stimulus that is the experimental end point. At some point the CS is presented with the stimulus (unconditioned stimulus, US) which will induce nausea/malaise/gastrointestinal illness (the unconditioned reaction, UR). A commonly used US in rats is intraperitoneal injection of lithium chloride, whereas the normal food or liquid will be paired with an injection of saline. At some time period after administration of the US or saline, the animal will be allowed access to the novel food or liquid (the CS) and the amount ingested measured, with a reduction in the amount ingested (the conditioned reaction, CR) by the animals receiving the US being an indication of genesis of

CTA/CFA. Studies can also be undertaken using solid food. For example, in the house musk shrew studies were undertaken using two different flavors of cat food (tuna or chicken) and pairing one with an emetic challenge (lithium chloride, motion exposure, nicotine) and the other with saline or a sham procedure. The induction of a conditioned food avoidance was tested by presenting animals simultaneously with both foods on a later occasion and measuring the amount of each ingested, with a positive CFA being indicated by aversion to the food paired with the emetic challenge (Smith, Friedman & Andrews, 2001). Although all three substances induced CFA, only nicotine and motion induced vomiting, providing further support for the proposal that CFA and CTA do not depend on the induction of vomiting itself.

The basic CTA/CFA technique can be readily adapted to a wide range of species including aquatic invertebrates such as the cuttlefish (*Sepia officinalis*; Darmaillacq et al., 2004), fish, birds, and mammals in the natural habitat, and in the case of the latter adapted as a method for predator control (Gustavson et al., 1974). Irrespective of their relevance to the measurement of nausea, CFA/CTA are a powerful paradigm for the study of learning and memory (Welzl, D'Adamo & Lipp, 2001).

In the previous section the significance of distinguishing between a conditioned aversion and an avoidance was highlighted, and to ensure correct interpretation of CTA/CFA studies it would appear necessary to investigate the rejection responses induced by intra-oral infusion of the flavor paired with the toxin. However, this is rarely done.

Laboratory Species in Which CFA/CTA Has Been Demonstrated and Stimuli for Induction

The vast majority of studies have been performed using the rat, but there is evidence for the induction of learned flavor avoidance (not necessarily aversion) in both species with an emetic reflex including humans and species lacking an emetic reflex such as the mouse and hamster. Table 8.1 summarizes the variety of mammalian species investigated and the stimuli used to induce the CFA. Of particular interest is the diversity of stimuli, which include motion, radiation, anticancer drugs, hormones, and intragastric irritants. Thus, CTA/CFA models do have the potential to be useful in identification of substances likely to have an emetic liability or to have antiemetic potential if experiments are appropriately controlled and results interpreted correctly.

Effects of Anti-Emetic Agents and Nerve Lesions

Pathway Lesions   Researchers studying the pathways involved in CTA/CFA have in general made the assumption that where evidence existed from an emetic species that a particular emetic stimulus acted via a particular pathway, then the same pathway was likely to be involved in the induction of CTA/CFA in a nonemetic species. However, Borison (1989) pointed out that "of the 150 agents listed as inducers of CTA, only 12 are identifiable by the writer as substances that act on the area postrema to induce vomiting." For the rat model

Table 8.1 Summary of Mammalian Species and Stimuli Used to Study Emesis, CFA, and Pica

Species	Stimulus	Emesis	CFA	Pica
Cat	Cytotoxic drugs:	Cisplatin (McCarthy & Borison, **1984**) Cyclophosphamide (Fetting et al., **1982b**)		
	Intragastric irritants:	Copper sulfate (Kayashima & Hyama, **1976**)		
	Motion	(Crampton & Daunton, **1983**)	(Fox, Corcoran & Brizzee, **1990**)	
	Apomorphine	(Costello & Borison, **1977**)		
	Morphine	(Villablanca et al., **1984**)		
	Radiation	(Rabin et al., **1986b**)	(Rabin et al., **1986b**)	
	Nicotine	(Beleslin et al., **1981**)		
	Hormones and neurotransmitters:		Angiotensin II (Rabin et al., **1986a**)	
	Other:		Amphetamine (Rabin & Hunt, **1992**)	
Dog	Cytotoxic drugs:	Cisplatin (Gylys, Doran & Buyniski, **1979**) Cyclophosphamide (Amber et al., **1990**)		
	Intragastric irritants:	Ipecac (Gardner et al., **1996**) Copper sulfate (Kayashima & Hayama, **1975**)	LiCl (Vavilova & Kassil, **1984**)	
	Apomorphine	(Harrison, Lipe & Decker, **1972**)		
	Morphine	(Lefebvre, Willems & Bogaert, **1981**)		
	Radiation	(Cooper & Mattsson, **1979**)		
	Nicotine	(Vig, **1990**)		
	Hormones and neurotransmitters:	CCK (Levine et al., **1984**) Vasopressin (Wu et al., **1985**) Peptide YY (Smith et al., **1989**)		

Species	Stimulus		
Ferret	Cytotoxic drugs:	Cisplatin, cyclophosphamide (Andrews et al., 1990a)	LiCl (Rabin & Hunt, 1992)
	Intragastric irritants:	Copper sulfate, ipecac, NaCl, KCl (Andrews et al., 1990a)	
	Apomorphine	(Andrews et al., 1990a)	
	Morphine	(Barnes et al., 1991)	
	Radiation	(Andrews et al., 1990a)	
Guinea pig	Intragastric irritants:		LiCl (Braveman, 1974)
Hamster	Cytotoxic drugs:		Cyclophosphamide (Hobbs, Clingerman & Elkins, 1976)
	Intragastric irritants:		LiCl (Fox, 1977)
	Apomorphine		(Nowlis, Frank & Pfaffmann, 1980)
	Nicotine		(Etscorn et al., 1986)
	Other:		2-deoxy-D-glucose (Dibattista, 1988)
Human	Cytotoxic drugs:	Chemotherapy (Rudd & Andrews, 2005)	Chemotherapy (Schwartz, Jacobsen & Bovbjerg, 1996)
	Intragastric irritants:	Ipecac (Jackson & Smith, 1978) Copper sulfate (Liu et al., 2001)	Ipecac (Jackson & Smith, 1978)
	Motion	(Yates, Miller & Lucot, 1998)	(Arwas, Rolnick & Lubow, 1989)
	Apomorphine	(Schofferman, 1976)	
	Morphine	(Bailey et al., 1993)	
	Radiation	(Cordts, Yochmowitz & Hardy, 1987)	(Carrell et al., 1986)

(continued)

Table **8.1** (continued)

Species	Stimulus	Emesis	CFA	Pica
	Hormones and neurotransmitters:	CCK (Miaskiewicz, Stricker & Verbalis, 1989)		
	Other:	Pregnancy (Weigel & Weigel, 1989) Reduced intracranial pressure (Mokri, 2004)	Pregnancy (Bayley et al., 2002)	Pregnancy (Corbett, Ryan & Weinrich, 2003; Lopez, Ortega Soler & de Portela, 2004) Gastric bypass surgery (Kushner, Gleason & Shanta-Retelny, 2004)
Monkey	Cytotoxic drugs:	Cisplatin (Fukui et al., 1993)	Cyclophosphamide (Hikami, Hasegawa & Matsuzawa, 1990) LiCl (Bergman & Glowa, 1986) (Wilpizeski et al., 1987)	
	Intragastric irritants:	Copper sulfate (Fukui et al., 1993)		
	Motion	(Wilpizeski et al., 1987)		
	Radiation	(Brizzee, 1956)		
	Nicotine	(Spealman, 1983)		
	Hormones and neurotransmitters:	CCK (Perera et al., 1993)		
Mouse	Cytotoxic drugs:			Cisplatin (Yamamoto et al., 2002)
	Intragastric irritants:		LiCl (Risinger & Cunningham, 2000)	

Animal	Stimulus		
Quoll	Motion		*(Santucci et al., 2002)*
	Radiation	*(Kinney, Wright & Harding, 1993)*	
	Nicotine	*(Kimeldorf, Garcia & Rubadeau, 1960)*	
	Other:	*(Etscorn, 1980)*	
		Magnetic field (Lockwood et al, 2003)	
		Thiabendazole (O'Donnell, Webb & Shine, 2010)	
Rat	Cytotoxic drugs:	*Cisplatin (Rudd, Ngan & Wai, 1998)*	*Cisplatin (Takeda et al., 1993a)*
		Cyclophosphamide (Ader, 1976)	
	Intragastric irritants:	*Ipecac (Rudd, Ngan &Wai, 1998)*	*LiCl, Copper sulfate (Hasegawa et al., 1992)*
		Copper sulfate (Coil et al., 1978)	
		LiCl (Coil et al., 1978)	
	Motion	*(Hutchison Jr, 1973)*	*(Mitchell, Laycock & Stephens, 1977)*
	Apomorphine	*(Krane, Sinnamon & Thomas, 1976)*	*(Hasegawa et al., 1992)*
	Morphine		*(Aung et al., 2004)*
	Radiation	*(Garcia, Kimeldorf & Koelling, 1955)*	*(Yamamoto, Takeda & Yamatodani. 2002)*
	Nicotine	*(Etscorn et al., 1987)*	

(continued)

Table 8.1 (continued)

Species	Stimulus	Emesis	CFA	Pica
	Hormones and neurotransmitters:		NPY (Sipols et al., 1992) CCK (Ervin et al., 1995)	NPY (Woods et al., 1998) CCK (McCutcheon, Ballard & McCaffrey, 1992)
	Other:		Fat oxidation inhibitors (Singer et al., 1999) 2-deoxy-D-glucose (Stephan, Smith & Fisher, 1999) Magnetic field (Houpt et al., 2003)	2-deoxy-D-glucose (Watson et al., 1987) Rolipram, roflumilast, cilomilast, EPPA-1 (Davis et al., 2009)
House Musk Shrew (Suncus murinus)	Cytotoxic drugs:	Cisplatin, cyclophosphamide (Matsuki et al., 1988)		
	Intragastric irritants:	Copper sulfate, ipecac (Ueno, Matsuki & Saito, 1987) LiCl (Parker et al., 2004)	LiCl (Smith, Friedman & Andrews, 2001)	
	Motion	(Ueno, Matsuki & Saito, 1988)	(Smith, Friedman & Andrews, 2001)	
	Radiation	(Torii et al., 1993)		
	Nicotine	(Ueno, Matsuki & Saito, 1987)	(Smith, Friedman & Andrews, 2001)	
	Hormones and neurotransmitters:	Vasopressin (Ikegaya & Matsuki, 2002)		

Modified and used with permission from Andrews and Horn, 2006.

of CTA/CFA to have utility for identification of anti-nausea/emetic drugs, it is important to know which pathways are involved in the response to which stimulus and thus studies have investigated the effects of either area postrema or abdominal innervation on the induction of CTA. With regard to the area postrema there are consistent data that a normal response to systemic lithium chloride requires an intact area postrema, and there is also evidence implicating the area postrema in the response to systemic copper sulfate and xylazine (see Grant, 1987, for refs. and review; Fox, 1992). Interestingly, both apomorphine and morphine, which are known to induce emesis via the area postrema, induce CTAs by an action either independent of the area postrema or not entirely dependent on the area postrema (Rausschenburger, 1979, cited in Borison, 1989; Blair & Amit, 1981; van der Kooy, Swerdlow & Koob, 1983). Evidence for an involvement of the abdominal visceral innervation (vagus and splanchnic nerves) in CTA produced by intragastric copper sulfate is equivocal, although there is clear evidence for involvement in emesis (see Grant, 1987). It should be noted that recent studies of CTA have focused on the use of pharmacological agents to attempt to block the response and have not reinvestigated the involvement of pathways known to be involved in emesis in other species. Furthermore, the influence of lesions on induction of CTA/CFA has not been investigated in studies where a taste reactivity test has also been investigated to study the rejection reaction and thus establish a clearer distinction to be drawn between *aversion* and *avoidance*. In addition, the analysis is confounded by comparison with emetic species as even between such species (e.g., cat and ferret) there are reported differences in the relative roles of the vagus and area postrema in mediating the emetic response to stimuli such as radiation. CFA has been demonstrated in the dog, cat, ferret, and *Suncus*, all species with a clear emetic response. It can be argued that there is a need to study the effect of area postrema ablation and peripheral nerve lesions on the development of CTA/CFA, oral rejection responses, and induction of the emetic response in the same species to identify to what extent emetic pathways are involved in both phenomena.

Pharmacological Agents   The above discussion highlights a number of issues that may confound the interpretation of the results from CTA/CFA studies (especially in the rat) and which need to be borne in mind when considering whether such studies may predict an anti-nausea/emetic effect of a particular drug or indeed predict whether a substance is likely to induce nausea/emesis in another species including humans. In addition to the issues related to the interpretation of the experimental design, the results obtained using pharmacological agents also need careful interpretation to ensure that differences between blockade of the input pathway, the central integrative emetic mechanisms, and the mechanisms involved in the establishment and subsequent expression of the learned aversion can be identified. This section reviews some of the studies that have used CTA/CFA as a model to investigate pharmacological and other interventions for their potential to treat nausea/emesis.

However, as will become apparent, there is a weight of evidence that drugs that have efficacy against either nausea or emesis in humans and/or animals do not have an effect on either the expression of, or establishment of, conditioned taste avoidance learning in rats (Parker, 2006). This section does not deal with agents such as GLP-1 receptor antagonists, which when injected intracerberoventricularly block lithium chloride–induced conditioned taste aversion in the rat (Seeley et al., 2000). At present there are no data on the anti-nausea/emesis effects in models of emesis. GLP-1 receptor antagonists could have considerable anti-nausea/emesis potential if suitable small-molecule antagonists can be identified, as in the above study the GLP-1 receptor antagonist also blocked the pica and reduced food intake induced by lithium chloride.

Dopamine Receptor Antagonists   Dopamine D_2 receptors and the area postrema have been implicated in apomorphine-induced emesis in humans, ferrets, and dogs (Yoshikawa, Yoshida & Oka, 2001). However, in the rat apomorphine-induced CTA is neither abolished by area postrema ablation nor by the D_2 receptor antagonist domperidone, which does block the emetic response to apomorphine (Pratt & Stolerman, 1984). Apomorphine-induced CTA was blocked by the dopamine antagonist pimozide indicating an involvement of dopamine receptors although not those involved in the emetic response. The site at which pimozide is acting has not been determined. It appears unlikely that apomorphine-induced CTA provides a useful model in which to investigate the role of D_2 receptors in either nausea or emesis; however, studies in the ferret have implicated D_3 but not D_4 receptors in the emetic pathway (Yoshikawa, Yoshida & Oka, 2001; Osinski et al., 2005) and the involvement (if any) of these receptors in CTA needs investigation.

5-Hydroxytryptamine$_3$ Receptor Antagonists   5-HT$_3$ receptor antagonists such as ondansetron (GR38032F) can block the acute emetic response to both the anticancer agent cisplatin and radiation in the ferret and reduce vomiting induced by the same stimuli in humans (see Rudd & Andrews, 2005 for refs.). In the rat ondansetron failed to affect the CTA response to cisplatin, lithium chloride, and ipecacuanha (Rudd, Ngan & Wai, 1998; Mele et al., 1992), although it did block the response to an amino-acid imbalanced diet, amphetamine, and apomorphine (Terry-Nathan, Gietzen & Rogers, 1995; McAllister & Pratt, 1998). The latter is of note because ondansetron does not block the emetic response to apomorphine in the ferret.

   Although ondansetron did not affect either the establishment or expression of the conditioned taste *avoidance* induced by lithium chloride, it does reduce both the establishment and expression of the conditioned aversive responses to lithium chloride assessed using the taste reactivity test (Limebeer & Parker, 2000). The disgust reaction to quinine was unaffected by ondansetron indicating that this effect was not due to a change in palatability of the conditioning stimulus flavor although this is potentially an issue with 5-HT$_3$ receptor antagonists, as serotonin has a role in taste bud signaling in rats and both 5-HT$_3$ and 5-HT$_{1A}$ receptors have been implicated (Kaya et al., 2004). A dissociation between conditioned aversion and avoidance has also been reported using a 5-HT$_{1A}$ receptor agonist, an observation of particular interest as such agonists have antiemetic effects in several animal models (e.g., Sanger & Andrews, 2006).

Neurokinin$_1$ Receptor Antagonists   The NK$_1$ receptor antagonist GR205171 has broad-spectrum antiemetic activity in the ferret (Gardner et al., 1996), and in contrast to ondansetron is capable of blocking apomorphine-induced emesis although having no affinity for dopamine receptors. GR205171 prevented the conditioned "aversion" to both apomorphine and amphetamine in the rat, although it must be noted that taste reactivity tests were not carried out (McAllister & Pratt, 1998). It should be noted that GR205171 has a relatively high affinity for the rat, ferret, and human NK$_1$ receptor, whereas other NK$_1$ receptor antagonists (e.g., CP-99,994, L-741671) have a high affinity for ferret and human receptors but 50- to 100-fold lower affinity for the rodent receptor (see Table 8.2 from Andrews & Rudd, 2004, for details). It is essential to take the species differences in compound affinities into account when interpreting results; if a compound other than GR205171 has been used it is conceivable that no effect would have been observed.

Cannabinoids Δ^9-Tetrahydrocannabinol (THC) attenuated the taste "aversion" induced by the anticancer agent cyclophosphamide in mice (Landauer, Balster & Harris, 1985) although not in rats (Revusky & Martin, 1988); but more recently, Limebeer and Parker (1999) showed that it also blocked the expression of "disgust reactions" (using the taste reactivity test) induced in the rat by cyclophosphamide. In addition, cannabidiol (a nonpsychoactive constituent of cannabis) affected both the establishment and expression of a conditioned disgust response to lithium chloride (Parker, Mechoulam & Schlievert, 2002), and a selective cannabinoid$_1$ (CB$_1$) receptor antagonist enhanced the conditioned disgust response to lithium chloride (Parker et al., 2003; Parker & Mechoulam, 2003). The latter observations are of particular interest as selective CB$_1$ receptor agonists have antiemetic effects in the ferret and *Suncus* (e.g., Van Sickle et al., 2001; Parker et al., 2004) and CB$_1$ receptor antagonists can facilitate the emetic response to an opioid (Van Sickle et al., 2001). The effects of the CB$_1$ antagonists in both rat and ferret implicate endogenous cannabinoids in the modulation of nausea.

Glucocorticoids   The synthetic glucocorticoid dexamethasone attenuated the taste aversion produced by a range of cytotoxic drugs including cisplatin and cyclophosphamide, radiation, copper sulfate, and lithium chloride in the rat (Revusky & Martin, 1988).While these studies are consistent with evidence for antiemetic effects of dexamethasone, the results must be interpreted with caution until comparable conditioned disgust/taste reactivity test studies are performed.

Table 8.2 Species Differences in the Pharmacology of Tachykinin NK$_1$ Receptors

Compound	NK$_1$ receptor affinity (nM)				
	Human	Ferret	Rat	Cat	Suncus murinus
CP99994	0.3[a]	1.7[a]	111[a]	0.5[b]	12.0[c]
CJ11974	0.2[d]	0.6[d]			
RP67580	56[a]	111[a]	3[a]		>1,000[e]
GR205171	0.03[f]	0.16[f]	0.32[f]		
GR203040	~0.04[g]	0.08[g]	2.5[g]		
L741671	0.03[a]	0.7[a]	64[a]		
L743310	0.06[a]	0.1[a]	17[a]		
L758298	2.8[h]	1.1[h]	33[h]		
L754030	0.1[h]	0.7[h]	4[h]		
PD154075	0.84[i]	3.4[i]	302[i]		
R116301	0.45[j]	8.3[j]	98[j]		

[a] K_i values against [^{125}I]-labelled Tyr^8-substance P (Tattersall et al. 1996)

[b] IC$_{50}$ values against [^{3}H]-substance P (Lucot et al. 1997)

[c] IC$_{50}$ value (Tattersall et al. 1995)

[d] K_i values against [^{3}H]-substance P (Tsuchiya et al. 2002)

[e] K_i values (Tattersall et al. 1995)

[f] K_i values [^{3}H]-substance P (Gardener et al. 1996)

[g] K_i values [^{3}H]-substance P (Beattie et al. 1995)

[h] IC$_{50}$ values against [^{125}I]-labelled substance P (Tattersall et al. 2000)

[i] IC$_{50}$ values against [^{125}I]Bolton-Hunter Substance P (Singh et al. 1997)

[j] K_i values against [^{3}H]-substance P (Megens et al. 2002)

Used with permission from Andrews and Rudd, 2004.

Advantages and Disadvantages of CTA/CFA—Summary

Advantages: mimics a natural learned behavior with a clear functional significance; occurs in a range of vertebrates and may occur in some invertebrates; occurs in animals with and without an emetic reflex; mimics a behavior that occurs in humans and is associated with the presence of nausea; can be induced by a single exposure to the toxin; gradation of response is possible by measurement of volume of liquid or weight of food ingested, but in essence an aversion is either present or not; potentially good face, construct, and predictive validity provided an aversion is demonstrated and not just avoidance.

Disadvantages: requires careful experimental design to distinguish between learned aversions and avoidance; should be combined with taste reactivity test to aid interpretation; appetitive and consummatory responses may confound interpretation; may be different between species with and without an emetic reflex; poor time resolution; results may depend on the exact paradigm used; potential antiemetic drugs tested in this model should be devoid of amnesic or psychotropic effects that could interfere with learning and memory; can be induced (in rats) by a range of psychoactive compounds some of which may be rewarding but do not induce nausea and vomiting in other species and some of which (e.g., scopolamine, benzodiazepines, tetrahydrocannabinol) are themselves antiemetic in other species; numerous factors may confound interpretation so considerable care is needed in design of control, especially when potential antiemetic agents are used; variable predictive value of antiemetic activity of drugs for use in humans.

Context Aversion Conditioning

What Is It?

This technique was developed to provide a model for the anticipatory nausea and vomiting (ANV) associated with anticancer chemotherapy. ANV is the nausea and vomiting triggered by the sights, smells, and sounds associated with chemotherapy, including the place where it was administered, and may be induced by stimuli such as the arrival of the appointment card for the next cycle of therapy, the sight of the oncologist including outside of the hospital, and the smell of the floor cleaner used in the oncology ward (Stockhorst, Klosterhalfen & Steingrüber, 1998). It is a form of a classically conditioned (aversive) response (Morrow et al., 2002b). It is related to the protective phenomena of CTA/CFA, as it would help an animal to avoid situations that in the past have made it ill, although in the wild illness would usually have been associated with the ingestion of a toxin rather than its intravenous administration (with the exception of snake bites!) as is usually the case for chemotherapy. In the case of context aversion conditioning the administration of an agent such as lithium chloride inducing illness (presumed to be nausea) is paired with transient exposure of the animal to a novel environment (Hall & Symonds, 2006). On subsequent exposure to this environment in the absence of further administration of the illness-inducing agent the animal will exhibit responses as if it had been given the agent.

Why Might It Be Indicative of Nausea?

The primary reason for assuming that the paradigm used in animals closely mimics the clinical experience is that it arguably reflects the human experience of nausea and perhaps facial expressions of disgust (e.g., tongue protrusion) associated with the sight or smell of a food that has previously caused nausea. In addition, context aversion conditioning in animals is affected by the behavioral interventions of "overshadowing" and "latent inhibition," which have some beneficial effects against ANV in humans (Symonds & Hall, 1999; Stockhorst et al., 1998; Klosterhalfen et al., 2005b; Hall & Symonds, 2006).

How Is It Measured?

Rodriguez et al. (2000) describe a detailed protocol for use with rats. In essence rats are adapted to the scheduled consumption of a sucrose solution and following pairing of exposure to one of two novel types of cage with administration of either saline or lithium chloride (note that the lithium chloride is not injected when they are in the novel environment but prior to placement) animals are returned to their home cage. The conditioning procedure is repeated over several days, and on the test day the consumption of sucrose is measured when the animals are placed in one of the novel cages. In the case of the cage where placement was preceded by injection of lithium chloride, consumption was reduced in comparison to animals given saline and exposed to the same environment. In a subsequent study Hall and Symonds (2006) showed that animals subjected to the context aversion procedure described above would gape (an oral behavior arguably indicative of nausea; see below and also section on CTA/CFA above) when saccharine was infused orally, providing further support for development of conditioned *aversion* rather than *avoidance*.

Other types of conditioned responses are described in the next section, but there appear to be no studies of other species or other stimuli using the paradigm described by Rodriguez et al. (2000). The emetic stimuli cisplatin, cyclophosphamide, and nicotine have been shown to induce place aversion as have lithium chloride, fenfluramine, and morphine withdrawal (see Parker & Joshi, 1998; Parker, 1998, 2003) although morphine itself, which can be emetic, does not. These studies indicate that animals will avoid a place (context) where they experienced an illness or unpleasant experience, but interpretation is partially confounded by the administration of the stimulus in the novel environment rather than prior to exposure as in the Rodriguez et al. (2000) study.

The involvement of the emetic pathways in context aversion conditioning has not been investigated using lesions, although the 5-HT$_3$ receptor antagonist ondansetron has been shown to attenuate the response (Symonds & Hall, 2000).

Advantages and Disadvantages of Context Aversion
Conditioning—Summary

Advantages: design approximates the clinical experience so potentially good face validity; relies on the recollection of an unpleasant experience by the animal and may mimic a natural behavior; susceptible to behavioral interventions effective in humans.

Disadvantages: requires a relatively complex conditioning procedure; poor temporal resolution; demonstration may be highly dependent on the experimental design; relatively little literature and information on pathways involved and their susceptibility to antiemetic agents used in humans.

Conditioned Gaping and Retching

What Is It and Why Might It Be Indicative of Nausea?

Conditioned gaping and retching is similar in some respects to both the conditioned taste aversion and conditioned place aversion responses discussed above, except that here the measure is a specific behavior, either gaping or occasionally retching (see Table 8.1 for a summary). Two types of conditioned responses are reported. The first type is a conditioned "emetic" response manifest as retching/vomiting (*Suncus*, coyote, wolf, blue jay, hawk) and accompanied by other behaviors such as gaping in *Suncus* or paw-shaking in the cat (Gustavson, 1977) when an animal is presented with a food that previously induced illness or was paired with a stimulus that induced illness. In addition, in the ferret, *Suncus*, chicken, and pigeon, emetic responses can be induced by returning the animal to a location where emesis or toxicosis had previously been induced (Riddle & Burns, 1931; Davey & Biederman, 1998; Parker & Kemp, 2001). And in the dog, Kyrlov, working in Pavlov's laboratory, observed that nausea (the term used by Kyrlov), secretion of saliva, and vomiting could all be induced by the "preliminaries of injection" after morphine was given over five or six days and in some cases could be induced by "seeing the experimenter" (Pavlov, 1927, p. 35).

The second type is reported in the rat and is a conditioned rejection reaction induced when an animal is given a flavor intra-orally some time after that flavor has been paired with a substance inducing illness (presumed to be nausea; e.g., Parker, Rana & Limebeer, 2008). Rejection reactions in the rat include paw treading, chin rubbing, tongue protrusion, and gaping, with the latter considered to be the most reliable (Parker, 2003; Parker & Limebeer, 2006; Parker & Mechoulam, 2003) (see Table 8.3). An electromyographic study investigating the patterns of activity in the pharyngeal muscles seen following intra-oral administration of either sucrose or quinine in the rat concluded that, "although rats do not have the capacity for a complete emetic action, the gape appears as an abbreviated version of this reflex at the buccal level" (Travers & Norgren, 1986). The pattern of muscular activity in the gape prevents the liquid being swallowed and also leads to its propulsion from the back to the front of the oral cavity from where it exits the body. It would be interesting to compare the activity in the oropharyngeal musculature during the gape, with that occurring during a gag, which also occurs in the rat. It is worth noting that in contrast to the rat, intra-oral quinine in the mouse is reported to evoke chin rubbing and reduction in licking with few gapes occurring (Travers & Travers, 2005).

These two types of conditioned response are thought to provide models of nausea largely because in similar settings humans show arguably comparable responses. For example, humans presented with a food that previously made them ill may show signs of disgust, push food away, exhibit tongue protrusion, and even gag. Although yawning may be associated with nausea (see Chapter 5, in this volume), gaping is not reported in humans. However, it remains an assumption that the sensory experience in the animal is the same as nausea in humans. This proposal is supported by the effect of antiemetics on these responses, with the majority of studies being in the rat and *Suncus*.

In the rat conditioned gaping is induced by emetic stimuli such as lithium chloride, cisplatin, cyclophosphamide, nicotine, apomorphine, fluoxetine, and

**Table 8.3 Definition of Disgust, Neutral, and Hedonic Reactions During
Intraoral Infusion of a Flavor**

Type of Response	Description
Disgust reactions	
Gape (g)	Rapid, large-amplitude opening of the mandible with retraction of the comers of the mouth
Chin rub(c)	Mouth or chin in direct contact with the floor or wall of the chamber and body projecting forward
Paw tread (pt)	Extension of one forepaw against floor or wall of chamber while other forepaw is retracting
Neutral reaction	
Passive drips (pd)	Solution passively falling from mouth
Hedonic reactions	
Mouth movement (mm)	Lower mandible movements without opening mouth
Tongue protrusion (tp)	Extending tongue out of the mouth
Paw lick(pl)	Licking flavoured solution from forepaws

Used with permission from Rana and Parker, 2008.

motion, all stimuli that evoke conditioned taste avoidance or conditioned place/context aversion (Parker & Limebeer, 2006; Parker, 2006; Limebeer, Litt & Parker, 2009; Rodriguez et al., 2000; Parker, Rana & Limebeer, 2008). Conditioned gaping to both intra-oral sucrose and to a novel context can also be induced by rolipram, a phosphodiesterase₄ inhibitor known to be capable of emesis induction in other species including humans (Rock et al., 2009). Using lithium chloride as a stimulus in the rat, it has been shown that ondansetron and palonosetron, 8-OH-DPAT (a 5-HT$_{1A}$ receptor agonist with antiemetic properties; see Sanger & Andrews, 2006 for refs.), and the cannabinoid receptor agonists Δ^9–THC and cannabidiol all affected the establishment and expression of conditioned gaping (Limebeer & Parker, 1999, 2000, 2003; Parker & Mechoulam, 2003; Limebeer, Litt & Parker, 2009). Conditioned taste avoidance was unaffected by these treatments, providing further support to the proposal by Parker and Limebeer (2006) that in the rat conditioned gaping may be a more selective measure of nausea than conditioned taste avoidance. For example, Parker, Rana, and Limebeer (2008) argue that conditioned taste avoidance is more likely to be a consequence of conditioned fear, whereas the conditioned disgust reactions (including gaping) are a result of conditioned nausea. The acquisition of lithium chloride–induced conditioned gaping is also reduced by lipopolysaccharide treatment (Chan et al., 2009).

In *Suncus*, using the conditioned retching/gaping reaction argued to be a model of ANV, Parker and Kemp (2001) demonstrated that Δ^9-THC blocked the expression of these behaviors without an effect on overall locomotor activity. This observation is consistent with other studies in which effects of cannabinoids against both vomiting and "nausea" have been reported (Van Sickle et al., 2001; 2003; Parker, Limebeer & Kwiatkowska, 2005).

Advantages and Disadvantages of Conditioned Gaping
and Retching—Summary

Advantages: design approximates the clinical experience, so potentially good face validity; relies on the recollection of an unpleasant experience by the animal and may mimic a natural behavior although it is difficult to see the survival advantage of actually vomiting resulting in loss of nutrition; susceptible to pharmacological treatments with antiemetic activity in animal models; required the presence of forebrain structures.

Disadvantages: requires a relatively complex conditioning procedure; poor temporal resolution; demonstration may be highly dependent on the experimental design; relatively little literature currently; relative paucity of information about pathways from lesion studies but see Rana and Parker (2008) and Chapter 4 in this volume.

Reduced Spontaneous Food Intake and Delayed Gastric Emptying

What Is It and Why Might It Be Indicative of Nausea?

The presence of nausea is accompanied by a reduced desire for food (appetite), loathing of food, and if feeding is ongoing when nausea begins, a progressive reduction of intake. Thus, a reduction of food intake in the context of an abnormal Behavioral Satiety Sequence (BSS; Halford, Wanninayake & Blundell, 1998) could arguably be used as a marker for the onset of nausea. In addition, nausea (and a reduction of food intake) is often associated with a delay in gastric emptying and gastric stasis although the interrelationships are unclear. A delay in gastric emptying is considered to be one of the early reflex responses to the recognition of an ingested toxin in species with and without an emetic reflex. For example, in the rat intragastric administration of solutions (e.g., hypertonic sodium and potassium chloride, copper sulfate), which would cause emesis in other species, results in a profound delay in gastric emptying (Andrews & Horn, 2006). In emetic species this delay in gastric emptying is proposed to confine any toxin to the stomach until such time as it can be ejected by vomiting while the retrograde giant contraction (RGC) serves to return already emptied contaminated material to the stomach for ejection by vomiting (Lang, 1990; see Chapter 5, in this volume). Although there are multiple confounding factors that make interpretation of measurements of food intake and gastric emptying difficult to ascribe to induction of nausea by a particular stimulus, they are discussed here, as they both provide a useful adjunct that aids in the interpretation of other measurements and in addition are readily applicable to human volunteer studies in a way that some others (e.g., pica, CTA) are not. In addition, in studies of CTA/CFA neither the impact of the conditioning stimulus nor the putative antiemetic effect on food intake and gastric motility are often taken into account when interpreting the results.

A final justification for considering reduced food intake as an indicator of nausea (or gastrointestinal malaise) comes from studies of herbivorous species, rats (Freeland & Janzen, 1974), koala bears (Garcia, Hankins & Coil, 1976), sheep (Aldrich et al., 1993), and brushtail and ringtail possums (Lawler et al., 1998), which ingest potentially toxic plant metabolites with their diet. Ingestion must be balanced to ensure adequate nutrition while keeping toxic metabolites to an "acceptable" level. It has been argued that this balance is maintained via the induction of an aversive response to further ingestion perhaps mediated via induction of "nausea" and there is some evidence from detailed studies in possums using a 5-HT$_3$ receptor antagonist to support this proposal (Lawler et al., 1998). Thus "nausea" may be involved in normal regulation of food intake, although of course in this context it does not induce an aversion to the food that forms an essential part of the diet but does lead to a temporary avoidance. This type of response could be involved in seasonal switching of diets to avoid times when certain foods contain a higher level of toxic metabolites (e.g., mantled howling monkey; Glander, 1994).

How Is It Measured?

Food intake can be measured either over a 24-hour or shorter period by direct weighing of the hopper, by an automated method (especially in rodents) so that the pattern of food and water intake can be determined, or by either method in animals trained to eat food in a single meal at a fixed time of day. Any of these methods could be combined with measurement of activity using infrared arrays or video-tracking and also it may be possible to video orofacial reactions during feeding. An insight into gastric emptying can be gained by postmortem analysis of wet and dry weight of gastric contents especially if combined with measurement of food intake (Liu et al., 2006) but this only provides a single time point, and imaging (e.g., Hultin, Lindsrom & Lehmann, 2005) and radio-labeling techniques are likely to provide more useful information in the future. In species such as the rat, which lack a vomiting reflex, gas accumulation has also been noted in the stomach following the emetic cytotoxic agent cisplatin leading to the suggestion that rats may also lack the "belch" (eructation) reflex (Malik et al., 2007). The gas accumulation was measured by a buoyancy test, but imaging and radio-labeling studies would also provide information. In humans, gastric gas accumulation is associated with dyspeptic symptoms including nausea.

In rats gastric distension in the noxious range is associated with dorsoflexion of the head, and this can be quantified by recording the electromyogram (EMG) of the neck muscles (Rouzade, Fioramonti & Bueno, 1998). This technique could be adapted to provide an insight into the sensation associated with the gastric stasis induced by cisplatin.

Species in Which It Has Been Demonstrated and Stimuli for Induction

For simplicity this section will be confined to the more commonly studied emetic agents and laboratory species.

Cisplatin and Other Cytotoxic Drugs   In the rat cisplatin induces a dose-related reduction in food intake measured over the first 24 hours after administration (Yamamoto et al., 2004; Liu et al., 2005). A reduction in food intake was also seen in the mouse and *Suncus*, although the latter is less sensitive than either the rat or mouse to cisplatin in this assay, requiring >20 mg/kg in contrast to the 1–6 mg/kg required in the rat (Yamamoto et al., 2004; Liu et al., 2005). In addition, in *Suncus* other "emetic" stimuli such as nicotine, copper sulfate, and lithium chloride failed to reduce food intake over a 24-hour period (Yamamoto et al., 2004) although this measurement period may have masked a short duration suppression followed by a period of compensatory hyperphagia. With a single "high" dose of cisplatin, in the rat the reduction in food intake reaches a nadir at 2 to 3 days and recovers over the subsequent 7 to 10 days (Malik et al., 2006; De Jonghe et al., 2009) (see Figure 8.4 above). Water intake does not follow the changes in food intake probably because of the secondary toxic effects on renal function of cisplatin in the rat. Studies using transplatin failed to show any effect on food intake in the rat.

Yamamoto et al., (2007) investigated other cytotoxic anticancer drugs in addition to cisplatin for their effects on food intake. Cyclophosphamide and actinomycin D both produced a dose-related reduction in food intake in the first 24 hours following administration, but in the case of cyclophosphamide food intake recovered to control levels by 3 days. With the higher dose of actinomycin, food intake continued to decline over 3 days. Higher doses of 5-FU and vincristine failed to produce a significant reduction in food intake, although in both cases an effect may have been obscured by the high variability of the consumption. This study also investigated kaolin consumption and as a result the authors concluded that while pica was related to the emetic potential of the agents the effect on food intake was not. This needs to be confirmed by studies using a wider range of substances and also investigating the relationship between kaolin intake and food consumption for each stimulus to see if they are correlated and hence potentially subject to the same controlling factor. Although gastric distension in mice (see Figure 8.8) induced by cisplatin administration was originally reported as a result of a "fortuitous" observation by an alert technician (Bradner & Schurig, 1981) and was also demonstrated in rats (Broomhead, Fairlie & Whitehouse, 1980; Roos, Fairlie & Whitehouse, 1981), very few recent studies measure the weight of gastric contents despite the fact that at the end of the study period cisplatin-treated animals are culled in all studies. The increase in the weight of gastric contents (both wet and dry) is dose related and marked by 24 hours after cisplatin, with increases of almost 400% being reported at the highest doses (9 mg/kg i.p.; Rubio-Pérez et al., 1992). Longer-term studies indicate that the weight may increase further reaching ~ 600% at 4 to 5 days before beginning to resolve (Aggarwal et al., 1994). Despite this degree of distension, it should be recalled that animals will also be eating food and may also be ingesting kaolin if available (Malik et al., 2007). The delay in gastric emptying is reported to begin within 6 hours of administration, but this needs to be investigated

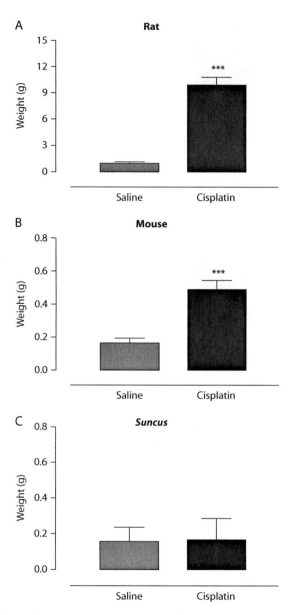

Figure 8.8 Wet weight of stomach contents at 48 h post–cisplatin treatment in A. rats (6 mg/kg; i.p.), B. mice (6 mg/kg; i.p.) and C. *Suncus* (20 mg/kg; i.p.). Results are mean ± S.E.M; $n = 6$ for rats and mice; $n = 8$–10 for *Suncus* (10 saline-treated and 8 cisplatin-treated with emesis). ***$P < 0.001$ vs. Saline-treated group. Reproduced with permission from Liu et al., 2005.

using more modern techniques as it may be possible to investigate the temporal relationship between induction of CTA/CFA, kaolin consumption, reduction of food intake, and the onset of delayed gastric emptying. For example, using radiological methods Cabezos et al. (2008) measured the changes in gastric emptying rate and intestinal transit for 3 days following two different doses of cisplatin (3 and 6 mg/kg i.p.; see Figure 8.9). The marked delay in gastric emptying observed over the first few days following cisplatin (especially at higher doses) resolves spontaneously if the animals are allowed to recover. No increased weight of gastric contents was seen at 7 days following a 6 mg/kg i.p. dose of cisplatin (Malik et al., 2008) although at 2 days the weight of gastric contents had increased from 2.32 ± 0.3g to 9.04 ± 0.8g (Malik et al., 2006).

While an increase in the weight of gastric contents following cisplatin has been reported in mouse and rat, this was not the case in *Suncus* (Liu et al., 2005; see Figure 8.8).

Other Stimuli   Among other stimuli with emetic potential that decrease "acute" food intake in the rat are cholecystokinin (McCann, Verbalis & Stricker, 1989), lithium chloride (Curtis et al., 1994, although see also Yamamoto et al., 2004, who failed to demonstrate an effect using a different protocol), whole body and abdominal X-radiation (Unno et al., 2002; Yamamoto, Takeda & Yamotadani, 2002), and nicotine (Yamamoto et al., 2004). Copper sulfate failed to reduce food intake although it did induce a weak increase in kaolin consumption (Yamamoto et al., 2004). Both CCK and lithium chloride inhibit gastric motility induced by food; but whereas the effect of CCK is blocked by vagal capsaicin treatment indicating involvement of vagal afferents, the response to lithium chloride was hardly affected (Flanagan, Verbalis & Stricker, 1989). All the above are able to reduce gastric emptying as can the free-radical generator pyrogallol (Sharma et al., 2000), which is also able to induce emesis in ferrets (Andrews, P.L.R. & Matsuki, N. unpublished observations). In sheep, rumination can be inhibited by digitalis, which is capable of inducing emesis in sensitive species, and this inhibition is abolished by area postrema ablation leading to the possibility that inhibition of rumination could be an indication of nausea in sheep (Bost et al., 1968).

Effects of Antiemetic Agents and Nerve Lesions

5-HT$_3$ Receptor Antagonists   Ondansetron had no effect on the radiation-induced reduction of food intake in the rat (Yamamoto, Takeda & Yamotadani, 2002) and had only a small but significant effect in ameliorating the reduced food intake in the first 24 hours following cisplatin (Malik et al., 2007). In another study using a higher dose of cisplatin (10 mg/kg i.p. vs. 6 mg/kg i.p.; Takeda et al., 1995b; Aung et al., 2003; Mehendale et al., 2004; 2005) there was found no effect of ondansetron, and this was also the case in a study using a lower (3 mg/kg, i.p.) dose of cisplatin (Rudd et al., 2002). Overall ondansetron has little ability to ameliorate the anorectic effects of cisplatin in the rat and this is also the case in the ferret (Percie du Sert, N., personal communication).

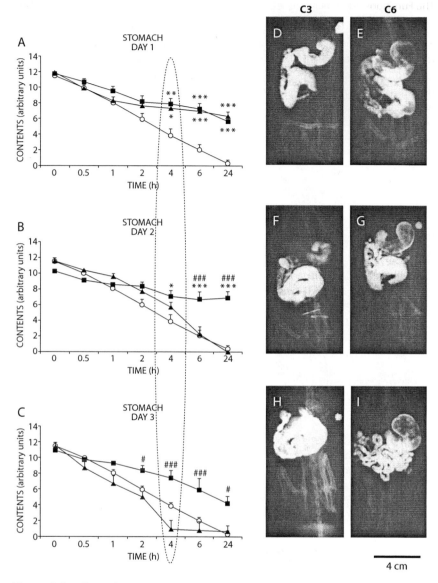

Figure 8.9 Effect of cisplatin on gastric emptying in the rat. Barium sulfate (2.5mL, 2 g mL^{-1}) was intragastrically administered immediately (A), or 24 (B), or 48 (C) hours after saline (4–5 mL kg^{-1}, i.p., open circles, $n = 4$ each experiment) or cisplatin at 3 (closed triangles), $n = 6$ each experiment) or 6 mg kg^{-1} (closed squares $n = 6$ each experiment), and X-rays were taken 0, 0.5, 1, 2, 4, 6 and 24 h after barium administration. Gastric emptying was measured by radiological methods (see text). Data represent the mean ± s.e. mean. * ($p < 0.05$), **($p < 0.005$), ***($p < 0.001$) vs. saline; # ($p < 0.05$), ### ($p < 0.001$) vs. cisplatin 3 mg kg^{-1} (two-way ANOVA followed by Bonferroni test). D, F, H and E, G, I: representative X-rays of rats treated with cisplatin at 3 (C3) or 6 mg kg^{-1} (C6) respectively, taken 4 h after barium administration, during the first (A), second (B) and third (C) days after cisplatin injection. Reproduced with permission from Cabezos et al., 2008.

This is in contrast to its effects in cancer patients, where an increase in food intake and appetite are reported possibly secondary to the reduction of nausea and vomiting (Hainsworth & Hesketh, 1992). Ondansetron also reduced the antifeedant effects of secondary metabolites of eucalyptus in marsupials, which has been ascribed to a conditioned aversion (Lawler et al., 1998).

Although ondansetron has the potential to stimulate gastric emptying (Forster & Dockray, 1990) including the emptying of a liquid and a semisolid meal delayed by the administration of cisplatin a short time before the meal (Eeckhout & Vedder, 1988; Eeckhout, 1989; Ozaki & Sukamoto, 1999), the solid and compacted nature of the gastric contents in cisplatin-treated animals on their normal pelleted diet probably accounts for the lack of effect of ondansetron reported in such studies (Malik et al., 2007).

NK_1 receptor Antagonists   The NK_1 receptor antagonist GR205171 decreased the cisplatin-induced reduction in food intake over 2 days following cisplatin in rats although the effect was not significant on day 1 alone (Malik et al., 2007). In contrast to the effect of ondansetron, GR205171 reduced the weight of gastric contents by 36% in cisplatin-treated animals eating a normal pelleted diet when contents were measured pos-mortem 2 days following cisplatin (Malik et al., 2007).

Dexamethasone   Analysis of the effects of dexamethasone on cisplatin-induced reduction in food intake is complicated by a reduction of food intake induced by dexamethasone given alone. However, it is argued that as the effects of cisplatin and dexamethasone are not additive, dexamethasone may have some beneficial effect (Malik et al., 2007). In the same study dexamethasone reduced the cisplatin-induced increase in the weight of gastric contents by 43%, although a study using a lower dose of dexamethasone and a higher dose of cisplatin failed to observe an effect (Rubio-Pérez et al., 1992).

Metoclopramide   This is an antiemetic and prokinetic agent with dopamine D_2 and 5-HT_3 receptor antagonist effects depending on the dose, and 5-HT_4 receptor agonist effects. Metoclopramide can stimulate the emptying of a liquid test meal delayed by cisplatin (Eeckhout & Vedder, 1988; Eeckhout, 1989) in rats fed on their normal pelleted food. When a lower dose (4.5 mg/kg, i.p.) of cisplatin is used, the weight of gastric contents is reduced by metoclopramide (Roos, Fairlie & Whitehouse, 1981). It was without significant effect on the weight of gastric contents when a higher dose of cisplatin was used (6 mg/kg, i.p., Roos, Fairlie & Whitehouse, 1981; 9 mg/kg i.p., Rubio-Pérez et al., 1992).

Other Treatments   A number of studies have used the delay in gastric emptying induced by cisplatin as a model to test the effect of natural products using the emptying of a semisolid test meal. For example extract of ginger (Sharma & Gupta, 1998) and ferulic acid, a plant derived antioxidant/anti-inflammatory (6 mg/kg, i.p., Badary et al., 2006), both reduce the retardant effect of cisplatin, with the effects being comparable to ondansetron used as a positive control, although on a mg/kg basis the potency of ondansetron was considerably higher in both cases. Although food intake was not measured, another plant extract (from *Scutellaria baicalensis*) with antioxidant properties did not affect the cisplatin-induced reduction in food intake but it did reduce the associated pica (Aung et al., 2003). Delayed gastric emptying and reduced food intake induced by cisplatin were both reduced in mice by administration of the gastric hormone ghrelin, which also stimulated food intake in cisplatin-treated rats (Liu et al., 2006).

Lesions

The interpretation of the effect of abdominal nerve lesions on reduction in food intake and delayed gastric emptying induced by emetic agents is confounded by the complex involvement of the vagus in the regulation of normal food intake and gastric emptying. Cisplatin-induced reduction of food intake in the rat was ameliorated by section of the common hepatic branch of the vagus (as is also the case for pica; De Jonghe & Horn, 2008) but not by section of either the gastric or celiac branches. Vagal capsaicin treatment had no effect on the reduction of food intake measured in the first 24 hours after abdominal X-radiation in the rat, but it did block the reduction on the subsequent three days (Unno et al., 2002). Interpretation of the effects of area postrema ablation on food intake is potentially confounded by the possibility of collateral damage to the subjacent nucleus tractus solitarius, where abdominal vagal afferents terminate. Area postrema ablation in the rat abolished the CTA, reduction in behavior, and inhibition of gastric emptying induced by lithium chloride, but did not affect the accompanying anorexia (Curtis et al., 1994). This combination of effects argues that "nausea" is not required for lithium chloride to induce a reduction in food intake.

Advantages and Disadvantages of Food Intake and Gastric
Emptying Measurement—Summary

Advantages: relatively easy to measure total food consumption over a period of time, although meal patterns may be more difficult to measure; food and water intake is a normal component of most experimental protocols; dose-related responses; potentially good time resolution; food intake is a natural behavior requiring a degree of motivation; food intake can be readily combined with other measures; noninvasive (depending on techniques used); mimics clinical observations; studied extensively, and a wealth of information available on factors regulating food intake and gastric emptying; occurs in species with and without an emetic reflex; amenable to treatment with drugs known to have antiemetic effects.

Disadvantages: nonspecific to substances inducing nausea and vomiting; multiple confounding factors (especially substances with direct effects on gastric motility); linkage to nausea is inferred from studies in humans; no data on involvement of higher regions of the brain and delay in gastric emptying could be a local effect on the gut and/or due to a brainstem reflex.

Behavior

What Is It?

This section reviews behaviors that occur following administration of a substance known or presumed to be capable of inducing nausea in humans and vomiting in animals with an emetic reflex. The period of interest is the time following administration of the substance and the time of onset of retching and vomiting as this is the time during which the sensation of nausea (if present) is most likely to be present and to manifest externally as a change in behavior. Wilpizeski et al. (1985) commented, "Because the occurrence of sickness cannot be based on subjective states conveyed by language, the criteria must be behavioural." From a theoretical perspective nausea could manifest in multiple ways:

1. the presence of a species-unique novel behavior only expressed when the animal experiences nausea or an equivalent sensation;
2. a reduction or absence of one or more normal behaviors with the magnitude of this effect arguably increasing as emesis approaches or occurring in cycles; and
3. an increase in the incidence of one or more natural behaviors with the magnitude of this effect arguably increasing as emesis approaches or occurring in cycles.

In the context of identification of antinausea (or antiemetic) drugs, it does not matter if the behavior under study in the animal is not actually a direct reflection of nausea (or emesis) itself or indeed anything that resembles it, provided that it is predictive of nausea in humans. For example foot-tapping in gerbils is an excellent model in which to study NK_1 receptor antagonist activity with the target disorders including pain and emesis and not foot-tapping (Rupniak & Williams, 1994).

Why Might It Be Indicative of Nausea?

If an animal is experiencing a sensation such as nausea, then it might be expected that there should be some external manifestation of this internal state apparent as some change in behavior. While this is not an unreasonable assumption, the problem is that while it is possible to measure behaviors we cannot know what the animal is experiencing when exhibiting a particular behavior(s) so that the two can be correlated and one used as a surrogate marker for the other. Even in humans where there is a greater degree of certainty about the sensory experience, we do not have quantitative descriptions of the behavioral changes that occur in the period between administration of an emetic and onset of vomiting (however, see Chapter 9, in this volume, for "Nausea Profile"). Despite these problems there have been several attempts to characterize the behavioral changes occurring prior to emesis in several species; and while there will always be uncertainty about the significance of any changes, it could be argued that any deviations from normal behavior induced by an emetic agent are undesirable and hence should be blocked together with retching and vomiting by an agent intended to be investigated for anti-nausea/emesis potential in humans. In addition, when attempting to reduce emetic liability as a side effect of a drug, assessment of behavior is important as it may provide insights into other liabilities.

How Is It Measured?

The ideal situation is an automated one that captures and analyzes all the behaviors automatically, but unfortunately no such system is available, and a full description relies at some point on the involvement of a trained observer. Depending on the species, locomotor activity (including speed of walking, rearing, time spent in particular parts of a cage), food consumption, and water intake can all be measured automatically and can be supplemented by real-time recording of electrocardiogram (EKG; from which heart rate can be derived), blood pressure, core temperature, intra-abdominal pressure (from which respiration rate can be derived as well as episodes of retching and vomiting and of defecation), and electrogastrogram (EGG) using telemetry. However, in order to describe individual behaviors occurring at a specific time it is necessary for the animals to be under direct observation (ideally not detectable by the animal) and/or recorded by video for off-line analysis ideally by an observer blinded to the experimental procedure using a checklist of well defined behaviors. Although video-recording has many advantages (e.g., the number of animals that can be studied in parallel is limited by the number of cameras and not the number of observers), the position of the camera is crucial and ideally more than one should be used. For long periods of observation such as the 3 days required for study of the delayed phase of cisplatin-induced emesis in the ferret, videorecording is essential (in early studies direct observation was used; Rudd, personal communication). Attempts have been made to reduce the recording time by using recorders triggered by motion detectors, but this strategy risks missing small, but perhaps significant, changes in behavior such as facial expressions (e.g., "slit-eyes" in the ferret following cytotoxic drugs; Hawthorn, Ostler & Andrews, 1988).

In addition to studying the effect of an emetic agent on behavior, a number of studies have also investigated the effect of antiemetics on these emetic-induced behaviors to obtain an insight into potential antinausea effects. However, Lau et al. (2005a) have pointed out that many such studies have not investigated the effect of the antiemetic alone on behavior, and hence the effects of emetic-induced behaviors may not be an accurate description of their effects.

As with all studies of behavior the conditions under which the studies are performed can have a major influence on the behaviors observed. For example, in ferret studies although individual research groups observe the animals individually in cages of a particular size, the cage sizes vary between groups (when they are given), which makes comparisons of behaviors difficult.

A common behavior reported is backward walking, but it may be more difficult for the animal to fully exhibit this behavior in a small cage; and burrowing is unlikely to occur if there is no suitable material in the observation cage, with the possibility that the animal may manifest some other behavior. It is essential that future behavioral studies report the experimental and environmental conditions in detail to allow more valid comparison between laboratories.

The method for scoring behaviors is also important to take into account. Some authors use the presence or absence of a behavior irrespective of the incidence, while others quantify individual behaviors in a particular time period. The latter method is preferable as it will more accurately characterize the dose-response relationships between the behaviors and emesis for an emetic agent and for the effects of a potential antiemetic agent. In the majority of studies behavioral scores have been aggregated over quite long time periods giving poor resolution and making it difficult to assess whether behaviors may occur in "waves" as does nausea in humans, or if behaviors increase in intensity as emesis approaches, or the probability of a particular behavior increases in the periemetic period. There is also a danger in a simple aggregation of behavioral scores (i.e., treating each behavior as equivalent) that subtle changes will be missed.

The veterinary literature now contains several examples of questionnaires developed to measure pain and health-related quality of life in dogs and provide valuable lessons for the development of observer-based scoring systems for use in laboratory animals (Wiseman-Orr et al., 2004; 2006).

Species In Which It Has Been Studied, Stimuli for Induction, and Effects of Antiemetics

Vomiting occurs in representative fish (e.g., dogfish, Andrews, Sims & Young, 1998; rays, Sims, Andrews & Young, 2000; reef shark, Brunnschweiler et al., 2005; killifish, Gerhart, 1991; trout, Tiersch & Griffith, 1988); amphibia (e.g., frog, Naitoh, Wassersug & Leslie, 1989; salamander, Naitoh & Wassersug, 1992); reptiles (e.g., salt water crocodile, Andrews et al., 2000); and birds (e.g., pigeon, Tanihata et al., 2000) and there are descriptions of behavioral changes accompanying emesis, with oral-related behaviors being most frequently mentioned. As species other than mammals are used relatively infrequently for the investigation of emesis and particularly for the identification of antiemetic drugs, this section will focus on studies of mammals with an emetic reflex used in laboratory-based investigations.

House Musk Shrew (*Suncus murinus*)   Although *Suncus* has become increasingly used as a model for the study of emesis, there are relatively few systematic descriptions of emesis-associated behaviors in this species. Lau, Rudd, and Yew (2005) investigated the behavioral responses to cisplatin-induced emesis and failed to find any change in spontaneous locomotor activity. In addition, cisplatin did not induce backward walking, lip-licking, burrowing, yawning, overt salivation, or curling up. Lip-licking, overt salivation, and mouth scratching have been observed in *Suncus* in response to the PDE$_4$ inhibitor rolipram (Andrews, P.L.R. & Woods, A.J., unpublished observations).

There have been a number of studies in the least shrew (*Cryptotis parva*) of locomotor activity and behaviors such as scratching and head twitching, but these have been in relation to investigation of cannabinoid receptors rather than in specific relation to emesis (Darmani et al., 2003a; Darmani et al., 2003b; Darmani & Johnson, 2004; Darmani & Crim, 2005).

Ferret (*Mustela putorius furo L.*) The ferret has probably been the animal subject to most behavioral investigations because of the desire to know whether it can be used as a model for nausea as well as for vomiting, with the behavioral effects of cisplatin (Bermudez et al., 1988; Lau et al., 2005a), cyclophosphamide (Hawthorn & Cunningham, 1990), radiation (King, 1988; King & Landauer, 1990), apomorphine (Osinski et al., 2003; Lau et al., 2005b), loperamide (Osinski et al., 2003; Zaman et al., 2000), and phosphodiesterase$_4$ (PDE$_4$) inhibitors (Montana et al., 1998; Robichaud et al., 2001) being the most extensively reported. It is notable that among the various studies and stimuli there is a remarkable consistency about the types of behavior to be induced or increased in incidence in ferrets prior to the onset of retching or vomiting reported in each study.

The frequently reported behaviors in the ferret are:

- Backward walking
- Burrowing in cage bedding
- Licking/lip-licking
- Gagging—a single abdominal contraction accompanied by a sharp cough-like noise
- Clawing at the mouth/mouth scratching—scratching of the hard palate or peri-oral region with one or occasionally both of the forepaws
- Flopping—an extended motionless prone position
- Reduction of overall locomotor activity (but note that apomorphine can increase activity, see Lau et al., 2005b)
- Defecation—ferrets usually defecate in the same corner of the cage even when housed in a group
- Overt salivation
- Hyperventilation/panting
- Curling up

The first three are reported consistently although they also occur in animals not exposed to an emetic stimulus. Of the remaining behaviors, gagging, overt salivation, belly flopping, panting, and mouth scratching are not normally encountered in healthy ferrets. It is of interest that "lying on the belly" is a "typical sign of nausea in rats" although not observed in mice (Welzl, D'Adamo & Lipp, 2001). Interestingly the "lying-on-belly" behavior induced by intraperitoneal injection of lithium chloride was abolished by area postrema ablation in the rat (Bernstein et al., 1992). Salivation is a normal prodrome of emesis reported in humans and dogs, it may be a stimulus for intense lip-licking and the intense production of saliva (especially if viscid) that is unable to be cleared from the buccal cavity by swallowing, and it may also provoke gagging. Increased defecation (and posturing to defecate) has been noted particularly with cisplatin (Bermudez et al., 1988) and X-radiation (King, 1988; King & Landauer, 1990) and is likely to be a stimulus-specific response rather than related to "nausea."

In general authors have quantified each type of behavior, and either report the effect of an emetic agent on an individual behavior or on the sum of a cluster of behaviors used to derive a global "nausea behavior score or index." Patterns of behavior have been studied for the centrally acting emetic loperamide, but a difficulty with studying agents having a relatively short latency such as loperamide is that the latency of onset of the behaviors, retching and vomiting, are not significantly different and the latency to onset of emesis is short (6.0 ± 1.2 min; Zaman et al., 2000) so there is little time to study the development of behaviors. The analysis of behaviors prior to the onset of emesis is probably only really applicable to agents such as cisplatin where the latency is one to two hours. Figure 8.10 plots some of the behaviors in ferrets treated with either cisplatin or vehicle illustrates the complexity of such studies.

Using the overall behavioral score approach, there is evidence for a dose-related increase in "nausea" behaviors for apomorphine, loperamide, (-) nicotine, copper sulfate, rolipram, cyclophosphamide and an increase in "nausea" behaviors in comparison to control for X-radiation and cisplatin . It should be noted that there has been very little analysis of the temporal pattern and incidence of the above behaviors in relation to the onset of the first or subsequent emetic episodes, so it is not known if the intensity of any of them increases as emesis approaches although if they are indicators of nausea this might be expected. Analysis has focused on summing scores for each behavior and treating each behavior as equivalent. More sophisticated analysis should be undertaken using "clusters" of behaviors.

There have been limited studies investigating the effect of pharmacological interventions on the above behaviors; however, Lau et al. (2005a) have noted that any effects may be overestimated, as some studies do not include a control group in which the effect of the antiemetic on normal behavior was investigated. While the $5\text{-}HT_3$ receptor antagonist ondansetron was without effect on baseline behaviors, the NK_1 receptor antagonist (CP-99,994) reduced locomotor activity, lip-licking, and burrowing. The result with ondansetron contrasts with the report by Bermudez et al. (1988) that in cisplatin-treated animals given the $5\text{-}HT_3$ receptor antagonist granisetron, three of four animals "showed near-normal behavior" but the behaviors were not quantified. Using total body X-radiation as a stimulus, Hawthorn, J. and Andrews, P.L.R. (unpublished observations, 1989) found that ondansetron reduced the "nausea score" by about 45%, although the score was significantly higher than in unirradiated animals either with or without ondansetron. Also, the benzamide batanopride protects against the radiation-induced decrement in locomotor activity and

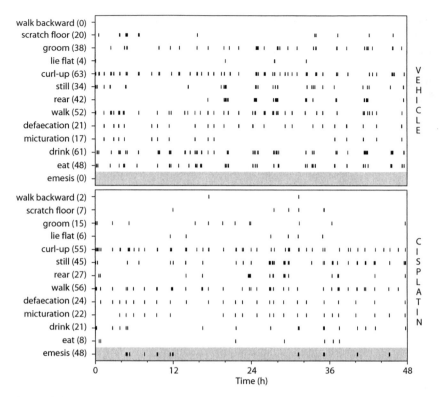

Figure 8.10 Illustration of the complexity of analysis of behavior following administration of an emetic agent in the ferret over a period of 48 hours. The upper panel shows the temporal distribution of behaviors in an animal treated with intraperitoneal saline and the lower panel an animal treated with cisplatin (5mg/kg, i.p.). The shading indicates the row showing emetic episodes and for each behavior the total number of episodes is shown in parentheses. From Percie du Sert and Andrews, unpublished observations.

the increase in burrowing although lip-licking was unaffected (King & Landauer, 1990). In cyclophosphamide-treated animals the "nausea score" was reduced by either ondansetron or dexamethasone (Hawthorn & Cunningham, 1990).

Two centrally acting emetics, apomorphine (dopamine receptor agonist) and loperamide (opioid receptor agonist), have also been studied in some detail. Using the NK₁ receptor antagonist CP-99,994, Zaman et al. (2000) abolished emesis and licking, mouth scratching, wet dog shakes, and gagging induced by loperamide. CP-100,263 the enantiomer of CP-99,994 was without effect. Lau et al. (2005b) were unable to demonstrate an increase in lip-licking, rearing, burrowing, backward walking, curling up, or defecation in response to apomorphine (250 μg/kg, s.c.), although it did induce emesis and increase locomotor activity. The emesis, but not the increase in locomotor activity was blocked by domperidone. Hawthorn, J. and Andrews, P.L.R. (1989, unpublished observations) found a small but significant ($p < 0.005$) increase in the overall "nausea score" induced by 100μg/kg s.c. apomorphine when compared to both control values and a lower dose (10 μg/kg, s.c.) of apomorphine (control 2.6 ± 0.2; apomorphine 10 μg/kg, s.c. 2.6 ± 0.4; apomorphine 100 μg/kg, s.c. 4.3 ± 0.4).

Cat (*Felis domesticus*)   The main descriptions of emesis-associated behavior in the cat come from studies of motion sickness where symptom scales have been used (Suri, Crampton & Daunton, 1979; Lucot, 1998) based on a similar scale for humans. The Suri et al. (1979) scale is as follows:

- Qualifying Symptoms (1 point per symptom): Salivation I—excessive licking and swallowing; drowsiness—drowsy or sleep demeanor, with eyes partially or fully closed; unusual postures maintained for at least one minute.
- Minimal motion sickness (2 points per symptom): Salivation II—several drops of saliva; panting.
- Minor motion sickness (4 points): Salivation III—copious saliva, foamy strings hanging from the mouth.
- Major motion sickness (8 points per symptom): urination; defecation.
- Pathognomic motion sickness (16 points): vomiting or retching

It should be noted that this scale was developed to assess motion sickness as a specific entity and not to be a nausea scale. The validity of inclusion of either urination or defecation in an emesis/nausea scoring system is questionable, and as Lucot (1998) notes, this scale primarily reflects efferent parasympathetic nervous system activation and hence drugs affecting this system can give rise to both false positive and negative conclusions when assessing their impact on symptoms associated with emesis. In their seminal review of the *Physiology and Pharmacology of Vomiting* published in 1953, Borison and Wang noted that "salivation associated with swallowing and frequent rhythmic forward licking in cats and dogs have long been considered manifestations of nausea." They also reported that another sign of imminent vomiting in the cat was a "peculiar deep-throated vocalisation which is not unlike its mating call," but there do not appear to be other reports of this behavior although it could be similar to the "gagging" reported in ferrets that is accompanied by vocalization. Borison and Wang (1953) commented in passing that all the signs of "nausea" with the exception of the distress cry can be elicited in the decerebrate cat in response to emetic stimuli indicating that they do not involve "higher" brain regions and hence are likely to be components of the reflex response to activation of the emetic pathways (see Chapter 4, in this volume).

Suri, Crampton, and Daunton (1979) used the motion sickness symptom scale to evaluate scopolamine and d-amphetamine, but the inclusion of emesis in the scores makes assessment of the impact on behaviors difficult.

Lucot (1998) excluded the emetic scores in his study of N-methyl-D-aspartate antagonists, and although a reduction occurred in the symptom score it was not statistically significant. Reductions in the symptom score were also reported using scopolamine and a 5-HT_{1A} receptor agonist but not with an NK_1 receptor antagonist even at doses that blocked vomiting in response to motion (Lucot, 1998).

Dog (*Canis familiaris*)   In 1925, Keeton reported that in the dog licking the nose was evidence of nausea, and a quotation from another contemporary report from Pavlov's (1927) studies with morphine and conditioned responses states:

> The dog has been injected with morphine on previous occasions, and is now held quietly on the table by an attendant who has never had anything to do with injecting the morphine. When the experimenter approaches, the dog gets restless and moistens its lips, and as soon as the experimenter touches the animal, severe nausea and profuse secretion of saliva begin.(p. 36)

Unfortunately no description of what constitutes nausea is given. Schrager and Ivy (1928) investigated the effects of gall-bladder distension and commented, "Salivation, denoting nausea, occurred in approximately 40 per cent of the dogs," and Grossman et al. (1945) used duodenal distension to induce nausea but did not give a description although they noted that it was accompanied by an inhibition of histamine-induced acid secretion as can occur with apomorphine, emetine, and quinine in emetic and subemetic doses in the dog (Atkinson & Ivy, 1938). In addition to salivation other symptoms associated with emesis in the dog include yawning, standing with the head drooping, and licking the nose (Borison & Wang, 1953). Chen et al. (2003) used licking tongue, closing eyes, yawning, belching, murmuring, rapid breathing, dry vomiting, liquid vomiting, and defecating to score the symptoms induced by vasopressin and demonstrate an effect of gastric electrical stimulation. A similar scoring system was used by Yu et al. (2009) to measure behaviors "suggesting" nausea induced by cisplatin in the dog. The behaviors included in an aggregated scoring scheme were: licking, nictation, belching, groaning, yawning, shortness of breath, movement.

Piglet (*Sus scrofa*)   The piglet has been used as a model for cisplatin-induced emesis with chewing-like activity recorded from the masseter muscle EMG and associated with intense salivation with viscous saliva and a generally prostrated state being described as "nausea-related behavior" (Milano et al., 1995; Grelot et al., 1996; 1998). In cisplatin-treated animals this behavior, which lasts 10–20 seconds, tracks emesis over a 60-hour period with 268 episodes of "nausea-related behavior" out of 433 (62%) being followed by an emetic episode (Milano et al., 1995). The same behavior was also reported following lipopolysaccharide administration (Girod, Bouvier & Grelot, 2000) in response to intrathecal morphine and in piglets with postoperative vomiting (Grelot et al., unpublished observations cited in Grelot et al., 1998, p. 1648). The NK_1 receptor antagonist GR205171 reduced this nausea-related behavior in both the acute and delayed phases of cisplatin emesis (Grelot et al., 1998).

Nonhuman Primates   In the marmoset (*Callithrix jacchus*) Costall, Domeney, and Naylor (1986) developed a "nausea" scoring system by assessing the following behaviors and allocating a point to each giving a maximum score of 7 for an individual animal with the scores being aggregated for all animals in a treatment group of 4 animals giving a possible total of 28:

- alteration in facial expression
- retraction of the ears
- salivation, tongue protrusion, and other mouthing movements
- nose rubbing on the perch
- hunched body posture
- drooped head and/or neck stretching
- slowness of movement

It should be noted that this system does not measure the magnitude or frequency of occurrence of these behaviors, only their presence or absence. Using the dopamine receptor agonist tetralin, a maximum score of 28 was obtained and this was reduced (14) by haloperidol and sulpiride, with the highest dose used reducing the score to zero.

Studies in the squirrel monkey (*Saimiri sciureus*) using oxotremorine (muscarininc receptor agonist), SKF 38393 (a selective D_1 receptor partial agonist), and the emetic ipecacuanha caused dose-related purposeless chewing that in some cases was accompanied by tongue protrusion (Rupniak, Tye & Iversen, 1990).

Squirrel monkeys have also been used for studies of motion sickness and a scoring system developed including "apparent sleep or behavioural encapsulation," "hyperactivity or pacing," and "licking or chewing" (Wilpizeski et al., 1985, p. 6) with the latency for consistent chewing being significantly shorter than for the onset of either retching or vomiting. The authors noted that animals that entered the state of profound behavioral encapsulation had the onset of vomiting delayed and interpreted the adoption of this behavior as an attempt to prevent emesis.

Radiation-induced emesis has been investigated in the monkey and preemetic behaviors noted include general malaise, yawning, grimacing, and exaggerated oral movements (Eldred & Trowbridge, 1954; Mattsson & Yochmowitz, 1980).

There is a growing body of evidence showing that in the wild, anthropoid apes (chimpanzees, bonobos, gorillas, and orangutans) communicate both vocally and by gestures (Pollick & de Waal, 2007). It would be interesting to know if an individual experiencing nausea following ingestion of a particular food was able to communicate this information to another member of the group, especially as geophagy has been reported in apes (Krishnamani & Mahaney, 2000).

Overall, the interpretation of behavioral data is fraught with difficulty. However, in attempting to identify novel chemical entities with potential antiemetic effects (e.g., against an anticancer chemotherapeutic agent), blockade of retching and vomiting *and* any behavioral changes associated with the chemotherapeutic agent would be a profile to encourage further studies but it would not guarantee efficacy against both nausea and vomiting. Additionally, studies with novel chemical entities intended for use in the treatment of diseases where current treatment is suboptimal sometimes identifies an emetic liability and when investigated some of the behaviors described above (especially in the dog and ferret) have been reported in addition to emesis. A precautionary interpretation would suggest a similar liability if administered to humans and indicate further research in animal models should seek other members of the chemical series, dosing, or formulation approaches to reduce both the behavioral and emetic liability before proceeding with caution to humans. A major difficulty in making a rational assessment of both the behavioral and emetic data from animal studies in which an emetic liability has been identified is that there is little information available in the public domain of the results of human studies that enable firm conclusions to be drawn about the degree of translation from the animal models to humans. Until either such data are available or we can be certain about the significance of the behaviors, induction of emesis should always be viewed as undesirable and the presence of any abnormal behaviors treated with caution.

Advantages and Disadvantages of Behavior—Summary

Advantages: potentially good time resolution; does not require additional intervention or preconditioning of the animal; animal is able to express any aspect of its behavioral repertoire providing the observation environment is suitable; can be quantified; some limited evidence that antiemetics may modify behaviors; can be studied in animals with and without an emetic reflex.

Disadvantages: interpretation is difficult and in some way relies on analogies with human behavior; behaviors may be highly species-specific; may be difficult to distinguish between nausea-related behaviors (assuming they exist) and those caused by a specific pharmacological effect of the drug under study; behaviors exhibited may depend on experimental conditions; different behaviors given equal weighting in most analyses despite no evidence that they are all (or any) are equivalent indices of nausea; pathways little studied.

The Nausea-Emesis Relationship in Animals

As was first discussed in Chapter 1 in this volume, for humans emesis and nausea are not on a simple continuum. The question is that if given an appropriate emetic stimulus an animal exhibits retching and vomiting, is it reasonable to assume that it must be experiencing or have experienced nausea? This issue is well illustrated by the following quotation: "However, when vomiting occurs, nausea can be inferred safely even in animals." (Stricker et al., 1988, p. 295). Using the occurrence of retching and vomiting to infer the presence of nausea in an animal is arguably invalid for a number of reasons:

- Retching and vomiting can be induced under general anesthesia and in decerebrate animals, where there is no evidence that the animal is experiencing any conscious sensation and, in addition, is not exhibiting any other than reflex changes in somatomotor behavior such as lip-licking and swallowing.
- Some mammalian species (e.g., rat, mouse, guinea pig, rabbit) do not have the ability to vomit, but it would be unwise to assume that they do not have nausea or some equivalent sensory experience.
- Vomiting is present in representative fish, amphibia, and reptiles where the cerebrum is less well developed than in mammals (and birds), raising the contentious possibility that they may not have any higher sensory experience equating to nausea (see Chapter 4, in this volume).
- In effect, vomiting is used by several species including birds and mammals as either a method for feeding the young or mates (e.g., penguins and African wild dogs) or as a way of purging indigestible material from the upper gastrointestinal tract (e.g., trichobezoars by cats and squid beaks by sperm whales). In these settings it is unlikely that nausea occurs.
- In humans there is abundant evidence that nausea is not inevitably followed by vomiting and that vomiting can occur in isolation with little or no preceding nausea such as occurs in patients with suddenly raised intracranial pressure.
- In humans both the 5-HT$_3$ and NK$_1$ receptor antagonists are more effective against vomiting induced by anticancer chemotherapy agents (Foubert & Vaessen, 2005; Hesketh, 2008) than against nausea, whereas if the two processes were directly linked the efficacy against both should be similar (see Chapter 14, in this volume).

Although using vomiting to indicate that an animal has or is experiencing "nausea" is unwise, it would be equally unwise in the process of investigating novel chemical entities (NCE) not to investigate the antinausea (and antiemetic) potential in a human study of a substance with efficacy against retching and vomiting in an appropriate animal model(s) of emesis assuming there were no safety issues. Conversely, if an NCE itself induces emesis in an appropriate animal model it would be wise to assume that it is likely to have a nausea and emesis liability in humans unless there is evidence to the contrary.

Do Animals Have Nausea and, If So, Can It Be Measured?

This chapter has reviewed a diverse range of techniques that have been claimed with varying degrees of certainty to be a measure of nausea in nonhuman animals, and now we have to attempt to answer the specific question of whether animals have nausea. Related to this question are the related questions of whether it can be measured and application of that knowledge.

The selected quotations below spanning over 50 years are relevant:

"It is impossible to determine whether nausea is experienced by experimental animals." (Borison & Wang, 1953, p. 194);

"As there is no way to directly validate the appropriateness of this behavioural model as an analogue to nausea, it remains an article of faith that taste aversion in the rat is an analogue to nausea in man." (Morrow, 1984a, p. 2271);

"One immediate discrepancy between studies with human subjects and those with animal subjects is that there is nothing that can be measured in an animal as nausea." (Lucot, 1998, p. 63);

"Nausea is a sensation and, as such, it can only be studied with assurance only in human subjects." (Stricker et al., 1988, p. 295); and

"Nausea cannot be studied in nonhumans." (Hornby, 2001, p. 106S)

Two broad conclusions can be drawn from these quotations, which are consistent with the analysis of publications presented above:

- Nausea cannot be measured *directly* in nonhuman animals and even if we assume it is present, its presence can only be indirectly inferred; rather as Robinson Crusoe inferred the presence of another human on his island from the footprint on the beach and although he might with a good knowledge of anthropometrics have been able to deduce a number of things about the person who made the footprint, he could never know what Man Friday was thinking when he made the footprint. From an animal welfare perspective it is best to adopt the precautionary principle and to assume that animals (at least mammals) are capable of suffering with nausea.

- The quotations do not deny the existence of nausea in animals, only whether it can be detected. What does having nausea (as opposed to another sensation) cause an animal to do that would be apparent to an observer? Among the mammals there is evidence for some conscious, unpleasant sensation categorized as distinct from pain, associated with administration of agents capable of inducing emesis (often when given at a higher dose than that inducing behavioral change) and which is capable of forming a memory of the experience leading to avoidance and aversive responses. The pivotal issue is one of "reporting" what is occurring or has occurred. Consider for a few minutes your own experience of nausea and your reactions that would be apparent to an external observer. A typical sequence would be: Awareness of an altered internal state—classification of that state as nausea as opposed to for example pain or headache—changed behavior at both subconscious (introversion, postural change) and conscious (go to bathroom, lie down, avoid eating) levels with possibly verbal communication of the experience. However, if we accept that it is possible to use one or more of the above behavioral indices as the equivalent of verbal reporting in humans, then a case can be made that nausea or an equivalent sensation does occur in mammals in general and with a greater degree of certainty in apes. This conclusion would be strengthened if the same pathways were present in animals and humans and that the pathways were shown to be activated by the same nausea-inducing stimuli. However, such an analysis awaits detailed imaging studies of the brain in humans experiencing nausea (see Chapter 4, in this volume, for discussion).

A key question is whether any of the measurements discussed above, together with the physiological indices discussed in the endocrine (plasma [AVP] or [OXY]—the latter in the rat) and autonomic nervous system (electrogastrogram; see Chapters 6, 5, and 7, in this volume) are specific measures of nausea and if so which measures are most reliable. These questions are inextricably linked to the reason why we are attempting to measure nausea. In essence there are three reasons why it may be necessary to measure nausea in animals: (1) to understand the mechanisms underlying the genesis of sensations and behavior; (2) identification of nauseogenic liability of novel chemical entities; and (3) identification of treatments for nausea in humans. These will be used as a basis to tackle the above questions and bring this chapter to a conclusion.

To Understand the Mechanisms Underlying the Genesis of Sensations and Behavior   Although this is often aimed at improving understanding of the assumed equivalent sensation in humans, from the perspective of the animal it is irrelevant whether it experiences the same sensation as a human. The issue for the animal is whether the sensation enables it to make the correct response to enhance its survival. This may mean that even if an animal is experiencing exactly the same sensation as a human then the behavioral (or indeed other including physiological responses such as the difference in AVP and OXY secretion between humans and rats) response may not necessarily be the same as in a human. In this context all measures have a degree of validity as they all contribute something to overall understanding. However, the appropriately controlled studies of conditioned aversion/avoidance to food or flavors provide good circumstantial evidence for the existence of a sensation in animals with at least the same functional consequence and adaptive value as in humans. Pica as measured by kaolin consumption in the laboratory is analogous to the widespread phenomenon of geophagia used both prophylactically to reduce the impact of toxic food that the animal is intended to ingest and as treatment to alleviate the effects of ingested toxins. It is likely that the latter response would be induced not only by nausea but also by more general visceral malaise or even pain. It is arguable whether a fine differentiation of the sensory experiences which may accompany toxin ingestion would enable the animal to make a more adaptive response. Arguably, behaviors that for their expression require the animal to recall and categorize an experience may be specific for the recollection of nausea (e.g., conditioned taste aversion). It would be unwise to assume that the presence of emesis in an animal capable of vomiting is a reliable indicator that the animal must have experienced nausea in the periemesis period as we know that humans can vomit without prior nausea and that antiemetics are not equally efficacious against nausea and vomiting. In addition many species vomit (or a very similar motor act) as part of their normal behavioral repertoire where it is highly unlikely that this is accompanied by nausea. A reduction in food intake, while likely to occur as an appropriate response in an animal with nausea, is not specific and this is also the case with the delay in gastric emptying, which often accompanies the reduction in food intake and which may itself contribute to the reduction in food intake. The potential biomarkers of a large elevation in plasma vasopressin (oxytocin in rodents) and characteristic changes in the electrogastrogram, while suggestive of the presence of nausea, are not specific; for example, given a plasma value for AVP or the frequency of the EGG, one could only make an estimate of the probability of the presence of nausea even in a human, but it would never be possible to be certain. However, this does not mean that other as yet unidentified biomarkers may not be predictive. Overall, there is a body of circumstantial evidence supporting the hypothesis that mammals have a sensory experience that has many of the characteristics (as assessed by the behavioral responses) of the sensation of nausea in humans. If we make this assumption then it should be possible to identify pathways in the brain that are common to mammals and are involved in genesis of this sensation. In view of the marked differences in the degree of encephalization between mammals there may be differences in the quality of the sensation. Further investigation of the existence of the pathways for processing potentially nauseogenic information in animals awaits brain imaging studies of these pathways in humans for comparison.

Identification of Nauseogenic Liability of Novel Chemical Entities   Nausea and vomiting are relatively common side effects of currently available medicines, with nausea listed as a side effect on over half of the Summaries of Product Characteristics in the Electronic Medicines Compendium (Lee, 2006). In addition, as is illustrated in Figure 8.1 above, nausea is also commonly encountered during the discovery and development of potential new drugs. There is a need for preclinical models to identify such a liability to reduce the high attrition rate and the time needed to reach market. Models may include in silico databases, microorganisms, invertebrates, and in vitro studies in animals as well as humans (see Holmes et al., 2009, for review), but this section will confine itself to the possible utility of the animal models described above, although it assumes that some compounds will have been excluded prior to in vivo animal studies.

    If a substance is to evoke nausea (and vomiting) it must either act directly or indirectly on one of the input pathways to the brain (see Chapters 4 and 5, in this volume) or on one of the pathways within the brain and to varying degrees most of the measurements reviewed above could contribute to identifying if one of these pathways is activated. Bearing in mind that it may be necessary to investigate a number of compounds in vivo, one strategy would be to adopt a stepped approach aimed at reducing the number of compounds tested and animals used, as the complexity of the test increases and degree of suffering and presumed sentience of the species used increases (see Figure 8. 11). For each test a range of doses would be used and criteria preset (probably based on the literature) for compound exclusion. This strategy could be applied for example as follows: Study 1, Mouse—Gastric motility and food intake; Study 2, Rat—Pica; Study 3, Ferret—emesis including measurement of plasma AVP and possible subemetic end points (e.g., EGG, retrograde giant contraction, proximal gastric relaxation, swallowing) using telemetry; Study 4, Human volunteers. The ideal screening cascade is a matter for debate and validation, so the above should only be taken as an indication to the approach that could be taken.

Identification of Treatments for Nausea in Humans   This aspect is the most difficult because in principle it requires that the animal respond to the drug or treatment producing the nausea in humans with the same sensory experience as humans, utilize the same neural (and other) pathways, and utilize the same neurotransmitters (and combination of cotransmitters) and receptors in that pathway so that potential novel treatments can be identified. There is no animal model that fulfills all these criteria, and apart from the currently insurmountable problem of knowing what an animal is experiencing, the lack of data in humans about pathways for nausea and their likely neurotransmitters limits refinement of current models. Differences between the degree of involvement of particular receptors even in the relatively conserved brain-stem pathways may contribute to the variable translation from models such as CTA in the rat to human (e.g., 5-HT_3 and NK_1 receptor antagonists). Translation further requires a knowledge of which species have human-like receptors so that the correct compounds can be identified (e.g., the ferret NK_1 receptor is more similar to the human receptor than the rat; see Andrews & Rudd, 2004, for review) and also species expressing the same receptor subunits as humans; for example, genes encoding the 5-HT_{3C}, 5-HT_{3D}, and 5-HT_{3E} receptor subunits are conserved in many mammalian species but are absent in rodents (Holbrook et al., 2009). These observations indicate the importance of knowledge of the molecular biology of transmitters (particularly peptides) and their receptors in the species of interest. The usual approach taken to the discovery of antiemetic drugs has been to use an animal model of vomiting, where possible using a model of the intended target stimulus such as motion or anticancer chemotherapy (usually using cisplatin as the challenge) as to investigate promising compounds (Holmes et al., 2009). Approaches to targeting pathways such as the area postrema and the gastric afferents using apomorphine and intragastric copper sulfate respectively have also been used. In all cases, although the blockade of emesis has been taken as an indication of likely efficacy against nausea, it has only been with clinical trials that it has been possible

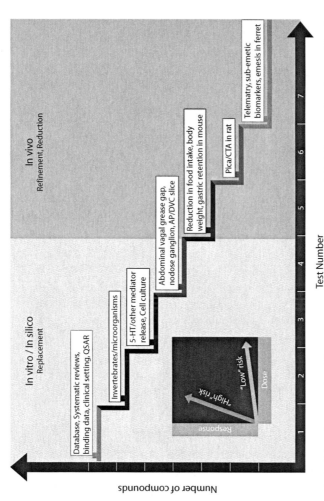

Figure 8.11 A hypothetical tiered approach to illustrate assessment of potential emetic liability of NCEs that could reduce animal use. This approach consists of a series of tests, starting with *in vitro/in silico* methods to assess emetic liability prior to progressing to conscious animal studies. Each test investigates the dose-response (e.g., *C. elegans* chemotaxis, neurotransmitter release, pica) relationships of the NCE (see inset). Such a weight-of-evidence approach would enable researchers to classify the emetic potential of an NCE as either relatively "high" or "low" risk over a series of *in vitro/in silico* tests. This should provide a more accurate overall indication of an NCE's potential to be emetic prior to undertaking any in vivo studies and may perhaps obviate their necessity. NCEs would be compared against a panel of compounds with known emetic liability in humans. An increasing probability of emetic liability in each test increases the probability of emetic liability being seen in humans. The *in vitro/in silico* studies would inform the in vivo studies and may enable studies to stop at a lower sentient species and potentially use less animals overall by reducing the number of compounds/doses tested in vivo. Reproduced with permission from Holmes et al., 2009.

to assess this with any degree of certainty. Systematic review and meta-analysis of the preclinical studies of the efficacy of 5-HT$_3$ receptor antagonists against cisplatin-induced emesis in the ferret is providing insights into the translation of the results from the animal model to humans as well as informing the design of future studies (Percie du Sert et al., 2010b). There are no animal models that allow direct investigation of the antinausea potential of an NCE, and the development of such models (if required) awaits improved understanding of nausea in humans. In the interim it is likely that models of emesis such as the ferret will continue to be used but will be refined by the use of simultaneous measurements of AVP and the EGG. However, it may be possible to develop further already established models of nausea and vomiting in humans using apomorphine, intragastric ipecac, and vection and hence obviate the need for animal models in this specific area (Holmes et al., 2009).

Chapter 9

The Measurement of Nausea in Humans

Very little has been written about the measurement of nausea in humans for several reasons. Perhaps the most obvious are the related issues that there is little agreement as to what nausea is, and that, because it is a subjective experience, only the person experiencing nausea can describe it. Another reason for the paucity of information about the measurement of nausea is that many investigators in this field write as if nausea were an all-or-none condition, like pregnancy, rather than an experience that also varies greatly in intensity— like pain or fatigue.

There have been several books published since 1995 with "Nausea" in the title, but only one discussed the assessment or measurement of nausea. That volume (Hawthorn, 1995) was aimed at nurses, and pointed out one reason why there is a need to measure nausea: "Usually the amount of nausea does not need to be evaluated, just establishing whether nausea is present or not is sufficient to determine treatment. However, for clinical trials assessing the efficacy of anti-emetics we need to be able to measure nausea to see if interventions are successful" (p. 7).

Before describing the tools available to measure nausea, this chapter will discuss some of the problems and complexities. Perhaps the most basic question has to do with the fact that nausea is a private sensation. How does one know that when a patient or research subject reports nausea he/she is referring to the same thing as the clinician/researcher thinks about when he/she thinks of nausea? Another important issue is the "point-in-time" when nausea is reported. Is nausea being reported in "real time" at the present moment or is nausea being rated for some time in the past day, week, or month? If the report of nausea is from the past, then all the factors that influence memory come into play. For example, has the individual experienced something unpleasant between the nausea episode and completing the nausea questionnaire? Or did the person experience something pleasurable between the nausea episode and completing a questionnaire? And, if possible, individual psychological characteristics such as whether the patient is a "sensitizer," one prone to report every bodily change, or a "repressor" of bodily sensations should be considered. Another psychological issue to consider is whether the patient is receiving secondary gain from reporting nausea symptoms. That is, does the patient receive desired attention, special diet, etc., as a result of reporting nausea, and do these gains reinforce the nausea?

Nausea in humans can be assessed using three basic methods: self-reports of nausea, behavioral indications of nausea, and physiological correlates of nausea. This chapter discusses the tools available within the three measurement approaches; discussion of their application to the study of nausea caused by different conditions in humans follows in Chapters 10–15. A detailed review of physiological biomarkers of nausea in humans and laboratory animals can be found in Chapters 5, 6, and 7, and Chapter 8 discusses the possible behavioral correlates of nausea in laboratory animals.

SELF-REPORTS OF NAUSEA

Am I Nauseous or Not?

Self-reports of nausea are the most basic method of assessing the presence or absence of nausea. The patient or research subject is simply asked whether nausea is present or absent, yes or no. This measure is not recommended because inherent in its use is the assumption that nausea is an all-or-none symptom rather than a complex syndrome. That subjects asked this question are often not provided a definition of nausea also compromises the usefulness of response data.

Visual Analogue Scale

A visual analogue scale (VAS) is usually a 100-mm-long line, sometimes horizontal and sometimes vertical, with the anchor ends labeled, for example, "no nausea" and "worst nausea I ever felt," or "no nausea" and "severe nausea." A score is determined by measuring the distance from the low end to the point marked by the patient. Some investigators have added discrete descriptive terms to the VAS such as "slight nausea," "mild nausea," "severe nausea," but Del Favero, Tonato, and Roila (1992) and others have pointed out that these additions do not seem to offer any advantage over the VAS without discrete descriptors. The VAS is often used to assess the intensity of nausea, and is sometimes used in combination with other measures (see, for example, Melzack et al., 1985.) A limitation of the use of a VAS is that the user assumes that nausea is a single dimensional sensation (see "Nausea Profile" below).

Self-Report Scales

Rhodes Index of Nausea and Vomiting (INV)

Rhodes, Watson, and Johnson (1984) describe the development of what they consider to be a reliable and valid measure of nausea and vomiting. The Rhodes INV is a 5-item, 5-point Likert-type questionnaire. Its purpose is to measure a patient's perception of the following: (1) duration of nausea, (2) frequency of nausea, (3) distress from nausea, (4) frequency of vomiting, and (5) amount of vomiting. The authors attempted to measure concurrent validity by asking family members of the patients to rate each of the five items along with the patients' rating. The authors reported good agreement between the ratings of patients and family members, but they admit that for the nausea items, one would expect agreement because the only way that the family members could rate the patient's nausea was by asking the patient.

Morrow's Assessment of Nausea and Emesis (MANE)

Morrow first described the MANE, a measure of both anticipatory and postchemotherapy nausea and vomiting, in 1984. He discussed its psychometric properties in a later article (Morrow, 1992). In the MANE frequency of anticipatory nausea, posttreatment nausea, anticipatory vomiting, and posttreatment vomiting are each assessed by a separate 4-point scale. Duration is quantified by having the patient write in the number of hours that the nausea and/or vomiting lasted. Severity of each response is assessed separately by a 6-point scale from "very mild" to "intolerable." The time during which the patient's nausea is at its worst is assessed by a 6-point scale from "during treatment" to "24 or more hours after treatment." The MANE is used by many researchers, but Muth et al. (1996) pointed out a shortcoming of this assessment tool in that it lacks a definition, operational or otherwise, of nausea. And the nausea experienced by one chemotherapy patient might be qualitatively different from that experienced by another patient, or by a fisherman suffering from seasickness.

Melzack et al. Nausea Questionnaire

Melzack et al. (1985) describe what they call a new approach to measuring nausea. Melzack had been studying pain for many years and in a pilot study of chemotherapy patients noted that many of the words used by the patients to describe their nausea were the same words used to describe pain in the McGill Pain Questionnaire. Therefore, in their 1985 study, the authors measured nausea of 25 chemotherapy patients using the descriptors and overall intensity scale of the McGill Pain Questionnaire along with an appropriate VAS. The authors reported finding a significant correlation between the Nausea Rating Index (NRI)-Affective (the patient ranking of the first five items in the questionnaire) and physicians' and nurses' estimates. The same was true for items 6–9. A significant correlation was found between the scores that make up the Nausea Questionnaire except for that between the NRI-Miscellaneous (items 6–9) and VAS scores.

Muth et al. Nausea Profile (NP)

The rationale behind the development of the NP was that nausea is probably not a simple symptom that is manifested in a similar manner across different individuals and situations. Rather, the authors conceptualized nausea as a complex syndrome with several dimensions, each of which could be measured. The NP was designed to measure the following three dimensions of nausea: (1) somatic distress, (2) GI distress, and (3) emotional distress. A total nausea score is also obtained. The initial study (Muth et al., 1996) consisted of four stages: descriptors were generated, categorized into three dimensions using factor analysis, and reevaluated to verify their reliability. In the final stage, the total nausea score from the NP was compared to VAS reports of nausea from subjects exposed to a rotating optokinetic drum to provoke nausea. The total NP score and the VAS score for nausea were highly correlated ($r = 0.71$, $p < 0.0 1$).

The Nausea Profile (NP) is a subjective symptom checklist used to describe the complex sensation of nausea. The NP can be used to evaluate an individual's nausea and how it changes over time as well as to compare the experience of nausea between individuals and situations. Figure 9.1 is a copy of the Nausea Profile questionnaire.

The subject or patient rates his or her experience of each of 17 descriptors on a scale of 0 (not at all) to 9 (severe). To score the NP: (1) sum the total points scored; (2) sum the points scored for questions 1, 3, 5, 9, 16, 17 (somatic distress); (3) sum the points scored for questions 4, 6, 13, 14, 15 (GI distress); and (4) sum the points scored for questions 2, 7, 8, 10, 11, 12 (emotional distress). Then calculate total nausea, somatic distress, GI distress, and emotional distress as follows: total nausea = (total of all items/153) x 100%; somatic distress = (total of somatic distress items/54) x 100%; GI distress = (total of GI distress items/45) x 100%; and emotional distress = (total of emotional distress items/54) x 100%.

BEHAVIORAL INDICATIONS OF NAUSEA

The rationale for using indirect measures of nausea is that a change in the patient or research subject's level of nausea will be manifested in observable changes in behavior. Two indirect measures of nausea that have been used in the past are measures of the patient's appetite (Heim & Queisser, 1982), and time interval until the patient is able to resume eating or drinking (Neidhart et al., 1981). Other indirect measures of nausea have included the patient's general well-being (Heim & Queisser, 1982), chart review of patient symptoms (Fetting et al., 1982a), and telephone follow-up with the patient in addition to the patient self-report (Orr & McKernan, 1981). As Morrow (1984a) has concluded, "While not a substitute for either self-report or observer-rated measures that relate more closely to the nausea or vomiting itself, indirect measures can, if they are not intrusive, yield valuable additional information" (p. 2271).

BIOMARKERS OF NAUSEA

There are several biomarkers that seem to change systematically with reports of nausea; but, since little is known about cause and effect, it is more appropriate

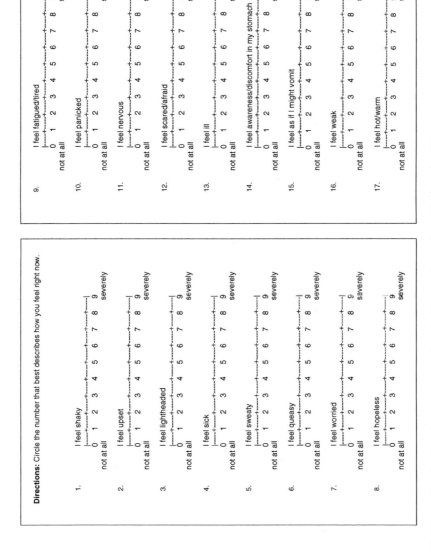

Figure 9.1 Nausea Profile Questionnaire. Reproduced with permission from Muth et al., 1996.

to refer to these changes as correlates of nausea rather than measures of nausea. Since these physiological changes that frequently accompany reports of nausea were discussed in Chapters 4–7 (in this volume), we will simply list them below showing the expected direction of change with increasing severity of nausea, along with methods of measurement and references.

Autonomic Nervous System Changes

As discussed in Chapter 5 (in this volume), an increase in sympathetic nervous system (SNS) activity often accompanies reports of nausea. The recording and analysis of skin conductance, a noninvasive measure of SNS activity, is described in Stern, Ray, and Quigley (2000, Chap. 13). Nausea is usually accompanied by a decrease in parasympathetic nervous system (PNS) activity or vagal tone. PNS activity can be measured noninvasively as a change in heart rate variability (see Stern, Ray & Quigley, 2000, Chap. 12).

Endocrine Changes

As reported in Chapter 6 (in this volume), the endocrine response that has been found to increase with reports of nausea and decrease as nausea subsides is vasopressin (Koch et al., 1990b). Vasopressin can be measured in blood samples and has the closest association with onset and offset of nausea of the hormones or neurotransmitters that have been measured during the acute onset of nausea during vection. Figure 9.2 is an example showing marked increases in plasma vasopressin that were observed along with gastric dysrhythmias and nausea provoked by exposure to a rotating optokinetic drum.

Gastric Changes

As described in Chapter 7 (in this volume), the two related measures of gastric myoelectric activity that correlate with increases in reports of nausea are decreases in normal 3 cpm activity and increases in tachygastria. These changes in gastric activity can be measured noninvasively using electrogastrography (EGG). Figure 9.3 shows an example of an abrupt loss of normal 3 cpm EGG activity in a pregnant woman with morning sickness. The figure shows that during the loss of 3 cpm rhythm, the subject experienced nausea. As the normal 3 cpm EGG pattern was reestablished, she reported the sensation of nausea had disappeared. Thus, the presence or absence of the 3 cpm rhythm correlated with the presence or absence of nausea.

   Correction of gastric dysrhythmias with the prokinetic agent domperidone has been observed in patients with chronic nausea and diabetic gastroparesis. (Figure 9.4). The upper two tracings in the figure show an EGG recording from a patient with bradygastria recorded at baseline (Month 0). She was then given 20 mg of domperidone by mouth four times per day. EGGs were repeated every two months. Nausea symptoms began to improve by Month 2, and by Month 4 the EGG recordings showed a clear 3 cpm pattern. The EGG recording at Month 6 shows normal 3 cpm EGG activity. During this 6-month

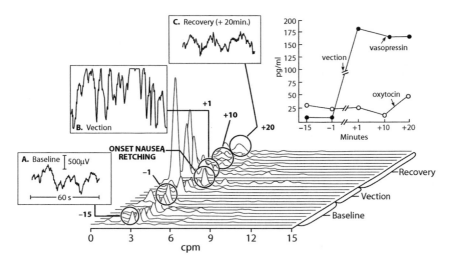

Figure 9.2 EGG changes and plasma vasopressin response during illusory self-motion and nausea induced by a rotating drum. The EGG rhythm strips are labeled (A) Baseline, (B) Vection, and (C) Recovery. Note that during (B) there are high amplitude 5–8 cpm EGG waves reflecting tachygastria at the onset of illusory self-motion. In contrast, the EGG at Baseline (A) and at Recovery (C) shows normal 3 cpm EGG rhythms. The spectral analysis shows the cycles per minute (cpm) in the EGG signal on the X-axis. The times of Baseline, Vection (illusory self-motion), and Recovery periods are indicated on the Y-axis. The Z-axis indicates the power of the various frequencies in the EGG signal. Note the peaks at 5 and 6 cpm at the time of nausea and retching during Vection. Finally, plasma vasopressin and oxytocin are shown in the inset. The X-axis indicates minutes before drum rotation and the 1-, 10-, and 20-minute periods after drum rotation have stopped. Note the dramatically increased levels of vasopressin immediately after drum rotation stopped and during the time of nausea and tachygastria. Reproduced with permission from Koch et al., 1990c.

period of time, the EGG signal converted to a normal 3 cpm pattern, presumably due to the effect of the drug on the stomach (or centers in the brain). The lower two tracings in Figure 9.4 are from the other diabetic patient with gastroparesis and nausea who had tachygastria at baseline (Month 0). The patient was treated with domperidone, and nausea resolved over time and a normal 3 cpm EGG signal was established (Month 6). The beneficial effect on symptoms and EGG rhythms in these two patients was sustained for 12 months. Regardless of whether the site of action was central or peripheral (the stomach), the observation revealed the correlation between the tachygastria and nausea at baseline and the reestablishment of the normal 3 cpm EGG activity that correlated with the resolution of the nausea.

These two clinical examples indicate that shifts in ongoing gastric electrical rhythm occur and that the shifts to abnormal rhythm (tachygastria, bradygastria, nonspecific dysrhythmias) are associated with nausea; whereas, shifts

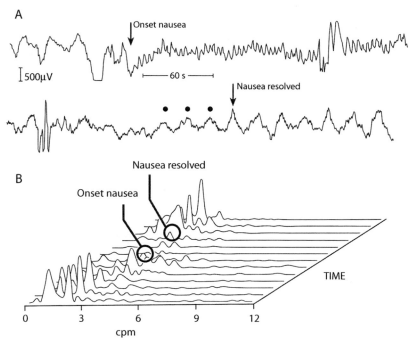

Figure 9.3 A. The tracing shows a continuous EGG recording for approximately 8 min. The EGG was recorded from a pregnant woman with morning sickness. At the beginning of the tracing, no nausea was reported. At the onset of nausea, there is loss of the 3 cpm EGG rhythm and start of a bradygastria (flatline) and the 16–17 per minute respiration signal. Several minutes later, nausea resolved as the 3 cpm normal EGG rhythm was reestablished. B. The running spectral analysis of the EGG signal recorded during the sudden onset of nausea is shown. Frequencies from 1 to 12 cpm are located on the X-axis, whereas time is on the Y-axis. The peaks represent the frequencies in the EGG signal. Note that at the time of onset of nausea there is loss of 3 cpm peaks and as nausea resolves, the normal 3 cpm signals return. These EGG recordings indicate that the sudden loss of the normal 3 cpm rhythm is associated with the onset of nausea. Modified and used with permission from Koch et al., 1990a.

from gastric dysrhythmias to the normal 3 cpm EGG pattern are associated with resolution of nausea. Gastric myoelectrical activity is an objective physiological measure (a "biomarker") that complements the "measurement" of the symptom of nausea. In fact, in many situations the onset of gastric dysrhythmias may be the cause of nausea symptoms, much as the onset of cardiac dysrhythmias (e.g., atrial fibrillation) is the cause of vague discomfort in the chest. The procedures for recording and analysis of the EGG are described in Chapters 4 and 5 in Koch and Stern (2004). Thus, control of gastric dysrhythmias is a potential therapeutic pathway for drug, diet, or device development in the treatment of nausea.

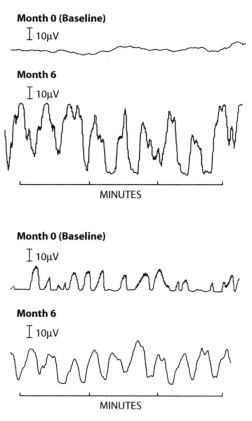

Figure 9.4 The effect of domperidone on bradygastria (upper two tracings) and tachygastria (lower two tracings) in two patients with nausea and diabetic gastroparesis is shown. The electrogastrogram (EGG) in the upper tracing shows a bradygastria pattern, a flatline signal with no rhythmic pattern, at Month 0. Domperidone (20 mg 4 times a day) was started and continued for 6 months. The EGG at 6 months shows clear and normal 3 cpm EGG activity. The lower tracing show a tachygastria at Month 0 before domperidone treatment; a 4–5 cpm tachygastria is seen. Domperidone was given for 6 months. Nausea resolved and the EGG recorded at Month 6 shows a normal 3 cpm EGG pattern. The eradication of nausea and the correction of the bradygastria and the tachygastria were attributed to treatment with domperidone.

CONCLUSIONS

As was stated at the beginning of this chapter, it is very difficult to measure nausea in humans for a variety of reasons. Behavioral measures are indirect. For example, loss of appetite might correlate highly with nausea for some people in some situations but, then again, it might not. Physiological correlates of nausea are just that, correlates. Some studies, particularly motion sickness studies, have reported significant correlations between autonomic nervous system and gastric myoelectric activity and nausea. But some subjects reported nausea and did not show the expected physiological changes, and others showed the physiological changes commonly associated with nausea and did not report experiencing nausea. The study of physiological markers of nausea is a promising area in need of additional research. Without it, only the patients or research subjects' self-reports are available. The issue of what nausea is should be considered before clinicians or researchers decide which self-report method to use to measure nausea. If one thinks of nausea as a simple symptom varying in severity, frequency, and duration for all people and in all nauseogenic situations, then one might use the Rhodes or MANE. If one thinks that nausea is a sensation very similar to pain, one might use Melzack's Nausea Questionnaire. But if one conceptualizes nausea as a complex syndrome with at least three dimensions, as do the authors of this volume, then one should use the Nausea Profile.

PART II: Management

Chapter 10

Diagnosis and Management
of Acute and Chronic Nausea

Acute nausea refers to nausea that is sudden in onset and resolves in 7–10 days. Nausea lasting more than 10 days is considered chronic nausea (Tack et al., 2006). Functional nausea is unexplained nausea in the setting of normal diagnostic tests. Fifteen percent of U.S. and Canadian adults have experienced nausea over a 3-month period (Frank et al., 2000). Additional statistics indicating the incidence of nausea are provided in Chapter 2 of this volume. Nausea is a component in the syndrome of functional dyspepsia, which affects almost 25% of the U.S. population (Camilleri et al., 2005). Symptoms of dysmotility-like functional dyspepsia include early satiety, fullness, epigastric discomfort, nausea, and vomiting. In this chapter the diagnosis and treatment of acute and chronic nausea are reviewed.

DEFINITIONS

Nausea is a sometimes difficult-to-describe sick or queasy sensation usually experienced in the epigastrium. Vomiting is the forceful expulsion of gastric content through the mouth. Nausea is often, but not always, linked with vomiting, but nausea generally precedes vomiting and vomiting usually cures nausea at least temporarily (Koch, 2001b). Vomiting should be differentiated from regurgitation and rumination. Regurgitation is the gentle but unpleasant return of liquids or solids from the stomach into the mouth that is experienced by patients with gastroesophageal reflux disease. Patients with motility disorders such as achalasia also experience regurgitation of esophageal contents. Rumination, in contrast, is the effortless return of solid foods from the stomach to the mouth in the absence of any noxious sensation such as heartburn or chest discomfort.

PATHOPHYSIOLOGY OF NAUSEA

Nausea remains poorly understood in terms of pathophysiologic and biopsychosocial mechanisms (see Chapters 4–7, in this volume). There are many different stimuli that evoke nausea. The critical neurohormonal circuits that mediate nausea are probably different depending on the nauseogenic stimulus. For example, the onset of severe and acute nausea during motion correlates with the onset of gastric dysrhythmias such as tachygastrias and the release of vasopressin from the posterior pituitary (Koch et al., 1990a). Vomiting but not nausea evoked by chemotherapy agents is reduced by specific 5-HT$_3$ receptor antagonists (Roscoe et al., 2000), and similarly nausea due to motion sickness is also not reduced (Levine et al., 2000). Women in the first trimester of pregnancy who report nausea often have gastric dysrhythmias (Koch et al., 1990b; Walsh et al., 1996), whereas estrogen and progesterone can induce gastric dysrhythmias and nausea in nonpregnant healthy women (Koch & Frissora, 2003). Nausea can be an atypical symptom associated with occult gastroesophageal reflux (Brzana & Koch, 1997). Nausea evoked by antral distention with balloons suggests that stretch of the gastric walls is another mechanism underlying this symptom (Owyang & Hasler, 2002). Gastric dysrhythmias are frequently present in patients with nausea, with or without gastroparesis (Koch, Hong & Xu, 2000; Parkman et al., 1997). Thus, causes of nausea include but are not limited to (1) central nervous system perturbations, (2) chemotherapy agents, (3) hormonal changes, and (4) mucosal and neuromuscular disorders of the stomach.

DIFFERENTIAL DIAGNOSIS

Many general diagnostic categories need to be considered when evaluating patients with unexplained nausea and vomiting (see Table 10.1). The evaluation of acute or chronic nausea can be straightforward, but at other times it is difficult. The differential diagnosis for acute and chronic nausea and vomiting is extensive, and the physician must review many categories of disease (Koch, 2006). In the approach outlined below in Table 10.1, 15 categories of disease causing acute and chronic nausea and vomiting are reviewed.

The work-up of chronic nausea and vomiting begins with a reasonable differential diagnosis of the diseases and disorders that may be causing these symptoms. The first distinction to make is whether or not the patient has a *specific abdominal pain* that accompanies the nausea and vomiting.

Thus, the first diagnostic category to consider is *mechanical obstruction*. Obstructions of the gastrointestinal tract from the pylorus to the duodenum to the small intestine to the colon are associated with abdominal pain located in the epigastrium or the periumbilical area or lower quadrants. Pain, which may be crampy in nature, precedes the onset of the nausea and vomiting in these patients with mechanical obstructions. The same is true if there are obstructions of the cystic duct, common bile duct, or pancreatic duct with stones. Therefore, careful attention to the quality, the timing, and the radiation of any *pain* in patients with nausea and vomiting is critically important. If a specific obstruction is identified, then specific treatment can be offered. In the realm of mechanical obstructions, the treatment is often very effective and definitive, whether by surgery, stent, balloon dilatation, or sphincterotomy.

Mucosal inflammation or peptic ulcer disease is another common cause of nausea and vomiting. That is, any mucosal irritation of the esophagus,

Table 10.1 Causes of Chronic Nausea and Vomiting

1. Mechanical Obstruction (pylorus, duodenum, small intestine, colon)
2. Mucosal Inflammation
3. Peritoneal Irritation
4. Carcinomas (gastric, ovarian, renal)
5. Metabolic/Endocrine Disorders (diabetes mellitus, hypothyroidism, hyperthyroidism, adrenal insufficiency)
6. Medications (anticholinergics, narcotics, L-dopa, progesterone, calcium channel blockers, chemotherapy agents, lubiprostone)
7. Chronic Mesenteric Ischemia
8. Post–Gastric Surgery (vagotomy/antrectomy, Roux-en-Y, fundoplication)
9. Intestinal Pseudo-Obstruction Syndromes
10. Myopathic Disorders (hollow viscous myopathy, scleroderma, muscular dystrophy)
11. Neuropathic Disorders (hollow viscous neuropathy, Parkinson's, paraneoplastic syndrome, Shy-Drager)
12. Central Nervous System Disorders (tumors, migraine, partial complex seizures)
13. Psychogenic Disorders (anorexia nervosa, bulimia)
14. Idiopathic Gastroparesis with or without Gastric Dysrhythmias
15. Cyclic Vomiting Syndrome

stomach, or duodenum, ranging from gastritis to erosions to frank ulceration, may be associated with nausea and vomiting. Some degree of burning discomfort is often times present as well. These diseases are usually easily identified with standard upper endoscopy. Treatments include proton pump inhibitors (PPI) and histamine$_2$ receptor antagonists.

Peritoneal irritation is an unusual cause of chronic nausea, but intra-abdominal abscesses, chronic peritoneal irritation with bacterial or fungal infections or carcinoma may present with nausea and vomiting.

Carcinomas of certain types may be especially nauseogenic. Infiltrating cancer of the stomach, for example, may present with nausea, vomiting, and gastroparesis. Other cancers that are nauseogenic include ovarian cancers, hypernephromas, and small cell cancers of the lungs with the paraneoplastic syndromes that are associated with gastroparesis.

Metabolic and endocrine disorders should be considered in the differential diagnosis of nausea and vomiting. Type 1 and Type 2 diabetes are straight-forward diagnoses in most cases. Almost 50% of patients with Type 1 or Type 2 diabetes mellitus (T2DM) have gastroparesis, and recent comprehensive reviews are available (Hasler, 2007; Intagliata & Koch, 2007). Patients with T2DM may have only subtle dyspepsia-like symptoms. Uremia and hypercalcemia are associated with nausea and vomiting and hypothyroidism is also associated with gastroparesis. In some patients with hyperthyroidism there may be loss of appetite and nausea. Adrenal insufficiency is a medical emergency in patients with nausea, vomiting, volume depletion, and low potassium.

While not specifically a metabolic or endocrine disorder per se, in the first trimester of pregnancy, nausea and vomiting occur in almost 80% of women (see Chapter 12 in this volume).

Medications can also be nauseogenic. Almost all medications have some percentage of nausea and vomiting associated with their use. NSAIDS are probably the most common. GI drugs such as PPIs, lubiprostone, and others have a high incidence of nausea (Johanson et al., 2008). Patients' medication lists should be examined, and drugs with a higher incidence of nausea, such as narcotics, cardiac antiarrhythmic drugs, estrogen, and progesterone should be identified.

Ischemic gastroparesis is an unusual type of gastroparesis that also may present with nausea and vomiting and very little pain. These patients have chronic mesenteric ischemia with 2 of 3 mesenteric arteries occluded, usually by atherosclerotic plaques. Only 50% of these patients have an abdominal bruit and weight loss. The gastroparesis can be totally corrected with vascular stents or bypass graft surgery (Liberski et al., 1990).

Gastric surgeries may be a source of nausea and vomiting. After vagotomy or after resection of any major region of the stomach, nausea and vomiting can be a major problem. Chronic nausea and vomiting and gastroparesis may occur after fundoplication. Fundic resection with esophageal resection and mobilization of the stomach and anastomosis of the stomach with the esophagus within the chest frequently results in nausea, vomiting, gastric dysrhythmia, and gastroparesis. Billroth I, Billroth II, and Roux-en-Y operations have all been associated with severe gastroparesis, nausea, and vomiting.

Intestinal pseudo-obstruction should be considered in patients who have gastroparesis and dilated small bowel or colon. These patients often have GERD. Thus, neuromuscular dysfunction of the entire GI tract from stomach to colon is present. Degenerative disorders of the enteric nerves, smooth muscles, or interstitial cells of Cajal may be primary mechanisms (Owyang & Hasler, 2002). Pseudo-obstruction may be secondary to systemic disorders such as scleroderma or amyloidosis.

Central nervous system disorders should be considered during differential diagnosis. Causes of nausea and vomiting from disorders outside the GI tract should be considered in the patient with chronic nausea and vomiting. These disorders include migraine, CNS infections, tumors, complex partial seizures, vestibular nerve lesions, and Parkinson's disease. Careful history and neurological examination will reveal these lesions. Referral to neurologists may be required.

Eating disorders such as anorexia nervosa, bulimia nervosa, and psychogenic vomiting occur in the population, but these patients rarely present to the gastroenterologist for evaluation and treatment. Thus, these are uncommon diagnoses to consider in a gastroenterology practice.

Idiopathic nausea and vomiting are another category to consider. In these patients the symptoms are chronic and vague epigastric discomfort, early satiety, and prolonged fullness are present, all of which may be incorporated into the vague symptom complex of functional dyspepsia (Stangellini, Tosetti &

Paternico, 1996). Within the group of patients with functional dyspepsia or unexplained nausea and vomiting, many have definable gastric neuromuscular disorders that range from gastric dysrhythmias like tachygastria to frank gastroparesis (Koch, 2003). Some of these patients also have abnormalities of gastric relaxation and others may have visceral hypersensitivity. To obtain a specific diagnosis in these patients, tests of gastric neuromuscular function are required.

CAVEATS IN THE NAUSEA HISTORY AND PHYSICAL EXAM

Is abdominal pain present? A key aspect in determining the cause of nausea is whether abdominal pain is present. Does the patient have a mechanical obstruction of the gastrointestinal or biliary-pancreatic tract? If pain is followed by bilious vomiting, mechanical obstruction of the small bowel must be excluded. The diagnostic approach in patients with nausea and pain should be based on the characteristics of the pain. Is the irritable bowel syndrome the source of pain? About 30% of patients with irritable bowel syndrome also have nausea and dyspepsia (Coresetti et al., 2004). Is there an abdominal wall syndrome that accounts for the pain (Carnett, 1926)?

Have occult gastroesophageal reflux disease (GERD) and gallbladder disease been considered? Atypical GERD may present with prominent nausea and little or no heartburn (Koch, 2000b), and nausea that is present on awakening is common. Gallbladder dysfunction and chronic cholecystitis may be difficult to diagnosis and association with postprandial nausea may not be clear-cut.

Have endocrine disorders been excluded? Metabolic causes of chronic nausea, such as Addison's disease, must be considered because severe cortisol deficiency is life-threatening. Hyperthyroidism and hypothyroidism may be overlooked. Fasting cortisol and thyroid-stimulating hormone levels should be obtained. Electrolytes, calcium, and magnesium levels should be measured.

Are neurologic symptoms present? If blurred vision or recurrent headaches are concurrent symptoms, a computerized axial tomographic (CAT) scan of the head, and neurology consultation should be considered. Patients with central nervous system diseases (e.g., partial complex seizures) may present with unexplained nausea.

THE PHYSICAL EXAM

The general examination may reveal signs of weight loss, dehydration, and poor nutrition. Inspection of dentition may show erosion of enamel associated with bulimia or chronic GERD. Abdominal examination will detect masses, organomegaly, and the areas of tenderness. The presence of abdominal distension and succession splash should be looked for. Auscultation of the abdomen may detect bruits that indicate stenosis of the mesenteric arteries. The presence of Carnett's sign should be determined, especially when healed incisions are noted on the abdominal wall (Carnett, 1926). As mentioned above, a neurologic examination may reveal nystagmus, facial weakness, ataxia, or other abnormalities.

AN APPROACH TO THE PATIENT WITH UNEXPLAINED ACUTE OR CHRONIC NAUSEA AND VOMITING

Acute Nausea and Vomiting

The entities from 1 to 11 listed in Table 10.1 may present as acute symptoms. A specific diagnosis should be made if possible. The most common causes of acute nausea and vomiting are viral infections (acute gastroenteritis) or food poisoning, and these are usually self-limited. If severe, intravenous hydration may be needed.

Chronic Nausea and Vomiting

Common causes of nausea and vomiting have usually been eliminated early in the evaluation by normal upper gastrointestinal (GI) series, CAT scans of the abdomen and head, and routine laboratory studies. Specific structural or neuromuscular diagnoses that are associated with nausea and vomiting are excluded, but the symptoms continue.

If a gastroenterologist is seeing the patient, then an upper endoscopy is usually performed to rule out mucosal diseases that may be undetected by radiographic studies. The presence of esophagitis may be significant because acid reflux may account for the nausea. Gastritis or duodenitis may be associated with nausea. In dyspepsia patients, gastric cancers are detected in less than 1% of the patients undergoing endoscopy (Delany et al., 2000). In patients with unexplained nausea and dyspepsia, the upper endoscopy shows mucosal abnormality in 50%–60% of the cases. Most patients referred for chronic nausea have already received acid-suppression therapy with proton pump inhibitors. On the other hand, 40%–50% of these symptomatic patients have normal upper endoscopy examination results. These patients frequently remain without a specific diagnosis. Gastric neuromuscular disorders should be considered next as a cause of the nausea.

BEYOND ENDOSCOPY: DIAGNOSING GASTRIC NEUROMUSCULAR DISORDERS

An objective diagnosis of neuromuscular disorders of the stomach can be established by the results of gastric emptying tests and electrogastrography. See Table 10.2 and Koch (2006).

Gastric Emptying Tests

Solid Phase Gastric Emptying Study

The most validated solid phase gastric emptying study uses Eggbeaters® with two pieces of white toast and jam. After an overnight fast, the subject ingests

Table 10.2 Categories of Pathophysiologic Abnormalities in Patients with Nausea and Vomiting based on EGG and Gastric Emptying

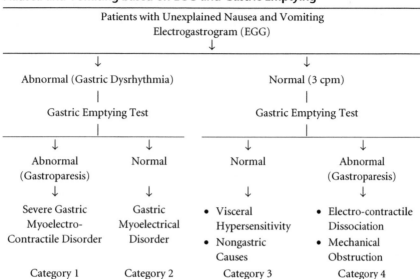

the meal in the nuclear medicine department. The eggs are cooked with technetium sulfur colloid. Scans are obtained at times 0, 1 hour, 2 hours, and 4 hours. In healthy subjects less than 10% of the meal remains after 4 hours. If more than 10% of the meal remains in the stomach after 4 hours, then the diagnosis of gastroparesis is made (Tougas et al., 2000). The *cause* of gastroparesis is not established by this test.

Wireless Manometry /pH Capsule

The Smartpill® capsule (Smartpill Corp, Buffalo, NY) measures intraluminal pH and pressure throughout the GI tract. This FDA-approved device is swallowed with a standard 250-calorie test meal. The time to empty this nondigestible solid from the stomach is approximately 5 hours in healthy subjects. If the time to empty the capsule is greater than 5 hours, then delayed gastric emptying is present (Kuo et al., 2008). Gastric pH and pressure data are also recorded by the capsule. Additional data on small bowel transit and colonic transit are available from the measurements.

Breath Tests

Breath tests using C13-labeled Spirulina and octanoic acid are available, but not yet approved by the FDA. These tests require the collection of breath samples over a 2-hour period after ingestion of the labeled test meal. Rate of gastric emptying is reflected in the measurement of C13 in timed breath samples. Breath tests require normal absorption of the foods from the small bowel, and normal liver and lung function to properly reflect the rate of gastric emptying of the test meal.

SPECT and MRI

SPECT and MRI images of the stomach can measure gastric emptying but are more complex procedures in that they involve CT scans performed in departments of radiology.

Electrogastrography

Electrical pacesetter rhythms occurring in the stomach are recorded as electro-gastrograms (EGGs; Koch & Stern, 2004). Electrodes are placed on the surface of the abdomen to record EGGs. Gastric electrical rhythms are filtered and recorded in an analog form as a raw EGG signal. The EGG signal is digitized and the frequency is analyzed with running spectral analysis with a commercially available and FDA-approved medical device. EGG rhythms range from the normal 2.5 to 3.75 cycles per minute (cpm) to abnormal rhythms such as bradygastria (0–2.5 cpm), tachygastria (3.75–10 cpm), and mixed gastric dysrhythmias, which include both tachygastria and bradygastria. For more information about electrogastrography, the reader is referred to Koch and Stern (2004).

EGG and gastric emptying tests are complementary in defining gastric neuromuscular disorders (Parkman et al., 1997; Brzana, Koch & Bingaman, 1998). By assessing the gastric electrical activity and the gastric emptying rates from individual patients, pathophysiological categories are defined (Koch, 2006):

1. Gastric dysrhythmia and gastroparesis
2. Gastric dysrhythmia and normal gastric emptying
3. Normal gastric electrical rhythm and normal gastric emptying
4. Normal gastric electrical rhythm and gastroparesis

By combining the results of the EGG and gastric emptying tests (Table 10.3), four pathophysiologic categories of gastric neuromuscular function and rational treatment approaches can be identified in the patient with nausea.

Category 1   These patients have severe neuromuscular dysfunction with gastric dysrhythmias such as tachygastria and gastroparesis. For example, patients with longstanding Type 1 or 2 diabetes mellitus may be in category 1. On the other hand, 20%–30% of patients with "functional dyspepsia" have gastric dysrhythmias and gastroparesis (Parkman et al., 1997). Patients in category 1 often have severe symptoms, require many drugs, and some may require venting gastrostomies and enteral feeding and gastric pacing, as discussed below.

Category 2   These patients have gastric dysrhythmias and *normal* gastric emptying rates. In a group of patients with functional dyspepsia, 40%–60% had gastric dysrhythmias and normal gastric empting (Koch & Bingaman, 1998). These patients had a significantly better response to the prokinetic agent cisapride compared with patients with normal EGG recordings (Bersherdas et al., 1998). Prokinetic agents such as cisapride and zelnorm have been withdrawn from the market.

Table 10.3 Treatment of Nausea and Vomiting Based on Gastric Electrical and Emptying Test Results

Category 1	Category 2	Category 3	Category 4
Test Results	*Test Results*	*Test Results*	*Test Results*
Gastric Dysrhythmia and Gastroparesis	Gastric Dysrhythmia and Normal Emptying	Normal Gastric Rhythm and Emptying	Normal Gastric Rhythm and Gastroparesis
Diagnosis	*Diagnosis*	*Diagnosis*	*Diagnosis*
Severe Gastric Myoelectric-Contractile Disorder	Gastric Myoelectrical Disorder	Visceral Hypersensitivity	†† Mechanical Obstruction • Electrocontractile Dissociation
Treatment	*Treatment*	*Treatment*	*Treatment*
Nausea/Vomiting Diet, Prokinetic Agents, G-tube/J-tube, Hyperalimentation, Acustimulation, Gastric Electrical Stimulation	Nausea/Vomiting Diet, Prokinetic Agents	Nausea/Vomiting Diet ? Neurosensory Agents, Tricyclic Agents, Drugs for Fundic/Antrum Relaxation † Further Workup for Nongastric Causes	†† Surgery • Nausea/Vomiting Diet • Prokinetic Agents

Modified and used with permission from Koch, 2006.
†† indicates a diagnosis of mechanical obstruction is treated with appropriate surgery.

Category 3   These patients have normal EGG rhythms and normal gastric emptying. In these patients, the normal endoscopy, normal gastric myoelectrical activity, and normal gastric emptying indicate that the nausea symptoms are likely due to visceral hypersensitivity or nongastric causes. In patients with normal EGG rhythms, normal gastric emptying, and unexplained nausea, visceral hypersensitivity may indeed be a tenable diagnosis. An uncontrolled trial of a tricyclic antidepressant such as amitriptyline alleviated nausea in approximately 70% of patients with unexplained nausea (Prakash et al., 1998).

Other nongastric diagnoses should also be considered. In these patients, a 24-hour pH study may confirm the relationship between nausea and GERD. A cholecystokinin-stimulated gallbladder emptying study scan may document gallbladder dysfunction in the absence of cholelithiasis. If postprandial abdominal discomfort and disturbed bowel function are components of the nausea, irritable bowel syndrome should be considered in these patients and treated appropriately. Central nervous system causes of nausea should also be reassessed.

Category 4   These patients have normal or high-amplitude 3-cpm EGG signals and gastroparesis. High amplitude, extraordinarily regular 3-cpm waves and gastroparesis are discordant findings, but have been reported in patients with mechanical obstructions of the stomach and duodenum (Brzana, Koch & Bingaman, 1998). Alternatively, patients with a normal-amplitude 3-cpm pattern and gastroparesis may have a form of electromechanical dissociation.

Further Questions to Consider in the Diagnosis of Unexplained Nausea and Vomiting

1. Is the patient describing vomiting or regurgitation or rumination?
2. Could the nausea be due to occult or atypical GERD? In such patients, early morning symptoms are common and substernal "burning" may or may not present in association with the nausea.
3. Is there a history of vascular disease? Is there an abdominal bruit?
4. Is constipation or irritable bowel syndrome present? Nausea, bloating, and abdominal discomfort may be due more to the IBS than the gastroparesis.
5. Is pylorospasm or subtotal small bowel obstruction the cause of "obstructive gastroparesis"?
6. In the patient with refractory symptoms, have psychosocial stresses, eating disorders, and rumination been considered?

TREATMENT APPROACHES FOR ACUTE AND CHRONIC NAUSEA

Knowledge of the neuromuscular function of the stomach is important for the physician and neurogastroenterologist when diagnosing and treating nausea and vomiting due to underlying neuromuscular disorders of the stomach.

Dietary Counseling

Patients with acute or chronic nausea and vomiting may benefit from dietary counseling. Patients with acute nausea and vomiting from gastroenteritis or food poisoning need to stay hydrated. The Nausea/Vomiting (Gastroparesis) Diet is designed with liquid and solid foods that are easy for the stomach to mix and empty (Table 10.4) (Koch, 2001b). The Nausea/Vomiting Diet is a 3-step diet with increasing work for the stomach as the diet is advanced.

The diet is important for patients with gastric neuromuscular disorders described above. Step 1 is primarily electrolyte solutions that are consumed in small amounts to avoid dehydration. Liquids require less gastric neuromuscular work to empty than solid foods. For those patients who tolerate step 1, step 2 may be tried next. Step 2 diet includes soups containing noodles or rice. Milk-based, creamy soups are avoided. A dissolvable or liquid multiple vitamin should be taken daily. Step 3 emphasizes starches and chicken and turkey breast meats. These solid foods require less gastric work to mix and

Table 10.4 Nausea and Vomiting Diet

Diet	Goal	Avoid
Step 1: **Sports drinks and bouillon** For severe nausea and vomiting: • Small volumes of salty liquids, with some caloric content to avoid dehydration • Multiple vitamin	1000–1500 cc/day in multiple servings (e.g., 12 120 cc servings over 12–14 hr) Patient can sip 30 cc at a time to reach approximately 120 cc/hr	Citrus drinks of all kinds; highly sweetened drinks
Step 2: **Soups** If sports drink or bouillon tolerated: • Soup with noodles or rice and crackers • Peanut butter, cheese, and crackers in small amounts • Caramels or other chewy confection • Ingest above foods in at least 6 small-volume meals/day • Protein drinks • Multiple vitamin	Approximately 1500 calories/day to avoid dehydration and maintain weight (often more realistic than weight gain)	Creamy, milk-based liquids
Step 3: **Starches, chicken, fish** If Step 2 is tolerated: • Noodles, pastas, potatoes (mashed or baked), rice, baked chicken breast, fish (all easily mixed and emptied by the stomach) • Ingest solids in at least 6 small-volume meals/day • Multiple vitamin	Common foods that patient finds interesting and satisfying and that evoke minimal nausea/vomiting symptoms	Fatty foods that delay gastric emptying; red meats and fresh vegetables that require considerable trituration; pulpy fibrous foods that promote formation of bezoars

Modified and used with permission from Koch, 2006.

empty than do fresh vegetables or red meats. Fried and greasy foods are avoided because fats delay gastric emptying.

Drug Therapy for Chronic Nausea

Some patients may need IV fluids, phenergan, or ondansetron to treat dehydration and to reduce nausea and vomiting, respectively. Few drugs have specific actions on the stomach's neuromuscular apparatus to improve stomach function and treat symptoms of nausea and vomiting (see Table 10.5). First-line GI drugs have effects on gastric contractility or gastric dysrhythmias and are used for patients in categories 1 and 2 (see Table 10.3). Nonspecific antinauseant and antiemetic drugs such as prochlorperazine, diphenylamine, and amitriptyline have variable effects on nausea from gastric neuromuscular disorders. Patients with severe nausea who cannot tolerate oral medications require sublingual, intravenous, or intramuscular antiemetic agents. These include metoclopramide, erythromycin, droperidol, and ondansetron and are primarily used for patients hospitalized with recalcitrant nausea and vomiting. In the United States cisapride and domperidone can be obtained via a

Table 10.5 Drugs Used to Treat Symptoms Associated with Gastroparesis and Gastric Neuromuscular Disorders

Drug	Mechanisms of Action	Dosage	Side Effects
Prokinetic Agents			
metoclopramide	Dopamine (D_2) receptor antagonist, 5-HT_3-receptor antagonist, 5-HT_4 agonist	5–20 mg before meals and at bedtime	Extrapyramidal symptoms, dystonic reactions, anxiety, drowsiness, hyperprolactinemia
cisapride (compassionate program only)	5-HT_4-receptor agonist	5–20 mg before meals	Cardiac dysrhythmias, diarrhea, abdominal discomfort
erythromycin	Motilin agonist	125–250 mg QID	Nausea, diarrhea, abdominal cramps, rash
domperidone (new drug application program)	D_2-receptor antagonist (peripheral)	10–20 mg before meals and at bedtime	Hyperprolactinemia
tegaserod (compassionate program only)	Partial $5HT_4$ agonist	6 mg BID or 2 mg TID	Diarrhea, abdominal pain
Neurosensory Agents			
droperidol	Central dopamine antagonist	2.5–5.0 mg, IV	Sedation, hypotension
alprazolam	CNS sites, benzodiazepine	0.5 mg TID	Drowsiness, lightheadedness
Clonidine	Central alpha-adrenergic agonist	0.1–0.3 mg BID	Dry mouth, drowsiness, dizziness
alosetron (n/a in USA)	$5HT_3$ antagonist	1.0 mg BID	Constipation, ischemic colitis

Table 10.5 (*continued*)

Drug	Mechanisms of Action	Dosage	Side Effects
Nondrug Therapies			
Gastroparesis Diet	Diet based on gastric emptying physiology	See Table 10.4	None
High Protein Drinks	Decreases gastric dysrhythmias	Unknown	None
Gastrostomy	Venting distended stomach	As needed	Skin infections
Jejunostomy	Nutritional support	As needed	Skin infections
Gastric Electrical Stimulation	Unknown		Pocket infections
Gastric Pacemakers	Decreases gastric dysrhythmia, increases rate of gastric emptying		Pocket infections
Total Parental Nutrition	Bypass paralyzed GI tract		Sepsis

compassionate clearance or IND program. Balloon dilation of the pylorus improves gastric emptying in patients with category 4 parameters of gastroparesis and normal 3 cpm EGG patterns (Noar, Koch & Levine, 2004).

Nondrug Treatments for Chronic Nausea

Acupuncture, acupressure, and acustimulation applied at P6 reduces: (1) nausea of pregnancy (Dundee et al., 1988), (2) nausea due to chemotherapy agents (Ezzo et al., 2005), (3) postoperative nausea and vomiting (Gan et al., 2004), and (4) the nausea of motion sickness (Hu, Stern & Koch, 1992; Stern et al., 2001b). For additional discussion of the use of the acupuncture procedure to reduce nausea, see the specific chapter of interest in this volume, e.g., Chapter 12, "Nausea of Pregnancy."

The alternative medicine approach to treatment of nausea with herbs may merit further study: powdered ginger (1 gram) given 1 hour before vection-induced motion sickness has been shown to decrease nausea associated with gastric dysrhythmias (Lien et al, 2003). Protein drinks decreased nausea of pregnancy (Jednak et al., 1999), motion sickness (Levine et al., 2004), and postchemotherapy treatment nausea (Levine et al., 2008). These protein-based meal approaches to therapy have not been evaluated for treatments of chronic nausea due to gastroparesis or gastric dysrhythmias.

Venting Gastrostomy

For category 1 patients with chronic nausea and vomiting, a venting gastrostomy may be placed to improve quality of life. The gastrostomy does not treat the underlying disorder but allows the patients to empty the dysfunctional stomach rather than suffer repeated episodes of severe emesis (AGA, 2001). A jejunal feeding tube for enteral nutrition is frequently needed to provide basic caloric support for these patients. Total parenteral nutrition via central intravenous catheters should be avoided if at all possible because of the frequent development of line sepsis.

Gastric Electrical Stimulation and Nausea

The development of gastric electrical stimulation (GES) with implantable devices has attracted the attention of gastrointestinal researchers and clinicians interested in normalizing gastric activity in patients with chronic nausea and gastroparesis unresponsive to drug therapy (Abell et al., 2003). GES was first used to reduce paralytic ileus by Bilgutay et al. in 1963, but it is still considered an investigative technique. There are numerous aspects of GES that must be studied further in order to determine the optimal combination of stimulation factors such as frequency, amplitude, pulse width, time on, time off, etc. Another complication is the issue of when stimulation should be applied: all the time or only after eating? And a largely unexplored area is the issue of what type of stimulation will best improve gastric emptying and reduce symptoms in a patient with a specific type of motility abnormality?

Three different electrical stimulation methods are currently being investigated:

1. Low-frequency stimulation (e.g., 3 cpm), long duration (300 ms)—gastric electrical pacing;
2. High-frequency (e.g., 12 cpm), short duration (300 microsec)—gastric electrical stimulation (GES); and
3. Sequential neural electrical stimulation with multiple pairs of electrodes.

The first method aims to entrain or reestablish a regular slow-wave rhythm by stimulating at or near the stomach's normal slow wave frequency, i.e., 3 cpm in humans. High-frequency gastric electrical stimulation has also been used to increase gastric emptying and reduce symptoms such as nausea. The last method, sequential neural electrical gastric stimulation, consists of a microprocessor-controlled sequential activation of a series of annular electrodes that encircle the distal two-thirds of the stomach and induce propagated contractions causing a forceful emptying of the gastric content. However, to date this procedure has only been tested with dogs (Mintchev et al., 1998; Zhu et al., 2007), and no publications have appeared in which patients were studied using this procedure. On the other hand, there have been several publications that have described the use of both low and high frequency gastric stimulation for medically refractory gastroparesis (Abell et al., 2003; McCallum et al., 1998; Lin et al., 1998). Examples of studies that used the two modes of stimulation follow.

Lin et al. (1998) conducted an early investigation of "low frequency" gastric stimulation using a 3 cpm stimulus to pace or entrain the normal slow wave in patients with gastroparesis. Electrodes were placed on the serosal surface of the stomach of 13 patients. After a baseline recording of 30 min, electrical stimulation was performed on each patient in a number of sessions with different stimulating parameters. The authors concluded that stimulation at a frequency up to 10% higher than the normal 3 cpm and with an amplitude of 4mA and a pulse width of 300 ms was able to entrain the gastric slow wave and normalize gastric dysrhythmias in patients with gastroparesis. In a similar study on nine additional patients, McCallum et al. (1998) found that electrical stimulation entrained all nine subjects and converted tachygastrias in two patients into regular 3 cpm slow waves. Following 1 month of outpatient electrical stimulation treatment, gastric emptying was significantly improved, symptoms of gastroparesis were significantly reduced, and eight of nine patients no longer required jejunostomy tube feeding.

Abell et al. (2003) reported the results of a multicenter investigation of "high frequency" GES on 33 diabetic patients with gastroparesis. All patients received continuous high-frequency (12 cpm) GES. The patients were randomly assigned to a double-blind crossover design with stimulation ON or OFF for 1-month periods. Patients reported that they could not feel the stimulation. After the initial 2 months the blind was broken and all patients were put in the ON mode and evaluated after 6 and 12 months. Outcome measures included the following: vomiting frequency, preference for the ON or OFF condition, upper GI symptoms, quality of life, gastric emptying, and adverse events. Results of the initial double-blind portion of the study showed that the patients reported a significant preference for the ON condition, and they vomited significantly less during the ON versus OFF periods. During the second part of the study, vomiting frequency decreased significantly at 6 and 12 months, and scores for GI symptoms and quality of life improved significantly at 6 and 12 months. However, it should be noted that gastric emptying did not improve significantly. The overall conclusion of this study was that high frequency GES improves GI symptoms but does not improve gastric emptying.

CONCLUSIONS

Nausea is a noxious and debilitating symptom with a broad differential diagnosis that remains challenging. In the evaluation of nausea and vomiting, structural diseases should be excluded. Consideration of gastric neuromuscular abnormalities provides the framework for establishing diagnoses and directing treatments for patients with nausea unexplained with standard tests. The therapeutic armamentarium for the treatment of nausea is small; better understanding of the pathophysiology of gastric neuromuscular disorders and their role in the production of nausea and vomiting is needed.

Chapter 11

Nausea of Diabetes

This chapter reviews the causes and treatment of nausea in patients with diabetes mellitus. Much remains unknown, but it is assumed that the symptom of nausea in many cases of diabetes is related to altered gastric neuromuscular (motility) function, usually but not always related to gastroparesis or delayed gastric emptying. The possible contribution of autonomic neuropathy, inadequate glycemic control, and psychological factors to gastric neuromuscular dysfunction and/or nausea will be considered. For a more complete discussion of the relationship of gastrointestinal function to diabetes mellitus, see Horowitz and Samsom (2004).

The World Health Organization estimates that 180 million people have diabetes (WHO, 2009). In the United States alone, it is estimated that diabetes affects nearly 23.6 million individuals, of whom 24% are believed to be undiagnosed (CDC, 2009a). Although linked by similar metabolic disorders resulting in hyperglycemia, patients with Type 2 diabetes are substantially different from patients with Type 1. Major risk factors for developing Type 2 diabetes include obesity, age, and physical inactivity. In Type 2 diabetes there is *relative* insulin deficiency and resistance compared to the *absolute* insulin deficiency characteristic of Type 1. Certain comorbidities like vascular disease, dyslipidemia, and hypertension are common in Type 2. As disease progresses in uncontrolled and unrecognized diabetes, most organs, including the GI tract, begin to show evidence of damage. Kim et al. (1991) found manometric abnormalities in 81 of 84 diabetic patients who successfully completed a 3-hour fast and 2-hour postprandial motility evaluation. Although Kim et al.'s findings support the view that nausea and other symptoms of diabetes are related to gastroparesis (e.g., Wegener et al., 1990), other investigators have found only a weak correlation between GI symptoms and decreased (Keshavarzian, Iber & Vaeth, 1987) or increased (Schwartz et al., 1996) rate of gastric emptying. In the next section factors that may affect gastroparesis and/or nausea in patients with diabetes mellitus are considered.

POSSIBLE CAUSES

Autonomic Neuropathy

Similarities in symptoms between postvagotomy patients with gastroparesis and diabetic patients with gastroparesis led to the hypothesis that vagal damage ("autovagotomy") from chronic hyperglycemia caused gastroparesis (Rundles, 1945; Kassander, 1958; Wooten & Meriwether, 1961). Studies have relied on heart rate variability or orthostatic blood pressure as a proxy by which to infer GI autonomic function. Determination of the relationship between autonomic neuropathy and gastroparesis is limited by at least two important factors: the indirect assessment of vagal activity in the GI tract and the confounding variables in gastric emptying tests in this population.

A study by Buysschaert et al. (1987) in diabetic patients (Note—if Type 1 or 2 diabetes is not specified, assume a mixed sample) showed that there is a higher prevalence of delayed emptying in patients with cardiac autonomic neuropathy (CAN). Migdalis et al. (2001) found that gastric emptying rate was slower in the group with CAN (n = 16) compared to the group without CAN (n = 18) and controls. Furthermore, a positive correlation was found between degree of autonomic dysfunction and gastric emptying rate for both solids and liquids. Sasaki et al. (1983) measured plasma gastrin in patients with Type 2 as a marker of vagal neuropathy. Fasting plasma gastrin was significantly higher in the diabetic group compared with controls, indicating that vagal neuropathy, as measured by elevated gastrin levels, occurs in diabetic patients. The authors did not indicate if the patients also reported nausea.

In contrast, other studies have not demonstrated a significant relationship between autonomic neuropathy and gastroparesis in diabetic patients. Horowitz et al. (1989) reported no significant relationship between delayed gastric emptying and total score for CAN in a group of Type 2 diabetes patients. Another study by Annese et al. (1999) concluded that the presence of CAN had a poor predictive value for GI neuromuscular disorders. In a postmortem study, Yoshida, Schuffler, and Sumi (1988) examined the abdominal vagus nerve and gastric wall in diabetic individuals with and without gastroparesis and found no morphological abnormalities in the vagus nerve or myenteric plexus of the stomachs compared to controls. The above studies indicate that gastroparesis often occurs in diabetic patients who show no evidence of autonomic nerve dysfunction. This suggests that other mechanisms must contribute to the pathogenesis of gastroparesis in these patients. Recent human studies show that patients with diabetes and gastroparesis have decreased ICCs and increased macros in the ENS.

In mouse models of diabetes, decreased stem cell factor is associated with decreased numbers of ICCs (Ördög, 2008). Increases in macrophages in the gastric wall in db/db and NOD mice result in decreased hemoxygenase-1 (HO-1) which is associated with increased oxidative stress, loss of ICCs and reduced nitric oxide, all of which results in decreased gastric emptying (Choi et al., 2008). Recent histological studies of full thickness specimens from the gastric wall of patients with diabetic gastroparesis reveal increased number of macrophages near ICCs and enteric neurons suggesting inflammatory processes may have a role in gastroparesis in humans (Lurken et al., 2008). Repopulation of the gastric wall with macrophages that increase HO-1 resulted in significant improvement of delayed gastric emptying (Kyoung et al., 2010).

Acute and Chronic Hyperglycemia

It has been demonstrated that hyperglycemia and gastroparesis are related (Aylett, 1962; MacGregor et al., 1976). Acutely elevated levels of blood glucose delay gastric emptying in patients with Type 1 diabetes and healthy subjects (Fraser et al., 1990; Schvarcz et al., 1997). Also, both Barnett and Owyang (1988) and Fraser, Horowitz, and Dent (1991) showed that gastric motility is abnormal in hyperglycemic states induced in healthy volunteers. Barnett and Owyang measured interdigestive gastric motility with manometry during hyperglycemia induced in healthy volunteers. They found that glucose levels >140 mg/dl significantly diminished antral contractions and inhibited MMC activity. Fraser, Horowitz, and Dent (1991) showed that acute hyperglycemia caused pyloric contractions and suppressed antral motility in healthy individuals. Hyperglycemia has also been shown to induce gastric dysrhythmias (tachygastria) in individuals with Type 1 diabetes (Jebbink et al., 1994) and several studies have demonstrated a strong correlation between tachygastria and nausea. These studies indicate that acute hyperglycemia produces effects on gastric neuromuscular function in healthy volunteers and patients with Type 1 diabetes that may provoke the sensation of nausea.

The effect of plasma glucose levels on gastric emptying in Type 2 diabetics has been studied infrequently. Horowitz et al. (1989) showed that the lag phase of solid emptying was significantly longer among those individuals with Type 2 and they had higher mean plasma glucose levels. In addition, the gastric half-emptying time for a liquid test meal was significantly correlated with plasma glucose concentrations ($r = 0.58$, $p < 0.01$). HbA1c levels did not correlate with delayed gastric emptying, suggesting acute hyperglycemia may be more important than chronic hyperglycemia for gastric emptying. Moldovan et al. (2005), however, found that individuals with Type 2 diabetes and delayed gastric emptying had higher plasma glucose and HbA1c levels when compared to diabetic patients with normal gastric emptying. Gastric emptying was measured before and after glucose control in hospitalized diabetic patients (Sogabe et al., 2005). After achieving adequate glycemic control over the course of a month, antral motility, gastric emptying, and upper GI symptoms including nausea were all significantly improved. On the other hand, Holzäpfel et al. (1999) reported that no change in gastric emptying was noted after mean plasma glucose was reduced during treatment for one week in 10 patients with Type 2 diabetes.

Other Factors

A variety of other factors may play a role in the pathogenesis of diabetic gastroparesis and nausea. The effects of diabetes on the enteric nervous system and interstitial cells of Cajal (ICC) have been studied in rodent models. ICC are networks of cells throughout the GI tract that induce rhythmicity (pacemaker function) and control the frequency of gastric smooth muscle contractions. Studies conducted in Type 1 rodent models by Ördög et al. (2000), and in patients with Type 1 diabetes by Forster et al. (2005), showed that diabetic gastroparesis is associated with an absence or decreased numbers of gastric ICC, which may be accompanied by gastric dysrhythmia and, theoretically, reports of nausea.

The pathogenesis of diabetic gastroparesis and its relationship to upper GI symptoms such as nausea involves numerous factors. It is probable that vagal neuropathy, hyperglycemia, and other factors all play a role.

SYMPTOMS

Kassander (1958) coined the phrase "gastroparesis diabeticorum" to describe the syndrome of gastric retention observed in 6 asymptomatic patients with Type 1 diabetes. Since then, a majority of research on diabetic gastroparesis has focused on individuals with Type 1 diabetes. The conventional patient with gastroparesis was considered to have advanced Type 1 diabetes with poorly controlled hyperglycemia (Feldman & Schiller, 1983). The impact of patients with Type 2 diabetes with upper GI symptoms such as nausea and gastroparesis on health care delivery and gastroenterology will become even more important as the number of patients with Type 2 diabetes continues to grow.

The prevalence of upper GI symptoms like nausea, early satiety, bloating, epigastric fullness, and abdominal pain in patients with Type 2 diabetes was unknown until recently. Current literature now shows that upper GI symptoms are common in Type 2, but some investigators (Maleki et al., 2000; Janatuinen et al., 1993), have found that the upper GI symptoms reported by diabetic patients are not more frequent than those reported by healthy control subjects. And Clouse and Lustman (1989), who studied the relationship of autonomic neuropathy in diabetic patients to GI symptoms, concluded that gastrointestinal symptoms occurring in diabetic patients are poorly related to neuropathic complications, and may often represent gastrointestinal syndromes commonly associated with psychiatric illness.

As mentioned previously, many studies have shown that upper GI symptoms are more likely to occur in diabetic patients compared with nondiabetic subjects (Bytzer et al., 2001; Enck et al., 1994; Ko et al., 1999; Spangeus et al., 1999; Ricci et al., 2000; Hammer et al., 2003; Mjörnheim et al., 2003; Rosztoczy et al., 2004). For example, a population-based study by Bytzer et al. (2001) of 423 patients with diabetes (95% with Type 2) revealed that GI symptoms were significantly more common in diabetic patients than the general population. "Poor" glycemic control was associated with higher rates of upper GI dysmotility symptoms. In a study by Ko et al. (1999), 70% of patients with Type 2 diabetes had higher rates of GI symptoms like diarrhea, constipation, and epigastric fullness compared with controls. Overall, 44.3% of these patients with Type 2 reported upper GI symptoms, such as epigastric fullness and early satiety, compared to 24.6% of controls. Duration of diabetes was the only independent variable that correlated with total GI symptoms score; BMI, age, fasting plasma glucose, and HbA1c (a measure of long-term control of blood glucose) did not correlate with GI symptoms. A Swedish study (Spangeus et al., 1999) of diabetic patients found that the frequency of heartburn and abdominal pain (the only two upper GI symptoms reported) occurred more often in the Type 2 patients cohort: 31.7% of patients with Type 2 complained of heartburn symptoms compared to only 14% of controls. Also, 28.3% of patients with Type 2 had abdominal pain more than once a month compared with 14% of controls. Enck et al. (1994) evaluated individuals in Germany with diabetes to determine the frequency of GI symptoms. Nausea was significantly more frequent among the group with Type 2 diabetes (11.8%) when compared with the control population (2.9%).

Ricci et al. (2000) evaluated the prevalence of upper GI symptoms in diabetics in a U.S. community. The prevalence of one or more upper GI symptoms in the past month was 50% in the diabetic group vs. 38% in controls. Specifically, significant differences were reported for the upper GI symptoms of bloating (21% in diabetic group vs. 15.2% in controls) and early satiety (32.2% in diabetic group vs. 20.2% in controls). Talley and colleagues (2001) used a questionnaire to study the impact of chronic gastrointestinal symptoms in diabetic individuals on health-related quality of life and compared their results to data from a group of healthy controls. The investigators concluded, not surprisingly, that the GI symptoms of their diabetic subjects impacted negatively on their health-related quality of life.

Delayed Gastric Emptying in Diabetes

The prevalence of delayed gastric emptying in Type 2 diabetes ranges from 30%–50% (Leatherdale et al.,1982; Sasaki et al., 1983; Horowitz et al, 1989; Chang et al., 1996; Annese et al., 1999) to as high as 70% in one group of symptomatic patients (Tung et al, 1997). These studies are limited by small sample sizes, presence of hyperglycemia during testing, and the variety of test meals and stomach imaging methods used. In one of the earliest studies of gastric emptying in 1982, Leatherdale et al. reported that patients with Type 2 diabetes had significantly delayed gastric emptying of a porridge meal. Sasaki et al. (1983) examined a group of obese Pima Native Americans with Type 2 and found gastric emptying of a water test meal was significantly slower in the diabetic group compared to obese controls.

Tung et al. (1997) showed that the prevalence of delayed gastric emptying in a randomly selected group of 20 individuals with Type 2 diabetes was 30% and comparable to patients with Type 1 diabetes. The percentage of a solid test meal remaining in the stomach at 100 minutes was significantly greater in the Type 2 group compared with controls. The emptying time for the liquid component of the meal was also significantly delayed. Annese et al. (1999) assessed gastric emptying rate in 25 patients with Type 2 diabetes. The patients had significantly slower half emptying time for the solid test meal (134.3 ± 35 min) compared with controls (85.5 ± 15.4 min). Another study by Moldovan et al. (2005) in patients with Type 2 (n = 23) and Type 1 diabetes (n = 13) used ultrasound to assess gastric emptying: 52.2% of the Type 2 group and 53.8% of the Type 1 group had delayed gastric emptying.

Tung et al. (1997) studied the prevalence of delayed gastric emptying in Type 2 patients specifically selected for presence of upper GI symptoms. The authors assessed gastric emptying rates of solid and liquid meals and indigestible markers in 20 individuals. Seventy percent of patients had delayed emptying of the solid meal and indigestible markers and 35% of patients had delayed emptying of the liquid meal. Chang et al. (1996) reported that 41 out of 70 male subjects (59%) with Type 2 diabetes and upper GI dysmotility symptoms had delayed emptying of solids. These two studies reveal a high prevalence of delayed gastric emptying in patients with Type 2 diabetes, nausea, and other upper GI symptoms.

Rapid Gastric Emptying in Type 2 Diabetic Patients

Rapid gastric emptying is a somewhat surprising finding in some Type 2, usually recently diagnosed, diabetic patients (Smith, 1996). Phillips, Schwartz, and McMahan (1992) examined the rate of gastric emptying of an oral glucose solution in recently diagnosed Type 2 diabetic individuals with no evidence of autonomic neuropathy. The patient group had significantly faster gastric emptying rates compared with controls. The average emptying rate was 3.3 kcal/min in the diabetic group and 1.6 kcal/min in the control group. The plasma glucose levels for the diabetic group showed a steeper rise initially and peaked later than the glucose curve for the control group. On the other hand, a study using a similar liquid glucose meal showed that gastric emptying rates in 16 patients with recently diagnosed Type 2 diabetes were slower compared to controls, but the difference was too small to have clinical significance (Jones et al., 1996).

Schwartz et al. (1996) evaluated solid gastric emptying in a recently diagnosed group with Type 2 diabetes. The average half emptying time in the diabetic group was approximately 45 min compared with 60 min in the control group ($p = 0.05$). The authors also reported a steeper rise in plasma glucose and a delayed glucose peak in the diabetic group.

Two studies using the double isotope technique in asymptomatic Type 2 diabetic patients with no evidence of autonomic neuropathy revealed rapid emptying with liquids (Frank et al., 1995) and solids (Bertin et al., 2001). Frank et al. found normal rates of emptying of solids, but significantly faster rates of liquid emptying in the diabetic patients. The time for 50% of liquid to empty from the stomach was 65 ± 7 minutes for the patients and 103 ± 13 minutes for controls. Bertin et al. assessed solid- and liquid-phase emptying in 13 obese Type 2 diabetic individuals. In direct contrast to Frank et al. they found no difference between liquid-phase emptying, but did find a significant difference in half emptying time of the solid meal, and rapid emptying was more common among the diabetic group. Weytjens et al. (1998) studied the gastric emptying rate of a liquid meal in patients with long-term Type 2 diabetes (mean duration of diabetes: 13 years). Seventy percent of the diabetic group had accelerated gastric emptying of a liquid meal. From 20 to 40 min after ingestion of the liquid meal, the diabetic group showed significantly greater liquid emptying than controls.

In summary, some patients with Type 2 diabetes have rapid, not delayed, gastric emptying. The patients with rapid gastric emptying generally had a much shorter duration of diabetes, and had no evidence of autonomic neuropathy. Rapid gastric emptying can produce upper GI symptoms of fullness, nausea, bloating, and abdominal discomfort, symptoms that are similar to those associated with gastroparesis.

Relationship Between Nausea and Other Upper GI Symptoms and Gastroparesis in Diabetic Patients

Many but not all studies reviewed above show that nausea and other upper GI symptoms occur with a higher frequency in people with diabetes than in healthy controls, but these symptoms are poorly correlated with delayed gastric emptying. For example, in a study by Annese et al. (1999), 43% of the patients with Type 2 diabetes and delayed gastric emptying were asymptomatic. In patients with long-standing Type 2 diabetes, Iber et al. (1993) reported no correlation between upper GI symptoms and delayed gastric emptying. Chang et al. (1998) studied a group of diabetic patients with upper GI symptoms suggestive of delayed gastric emptying. Gastric dysrhythmias, gastric emptying, and total symptom score improved after 8 weeks of treatment with cisapride, a prokinetic agent. However, there was no correlation between EGG changes, improvement of upper GI symptoms, or gastric emptying. In another study by Koch et al. (1989), improvement in upper GI symptoms was associated with restoration of a normal 3-cpm EGG rhythm, but not normalization of gastric emptying rate in patients with Type 1 diabetes mellitus treated with domperidone.

If improvement of symptoms does not necessarily correlate with normalization of gastric emptying, then it is likely that other mechanisms may produce symptoms; e.g., gastric dysrhythmias, fundic dysfunction, pylorospasm, or visceral hypersensitivity (see Figures 11.1 and 11.2). As Horowitz and colleagues (2002b) remarked, "it is appropriate to regard delay in gastric emptying more as a marker of gastroduodenal motor abnormality, rather than a direct cause of symptoms . . . the etiology of which is likely to be multifactorial." Visceral hyperalgesia or hypersensitivity may cause upper GI symptoms in some diabetic individuals who have neuronal impairment in peripheral and/or central nervous system (Zhao et al., 2006). Also, hyperglycemia may directly affect nerve function and sensation. In a study by Bytzer et al. (2002) of 1101 diabetic patients (956 patients had Type 2 diabetes), poor glycemic control was an independent risk factor for upper GI symptoms. As Maleki et al. (2000) pointed out, some patients with Type 2 diabetes may have unrelated functional GI disorders, common to the general population, that may explain their upper GI symptoms.

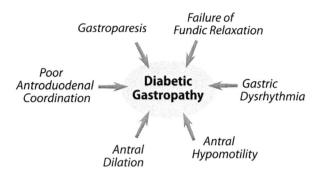

Figure 11.1 Diabetic gastropathy may encompass several neuromuscular disorders of the stomach. Although gastroparesis is the most recognizable abnormality within the general term of diabetic gastropathy, other areas of the stomach are often times dysfunctional in diabetic patients. These abnormalities include antral dilation and antral hypomotility, gastric dysrhythmia, and lack of antroduodenal coordination. In addition, diabetic subjects may have failure of the normal fundic relaxation in response to food. All of these neuromuscular problems can cause upper GI symptoms and represent underlying mechanisms for overall decreased gastric emptying, which can result in gastroparesis.

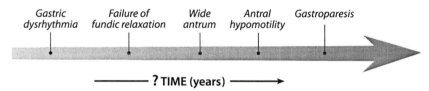

Figure 11.2 Spectrum of diabetic gastropathy. Although there are a variety of gastric neuromuscular abnormalities present in the diabetic stomach, it is unclear how or if these abnormalities progress over time. That is, subtle abnormalities such as gastric dysrhythmias may be an early indicator of dysfunction, whereas antral hypomotility and gastroparesis represent severe neuromuscular dysfunction.

However, as mentioned above, many patients with gastroparesis do not have upper GI symptoms. Kassander noted in 1958 that food retention occurred in asymptomatic diabetics and that gastroparesis was underappreciated. In an effort to learn more about the relationship between lack of symptoms and gastroparesis, Rathmann et al. (1991) measured cerebral evoked potentials during esophageal stimulation in Type 1 diabetes patients with delayed gastric emptying. Increased perception thresholds, as assessed by cerebral evoked potentials, were found in 7 of 10 patients with diabetes and gastric neuromuscular dysfunction. These results suggest that afferent sensory information may be processed differently in the nervous circuitry of some diabetic individuals, possibly due to afferent vagal nerve damage.

DIAGNOSIS OF THE NAUSEA OF DIABETES

Because upper GI symptoms such as nausea are typically poorly correlated with delayed gastric emptying, these symptoms in a diabetic patient warrant further investigation. An upper endoscopy or an upper GI series should be obtained in patients with nausea to exclude mucosal diseases and gastric or small bowel obstruction. If no obstruction is present and other standard causes of nausea and vomiting have been excluded (see Chapter 10, in this volume), then gastric neuromuscular function should be assessed. Gastric pacesetter potential function is assessed noninvasively with electrogastrogram (EGG) recordings (Koch, 2001a). EGG recordings are normally recorded during a baseline and then during a provocative test such as a water load test or satiety test. The presence of a tachygastria, bradygastria, or mixed gastric dysrhythmia or normal EGG signal is determined. Tachygastrias are associated with delayed gastric emptying and mixed gastric dysrhythmias with GERD and dyspepsia. Correction of the gastric dysrhythmia with domperidone resulted in improvement in symptoms (Koch et al., 1989). In an asymptomatic patient with poorly controlled glucose, a gastric emptying test should be performed. These patients may have a rapid or delayed gastric emptying rate. The altered gastric emptying may result in a marked mismatch with insulin or other antihyperglycemic therapy (Horowitz et al., 2002a).

There are a variety of methods to measure the rate of gastric emptying (see Parkman, Hasler & Fisher, 2004). Gastric scintigraphy is the standard for diagnosis of gastroparesis and emptying of solids, liquids, or both simultaneously using radioisotope-labeled foodstuffs is possible. Importantly, plasma glucose levels should be at least 200 mg/dL or lower and patients should discontinue any use of prokinetic or narcotic medication before testing. Gastric emptying is determined by scintigraphic imaging of the gastric contents during either a 2- or 4-hour test. A large, multicenter study done by Tougas et al. (2000) using Egg Beaters® to test gastric emptying in healthy volunteers concluded that gastric retention of $\leq 10\%$ at 4 hours was normal. Drawbacks to scintigraphy include radiation exposure, inaccessibility, and a lack of standardized interinstitutional meals and methods.

A breath test to evaluate gastric emptying measures the level of ^{13}C-labeled octanoate expired after ingestion of a test meal (see also Parkman, Hasler & Fisher, 2004). This method requires small intestinal absorption of the radiolabeled material, diffusion of the label into the blood stream, oxidization to $^{13}CO_2$ in the liver, and eventual transportation across the alveoli during respiration for measurement in the breath. Since the rate-limiting step in this process is gastric emptying, measured levels of expired $^{13}CO_2$ during respiration reflect rate of gastric emptying in diabetic patients (Ziegler et al., 1996). However, concurrent medical disorders affecting transport of the label, like small intestinal mucosal disease or respiratory disease, may alter the results. The advantage of this test is the ease of its performance and lack of radiation exposure.

Ultrasound has also been used to measure rate of gastric emptying. It has the advantage of real-time imaging to assess dynamic changes in gastric dimensions, antral contractility, and fundic accommodation. However, it requires user expertise and has a large amount of interobserver variability (see Parkman, Hasler & Fisher, 2004). Other methods to assess gastric motility currently being investigated include MRI and single photon emission computerized tomography (SPECT; Camilleri, 2006). A new, innovative encapsulated recording device, called SmartPill® (Kuo et al., 2006) measures gastric pH and pressure to determine gastric emptying rates and can be used in the ambulatory setting. The capsule is consumed with a standard test meal and the results are captured by a monitoring device.

For methods of measuring nausea in humans see Chapter 9 in this volume.

TREATMENT OF THE NAUSEA OF DIABETES

Once a diagnosis of diabetic gastroparesis or gastric dysrhythmia with nausea is made, a multidisciplinary approach should be undertaken to design a treatment plan that will encompass medical, nutritional, and lifestyle interventions to alleviate the nausea and other GI symptoms and improve glucose control. Given that hyperglycemia itself elicits gastric dysrhythmias and delays gastric emptying in patients with diabetes, the central goal of treatment should be to normalize glucose levels (Abell et al., 2006). See Figure 11.3.

Since the stomach regulates delivery of food and oral antihyperglycemic medication to the small intestine for absorption, it follows that abnormal gastric emptying will affect postprandial blood glucose levels (Kong & Horowitz, 1999). In some patients the emptying will actually be rapid. Knowledge of the gastric emptying rate is important when prescribing short-acting oral hypoglycemic agents or insulin to diabetic patients. In an investigation by Groop et al. (1989), absorption of glipizide, an oral anti-hyperglycemic agent in the sulfonylurea class that stimulates the release of insulin from beta cells in the pancreas, was reduced in a dose-dependent manner as higher levels of blood glucose were induced in healthy volunteers. At the highest plasma glucose levels, the concentration of glipizide in the blood was reduced by up to 50%. In the setting of gastroparesis, a mismatch may occur between doses of insulin or oral agents and postprandial plasma glucose levels (Kong & Horowitz, 1999). Increasing levels of hyperglycemia can worsen gastroparesis. Abell et al. (2006) suggest that patients with gastroparesis and uncontrolled blood glucose on oral therapy may benefit from the addition of basal, long-acting insulin, like insulin glargine, to prevent wide fluctuations in postprandial plasma glucose levels. In patients with gastroparesis, insulin is given after the meal to avoid postprandial hypoglycemia.

In patients with recently diagnosed Type 2 diabetes, administration of an oral proteinase inhibitor (Schwartz et al., 1994) or cholecystokinin-8 (CCK-8)

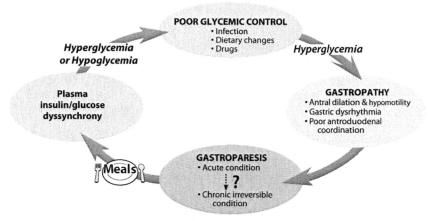

Figure 11.3 Glycemic control and the diabetic stomach. Poor glycemic control due to infection, dietary changes, or drugs (or gastroparesis) may result in hyperglycemia. Hyperglycemia itself can acutely stimulate gastric dysrhythmias and decrease antral contractions and antroduodenal coordination, all of which contributes to antral hypomotility in the acute hyperglycemia setting. Thus gastroparesis is induced acutely. It is unclear if recurrent acute hyperglycemic events are the mechanism that ultimately produces chronic irreversible gastroparesis. In the presence of acute (and) chronic gastroparesis, ingested meals are poorly mixed and emptied. Consequently the post-prandial glucose elevations that may be expected by the patient with known or unknown gastroparesis do not occur, but the insulin dose administered by the patient is not adjusted. In these patients, unanticipated hypoglycemic episodes are experienced in the postprandial period. These hypoglycemic events reflect the dyssynchrony between the insulin treatment and the actual postprandial plasma glucose in patients with gastroparesis. In this setting of dyssynchrony, poor glycemic control occurs repetitively on a daily and weekly basis and leads to repeated episodes of hyperglycemia and hypo-glycemia.

(Phillips, Schwartz & McMahan, 1993) significantly reduced postprandial glucose levels by delaying gastric emptying. This would be especially important if the patient had rapid gastric emptying. Gonlachanvit et al. (2003b) examined the effect of altering gastric emptying of a solid and liquid meal in 9 patients with Type 2 diabetes in a double-blind, randomized, placebo-controlled trial using erythromycin, morphine, and normal saline. Morphine treatment reduced gastric emptying and reduced the peak glucose levels during the first hour after the meal. In contrast, erythromycin increased gastric emptying rate and increased postprandial glucose levels and peak glucose levels com-pared with placebo. These studies indicate the role of gastric emptying in sub-sequent plasma glucose levels.

Other antidiabetogenic treatments that delay gastric emptying include pram-lintide (Thompson et al., 1997), an amylin analogue, and glucagon-like peptide 1 (GLP-1; Willms et al., 1996). Pramlintide significantly reduces postprandial glucose concentration and serum insulin levels. Gentilcore et al. (2006)

examined the effects of olive oil on gastric emptying and postprandial meta-bolic response in 6 individuals with Type 2 diabetes. Ingestion of 30 ml of olive oil 30 minutes before a meal significantly delayed gastric emptying, decreased plasma insulin and glucose, and increased levels of GLP-1. In mild to moderate diabetes, postprandial hyperglycemia contributes to the majority of the HbA1c profile (Monnier, Lapinski & Colette, 2003). Delay of the gastric emptying rate is an innovative approach that may improve control of hyperglycemia.

For patients with symptomatic diabetic gastroparesis, treatment is centered on prokinetic and antinausea therapy. Erythromycin, metoclopramide, domperidone, and cisapride are prokinetic agents used to treat patients with gastroparesis (Talley, 2003). Only erythromycin and metoclopramide are avail-able in the United States. Erythromycin stimulates antral contractions via motilin receptors and may help some patients with diabetes. Metoclopramide has been available for over 40 years for treatment of GERD and gastroparesis. Side effects of depression, Parkinson's-like movements, and tardive dyskinesia limit its long-term use. Acute hyperglycemia decreases the prokinetic effects of erythromycin (Petrakis et al., 1999). This underscores the importance of maintaining normal glucose control in diabetic patients with gastroparesis.

Evidence that chronic treatment with prokinetic agents directly improves glucose control in diabetic patients is scant. Erythromycin accelerates gastric emptying, and also independently increases insulin levels in patients, possibly by stimulating pancreatic beta cells (Ueno et al., 2000). Mosapride, a prokinetic serotonin 5-HT$_4$ receptor agonist, markedly improved gastric emptying, but only modestly improved glycemic control in Type 2 patients with upper GI symptoms (Asakawa et al., 2003). Studies in patients with Type 1 diabetes with delayed gastric emptying showed that acceleration of gastric emptying with cisapride did not improve glucose control (Horowitz et al., 2002a; Lehmann et al., 2003). Although evidence is limited in Type 2 diabetics, normalization of gastric motility may improve glycemic control by providing predictable delivery of nutrients to the duodenum. With knowledge of gastric emptying, antihyperglycemic treatment can be adjusted to match delivery of calories, and thereby better control glucose levels.

In patients with severe upper GI symptoms and gastroparesis, controlling plasma glucose will be difficult if the patient is unable to eat a consistent diet. Dietary recommendations for gastroparetic patients include the three-step gastroparesis diet (Koch, 2006). This diet focuses on small meals containing foods that are easier to digest (Gatorade®, soups, rice, chicken) and avoiding high fat foods and undigestible fiber.

The role of gastric electrical stimulation (GES) in diabetic patients with refractory gastroparesis remains undefined. GES studies have focused on individuals with Type 1 diabetes and gastroparesis or idiopathic gastroparesis. Interestingly, a prospective study in 17 patients with Type 1 diabetes and severe gastroparesis showed that GES not only improved upper GI symptoms and gastric emptying, but also significantly lowered HbA1c levels (van der Voort et al., 2005). A retrospective analysis of GES in patients with Type 1 diabetes showed that symptoms improved, and decreased HbA1c (lowered by 2.3%) was maintained over a 3-year period (Lin et al., 2006).

In a more recent retrospective study by Sawhney et al. (2007) the effects of a tricyclic antidepressant on 24 diabetics with nausea and vomiting were tested. The patients had previously failed to respond to prokinetic therapy. By chart review, 88% of the patient responded favorably to the tricyclic antidepressants. When the patients were questioned about the treatment, 68% responded that it was the most effective treatment that they had ever had for their diabetic-related nausea and vomiting.

CONCLUSIONS

The prevalence of nausea and other upper GI symptoms in the diabetic population is significant and will continue to increase with the worldwide increase in Type 1 and Type 2 diabetes. Nausea is a depressing and debilitating symptom. Nausea and upper GI symptoms are often overlooked but may reflect delayed or rapid gastric emptying. Large population-based, longitudinal studies are needed to learn more about the relationship of the nausea of diabetes to the following:

- Autonomic Neuropathy. Is sympathetic/parasympathetic balance relevant? Is central or peripheral neuropathy important?
- Gastric Neuromuscular Function. What is the role of decreased or increased rates of gastric emptying? What is the role of gastric electrical dysrhythmia?
- Blood Glucose Levels. What is the effect of acute and chronic, high and low blood glucose levels on gastric neuromuscular activity? What is the effect of hyperglycemia/hypoglycemia on other organs and/or neurotransmitters such as vasopressin? What measure(s) is most relevant?
- Psychological Factors. How can the factors that provoke the nausea of diabetes be separated from anxiety and depression, which can also provoke nausea, and which often times accompanies chronic disease?

Furthermore, a thorough understanding of the natural history and pathogenesis of the nausea of diabetes may allow for the development of therapeutic interventions that will more effectively treat the upper GI symptoms if not the underlying diabetes.

Chapter 12

Nausea During Pregnancy

Almost 80% of women have some degree of nausea in the first trimester of pregnancy (Gadsby, Barnie-Adshead & Jagger, 1993; Jewell & Young, 2002). A small subset of women with nausea and vomiting of pregnancy (NVP) develop severe unremitting symptoms termed hyperemesis gravidarum (HG). Several major issues remain unresolved, however, in understanding and treating NVP. First, the pathophysiology that might explain the symptoms is unknown. Second, because the pathophysiology remains unknown, there is no standard approach to the treatment of NVP, which varies along a spectrum from mild nausea to severe symptoms. Third, advances in understanding the pathophysiology and treatment of NVP have been limited in some degree by literature that indicates that NVP is protective for the fetus. Severe NVP is associated with lower risk of congenital heart disease compared with women with no nausea or with no treatment for nausea (Boneva et al., 1999). On the other hand, increasing evidence indicates that NVP is associated with less than optimal fetal weight gain; unappreciated maternal suffering from nausea and vomiting; and significant loss of social, family, and work-related functions (see Koch & Frissora, 2003, for more information).

Additional studies have addressed the association of NVP with physical and psychosocial disorders later in childhood. Martin, Wisenbaker, and Huttunen (1999) reported that children of mothers with NVP in the second and third trimester had lower sensory thresholds, higher levels of activity and emotional intensity, scored lower in task persistence at age 5 and were viewed as more careless in their school work at age 12. It was hypothesized that the prolonged nausea and vomiting interfered with proper fluid intake and nutrition, leading to a variety of blood chemistry alterations such as increased blood urea nitrogen and ketones. Furthermore, it was hypothesized that if dietary protein levels are reduced for weeks during gestation, then neural and/or behavioral effects may become apparent later in life. It should be noted that this study focused on women who had nausea lasting into the second and third trimesters. On the other hand, as noted above, in another retrospective study by Boneva et al. (1999) the most severe nausea of pregnancy was associated with lower risk for congenital heart defects. In this study the early onset of nausea of pregnancy and use of the antinausea medications were associated with a lower risk for congenital heart defects compared with women with: (a) the absence of nausea, and (b) nausea without medication treatment.

Thus, some degree of nausea may indicate the appropriate production of various pregnancy hormones or pregnancy-related growth factors that play a role in the development of the heart.

PATHOGENESIS

Is NVP during the first trimester pathological or is it beneficial for the mother and fetus? Profet (1988; 1992) stresses the adaptive value of morning or pregnancy sickness. Thus, the pregnant woman tends to avoid foods that may be teratogenic or contain abortifacient chemicals that occur in vegetables, caffeinated beverages, or alcohol. Such ingestive behaviors protect the developing fetus in the first trimester. Some investigators (e.g., Brown, Kahn & Hartman, 1997; Weigel et al., 2006) have questioned the validity of Profet's theory. On the other hand, support for the theory comes from Flaxman and Sherman (2000), who have done an extensive review of the literature and support the idea that pregnancy sickness is a mechanism that protects the mother and embryo. The evidence they present follows:

> (i) symptoms peak when organogenesis is most susceptible to chemical disruption (weeks 6–18), (ii) women who experience morning sickness are significantly less likely to miscarry than women who do not (9 of 9 studies), (iii) women who vomit suffer fewer miscarriages than those who experience nausea alone, and (iv) many pregnant women have aversion to alcoholic and non-alcoholic (mostly caffeinated) beverages and strong-tasting vegetables, especially during the first trimester. (p. 113)

Flaxman and Sherman (2000) also report that the greatest food aversions of pregnant women, according to their review of the literature, are meat, fish, poultry, and eggs. These products, particularly if not refrigerated, may well contain parasites and pathogens. And Haig (1993) has pointed out that it is particularly important for pregnant women to avoid food-borne microorganisms because they are immunosuppressed, he hypothesized, to avoid rejecting tissues of their own offspring. Olfactory sensitivity may also play a role in NVP (Blum, 2000; Hummel et al., 2002). Changes in taste sensitivity (Whitehead, Holden & Andrews, 1992) have also been suggested as contributing to NVP.

What is the pathogenesis of NVP? During the evolving development of the placenta and the embryo, and the evolving compensatory and adaptive responses of the mother's body, major neural, hormonal, and cardiovascular changes occur throughout a typical pregnancy. The pathogenesis of nausea as it develops in the first trimester may involve different pathophysiological mechanisms than vomiting. Metabolic and endocrine factors related to pregnancy affect the neuromuscular function of the gastrointestinal tract. Digestive activities are disturbed when gastroparesis or gastric dysrhythmias develop. Metabolic, endocrine, and gastrointestinal aspects of the pathogenesis of NVP are discussed below.

METABOLIC AND ENDOCRINE FACTORS

Human Chorionic Gonadotropin (hCG)

NVP is more common in women with hydatidiform mole and in mothers carrying babies with Down syndrome, conditions associated with elevated hCG. The peak concentrations and most rapid rise in hCG occur during the first 8 weeks of gestation, the time of increasing symptoms of NVP. In several studies, however, the concentration of hCG did not correlate with NVP (e.g., Fairweather, 1968). However, according to Goodwin (2000), hCG receptor mutations may confound the quantitative measures of hCG in NVP. Complex interactions among hCG, thyroid stimulating hormone (TSH), and steroid hormone synthesis (ovarian steroid metabolism) may underlie the NVP (Masson, Anthony & Chau, 1985). During thyrotoxicosis of pregnancy, hCG and nausea and vomiting are increased. The degree of hyperthyroidism also correlates with the severity of symptoms.

Estrogen and Progesterone

Estrogens are implicated in NVP because, according to Järnfelt-Samsioe, Samsioe, and Velinder (1983), women who experienced nausea after oral contraceptive use have higher incidences of NVP. Elevated urinary and circulating estrogen levels were also found in patients with NVP (Depue et al., 1987). Because subsequent studies found no relationship between estrogen levels and NVP, the role of estrogen in NVP remains unclear.

Progesterone, alone or in combination with estrogen, may have a role in NVP. Walsh et al. (1996) have suggested that since progesterone decreases smooth muscle contractions, it may cause gastric dysrhythmias and/or alter gastric emptying, thereby evoking nausea and vomiting. Progesterone levels peak during the first trimester of pregnancy as nausea and vomiting increase. Studies have not shown, however, a clear difference in progesterone levels in patients with or without NVP (Depue et al., 1987; Masson, Anthony & Chau, 1985). Walsh et al. (1996) reported that estrogen and progesterone at physiological levels elicited postprandial gastric dysrhythmias and nausea in healthy women. The disruption of gastrointestinal neuromuscular function, evoked by changes in a variety of hormones that are secreted during pregnancy, is one mechanism that may mediate nausea and vomiting related to pregnancy.

Prostaglandin E$_2$

A study by North, Whitehead, and Larkins (1991) evaluated prostaglandin E$_2$, IL-1β and TNFα levels in 18 women with NVP. Blood samples were taken within a 24-hour period when the subjects were either symptomatic or asymptomatic. The results showed that prostaglandin E$_2$ levels were higher (22.3 ± 4.6 ng/ml) during symptomatic periods compared with asymptomatic periods (16.8 ± 2.4 ng/ml). The IL-1β and TNFα levels were similar during symptomatic and asymptomatic periods. Synthesis of placental prostaglandin E_2 is stimulated by hCG and peaks during weeks 9–12 of gestation. Frissora and Harris (2001) have noted that high-dose estrogen birth control pills also induce nausea in nonpregnant women. Prostaglandin E_2 also induces gastric dysrhythmias (Sanders, Bauer & Publicover, 1983). Thus, fluxes in PGE_2 may be an important pathogenic mechanism of NVP.

Helicobacter Pylori

Helicobacter pylori was investigated as a pathogenic factor in NVP in a study by Wu et al. (2000). H. pylori seropositivity was present in 69% of pregnant women compared with about 50% in the general population. However, seropositivity did not correlate with GI symptoms. Therefore, H. pylori does not appear to be a factor in NVP.

ESOPHAGEAL AND GASTRIC NEUROMUSCULAR DYSFUNCTION AND NVP

The stomach and esophagus are intimately involved in nausea and vomiting elicited by diverse causes. Changes in neuromuscular function of the esophagus and stomach during NVP are reviewed below.

Esophagus

Normal esophageal peristalsis and a competent lower esophageal sphincter (LES) pressure maintain an alkaline pH in the esophagus for approximately 94% of the day. Gastric acid that is refluxed into the esophagus during the other 6% of the day is neutralized by esophageal peristaltic contractions that carry bicarbonate-rich saliva to the distal esophagus (Castell, Gedeon & Castell, 2002). Symptomatic gastroesophageal reflux is usually associated with heartburn, but in some patients acid reflux induces atypical symptoms such as nausea (Brzana & Koch, 1997). Thus, gastroesophageal reflux may be one of the pathogenic mechanisms underlying nausea during pregnancy.

LES pressures were measured by Van Thiel, Gavaler, and Stremple (1976) and Van Thiel et al. (1977) during gestation in asymptomatic pregnant women. The LES pressure was below normal during the first, second, and third trimesters, but returned to normal in the postpartum period. In another study, the LES pressure was found to be normal during the first 20 weeks of gestation (Fisher et al., 1978). Schulze and Christensen (1977) reported that in opossum treated with estrogen and progesterone to mimic pregnancy, LES pressure decreased significantly compared with non–hormone treated controls. Finally, when healthy female volunteers received progesterone with or without estrogen, LES pressure decreased significantly (Van Thiel, Gavaler & Stremple, 1976). LES pressure may be decreased early in pregnancy, but the predominant symptoms are nausea and vomiting, not heartburn and regurgitation, which tend to be common symptoms in the third trimester.

Stomach

Normal neuromuscular function of the stomach is associated with a good appetite and postprandial sensations of pleasant fullness. Abnormal gastric neuromuscular function is associated with postprandial nausea, bloating, discomfort, and vomiting. Normal gastric neuromuscular function and disturbances in neuromuscular function of the stomach in NVP are described below.

Normal Gastric Neuromuscular Function

The normal neuromuscular function of the stomach is to receive, mix, and empty ingested food (Lacy, Crowell & Koch, 2002). Reception or accommodation of food is accomplished by relaxation of the gastric fundus. Relaxation of the fundic muscle allows the volume of food to be accommodated without undue tension (and thus discomfort) on the gastric muscular wall. The ingested foods and liquids are then distributed from the fundus into the corpus and antrum of the stomach. The corpus and antrum of the stomach are the mixing chambers wherein recurrent gastric peristaltic waves triturate the solid foods into 1–2 mm pieces, a nutrient suspension termed chyme. When the chyme is of appropriate particle size, each gastric peristaltic contraction empties 2–4 ml aliquots of the chyme into the duodenum. The peristaltic contractions of the stomach are "paced" from the gastric pacemaker region located between the fundus and corpus on the greater curvature. From this area, spontaneous electrical activity comprised of depolarization and repolarization waves (pacesetter potentials or slow waves) migrate around the stomach and distally at a rate of 3 cycles per minute (cpm), the normal human gastric pacemaker frequency. Disturbances in gastric rhythmicity are associated with upper gastrointestinal symptoms, particularly nausea. Gastric dysrhythmias are termed bradygastrias (1–2.5 cpm) or tachygastrias (3.7–10.0 cpm) (Koch & Stern, 1993). Gastric dysrhythmias are described in detail in Chapter 7 in this volume.

Gastric Dysrhythmias and Nausea of Pregnancy

Koch et al. (1990a) recorded electrogastrograms (EGGs) in 32 pregnant women who had symptoms of "morning sickness." Bradygastrias and tachygastrias were recorded in 26 of the 32 women (see Figure 12.1). These women also had nausea scores of 70–80 mm on a visual analog scale that ranged from 0–300 mm. One woman had no nausea at the beginning of her EGG recording, but then experienced a wave of nausea, at which time the normal 3 cpm rhythm degenerated to a flatline or bradygastria pattern for several minutes. When the nausea resolved, the 3 cpm EGG rhythm reappeared (see Figure 9.3). Of interest, 6 of the 32 women had no nausea and their EGG recordings showed the normal 3 cpm EGG rhythm. Furthermore, several women were studied after delivery when they were symptom-free. Although these women had tachygastrias and nausea in the first trimester of pregnancy, normal 3-cpm EGG rhythms

A. **Tachygastria**

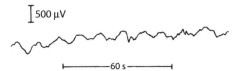

B. **Bradygastria (low-amplitude)**

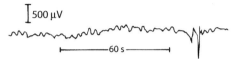

C. **Bradygastria (high-amplitude)**

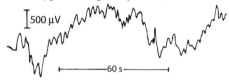

D. **Normal**

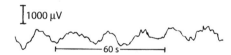

Figure 12.1 Electrogastrogram (EGG) rhythm strips recorded from women with the nausea and vomiting of pregnancy. Example of a 6 cpm tachygastria is shown in A, a low-amplitude (flatline) bradygastria in B, a high-amplitude bradygastria in C, and a normal 3 cpm EGG pattern in D. The women with the normal 3 cpm rhythm had no nausea on the morning of this recording, whereas the other women had mild to moderate nausea symptoms. Modified with permission from Koch et al., 1990a.

were recorded in the postpartum period. Thus, the presence of the normal 3-cpm EGG signal correlated with no nausea. The presence of gastric dysrhythmias recorded by the EGG suggests that these electrical abnormalities of the stomach have a role in the pathogenesis of the nausea of pregnancy.

The finding of gastric dysrhythmias during nausea in women with NVP was confirmed by Jednak et al. (1999). Moreover, nausea symptoms and gastric dysrhythmias were significantly reduced by treating the patients with high-protein meals. High-protein meals were beneficial whereas high-fat or high-carbohydrate meals did not reduce symptoms or gastric dysrhythmias. These data also confirm the linkage between the gastric dysrhythmias and the presence of nausea, since decreasing the dysrhythmias with the protein meal corresponded with a decrease in nausea (see Figures 12.2 and 12.3).

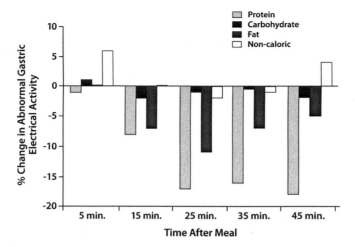

Figure 12.2 Change in abnormal gastric activity of pregnant women as a function of time since protein, carbohydrate, fat, and noncaloric meal. Redrawn with permission from Jednak et al., 1999.

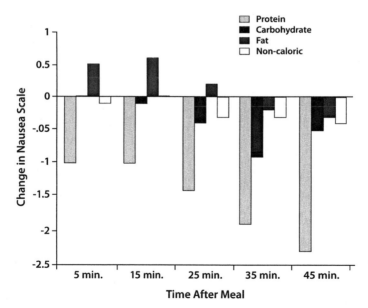

Figure 12.3 Change in nausea of pregnant women as a function of time since protein, carbohydrate, fat, and noncaloric meal. Redrawn with permission from Jednak et al., 1999.

Walsh et al. (1996) linked gastric dysrhythmias and estrogen/progesterone levels by the vaginal administration of estrogen and progesterone combinations in healthy women. In response to a test meal, the women treated with estrogen and progesterone had tachygastria and bradygastria EGG patterns, whereas women treated with placebo had normal 3-cpm responses to the test meal. It was concluded that estrogen and estrogen and progesterone combinations, at physiological plasma concentrations seen during pregnancy, disrupted normal gastric myoelectrical rhythms, possibly via prostaglandin mechanism, since indomethacin eradicated the dysrhythmias.

In a study by Riezzo et al. (1992), gastric electrical rhythms were recorded with EGG methods in patients with NVP. These patients were not having nausea at the time of the EGG recording and none of them had abnormal EGG rhythms such as tachygastria or bradygastria, confirming previous studies (Jednak et al., 1999; Koch et al., 1990a).

Hormones that affect stomach neuromuscular function are possible candidates for mediating NVP (Emond et al., 1999). Increasing levels of relaxin over the first trimester may link nausea and vomiting with gastric neuromuscular disturbances (Eddie et al., 1986). Leptin is an appetite-suppressing peptide that may have effects on the stomach. The relationships among the physiology of estrogen, progesterone, GNRH, and the enteric nervous system of the gastrointestinal tract was explored by Mathias and Clench (1998). Early in gestation the threshold for AVP release is decreased, and hCG may play a role in resetting the threshold for AVP release (Davison et al., 1984). And Xu et al. (1993) have observed that during motion sickness, increases in nausea and plasma vasopressin correlated with the percentage of tachygastria. Morphine infusions that induced nausea also increased plasma vasopressin levels, whereas morphine infusions that did not elicit nausea elicited no change in vasopressin levels (Koch et al., 1996a; Davison et al., 1988). Thus, increases in vasopressin in the first trimester may have a role in NVP.

In summary, pathogenic mechanisms of NVP are gastric dysrhythmias evoked by changes in estrogen and progesterone (or other hormones such as vasopressin) in the first trimester. The specific hormones that evoke gastric dysrhythmias are unknown, and treatment of gastric dysrhythmias and effects of this treatment on nausea requires more study.

PSYCHOSOCIAL FACTORS

Because women who reported unwanted pregnancies experienced greater NVP (FitzGerald, 1984), it was thought that psychological factors were the cause of NVP. This explanation was not supported by other studies. For example, DiIorio (1985) studied the incidence of nausea and vomiting during the first trimester in teenagers and found that the greater the desire to be pregnant, the greater the NVP. Additionally, psychosocial problems may evolve secondary to the nausea and vomiting that lasts for weeks. Atanackovic, Wolpin, and Koren (2001) reviewed the need for hospital care (emergency room, one-day observations, or hospitalization) in women with NVP; 43% of the patients needed hospital care due to the severity of vomiting (>5 times/day), the unsuccessful effect of multiple antiemetic medications, and being depressed and feeling that these symptoms had adversely affected their partner's daily life. Thus, psychosocial issues are present that need to be addressed, especially in patients with severe NVP.

DIFFERENTIAL DIAGNOSIS OF NAUSEA AND VOMITING DURING PREGNANCY

The term "morning sickness" should probably be abandoned because the nausea and/or vomiting that occurs in the first trimester can occur throughout the day (Whitehead, Andrews & Chamberlain, 1992). The differential diagnosis for nausea and vomiting is extensive and the range of causes should be reviewed in each patient (Koch, 1998), even in the woman with a known pregnancy. (See Chapter 10 for in-depth review of diagnosis and treatment of acute and chronic nausea and vomiting.)

If the patient with NVP has heartburn or regurgitation in the first trimester, then gastroesophageal reflux is present and should be treated. Epigastric burning pain may indicate peptic ulcer disease, not NVP. In NVP, the vomitus may contain yellow or even bile-stained secretions or recently ingested food, but there should be no severe periumbilical pain and recurrent voluminous bilious vomitus that may be indicative of partial or complete small bowel obstruction.

In the patient with NVP, there should be no abdominal pain. However, recurrent vomiting or retching may lead to painful abdominal muscles and ribs. If there is right upper quadrant pain that is worse after eating fatty meals, acute and chronic cholecystitis should be considered. Pain that radiates from the epigastrium through to the back suggests pancreatic disease. Severe constipation and the irritable bowel syndrome may also be associated with lower abdominal pain, abdominal bloating, and some degree of nausea. In patients with neurological disorders, vomiting usually predominates and may be projectile.

By reviewing the symptoms and appreciating the absence of abdominal pain, bilious vomiting, change in bowel habit, and other alarm symptoms, a clinical diagnosis of NVP is commonly established. There is a spectrum of NVP and some patients may be very ill at presentation.

Physical Examination

On examination, the patient with NVP will usually have normal vital signs. Dehydration and orthostatic hypotension may develop in severe cases and is discussed in the section on hyperemesis gravidarum. Because nausea and vomiting develops early in the first trimester, there is no physical evidence of the pregnancy. However, the physician should look for signs that may indicate that the nausea and vomiting is due to causes other than pregnancy.

An examination of the abdomen for rebound tenderness or palpable masses should be performed. A succussion splash, indicative of gastric stasis, would be very unusual in a patient with NVP (Koch, 2000a; Hasler et al., 1995b). A careful neurologic exam may be indicated in patients with protracted vomiting.

Laboratory Tests

A positive pregnancy test may be the only laboratory test needed to diagnose the cause of nausea and vomiting. Thus, these women have NVP rather than nausea and vomiting secondary to some other entity. Additional laboratory tests may be helpful, however. An elevated white blood count raises concern about cholecystitis, pancreatitis, or urinary tract infection (with pyelonephritis) that may be causing the nausea and vomiting. An elevated fasting glucose level reveals diabetes mellitus. Hyperglycemia (over 240 mg/dl) is associated with gastric dysrhythmias and decreased antral contractility (Hasler et al., 1995b). A liver panel may also be useful as mild elevations in liver enzymes in patients with chronic Hepatitis C virus are associated with a high incidence of nausea (Riley et al., 2001). Increased thyroid stimulating hormone level indicates hypothyroidism, another endocrine entity associated with nausea and vomiting. Increased thyroxine indicates hyperthyroidism, which is also associated with NVP. Urinalysis should be obtained and glucose, protein, or white cells in the urine should be dealt with specifically.

Management of Secondary Symptoms in NVP Patients

In the patient with NVP who has additional symptoms such as heartburn and regurgitation, lifestyle advice, antacids, or an H_2 receptor antagonist should be offered. If RUQ or epigastric pain suggestive of gallbladder or pancreatic disease is present, then an abdominal ultrasound should be obtained. Ultrasound studies are not deleterious to the human embryo or fetus (Edwards, 1994). Positive ultrasound findings of cholecystitis or pancreatitis are managed in the standard manner. Studies requiring radiation should be avoided.

For patients with hematemesis, abdominal pain, and nausea and vomiting, an upper endoscopy may be indicated. According to Cappell, Sidhom, and Colon (1996), upper endoscopy can be performed safely during pregnancy without adverse effects on the mother or on fetal outcome. Depending on the illness of the mother and other issues, fetal monitoring may be indicated when conscious sedation is used for the endoscopic procedures.

AN APPROACH TO THE TREATMENT OF NAUSEA AND VOMITING OF PREGNANCY

After excluding secondary causes of nausea and vomiting, the approach to treatment of NVP should center around relieving suffering of the individual patient while assessing the safety of the drug or nondrug treatments for the mother and the fetus (see for example Badell, Ramin, & Smith, 2006). In some women, the nausea is mild and tolerable and no treatment is necessary. In many others, there is considerable suffering. Nausea is much more disabling than vomiting, and thus, treatments should be focused on approaches to decrease nausea. Because the exact cause of the NVP is unknown, treatments are essentially empiric and supportive since symptoms diminish in most (but not all) women during the second trimester.

Diet Therapies

For patients with diabetic gastropathy, idiopathic gastroparesis, or other chronic nausea conditions, a gastroparesis or nausea and vomiting diet may be recommended (Koch, 2000a). (See Chapter 10 in this volume, for "Nausea and Vomiting Diet.") Such a diet may benefit women with NVP, but no formal studies have been carried out. The nausea/vomiting diet is a three-step diet that emphasizes salty liquids, soups, starches, and chicken breast meat for protein sources. Fatty foods are avoided because they delay gastric emptying, and vegetables or fibrous foods are avoided because they may form bezoars in patients with gastroparesis. The NVP literature is replete with similar supportive measures that encourage small frequent feedings of mainly carbohydrate foods, liquids in small amounts, and the avoidance of iron tablets or other irritating substances.

Protein-containing snacks have also been suggested. Jednak et al. (1999) showed that a high-protein meal in women with NVP significantly decreased nausea and gastric dysrhythmias when compared with a high fat or high carbohydrate meal. High protein liquids also decrease the nausea associated with motion sickness and cancer chemotherapy treatment (Levine et al., 2004; 2008). Rational selection of foods as a "nutraceutical" treatment approach to symptoms would appear to be very desirable for the nausea of pregnancy (Pepper & Craig-Roberts, 2006).

Complementary Therapies: Acupressure, Acustimulation, and Acupuncture

Acupressure

Acupressure at P6 (Neiguan) has been used to decrease nausea due to cancer chemotherapy agents and postoperative situations. Results of using acupressure to relieve the nausea of the first trimester of pregnancy have been equivocal (Aikins Murphy, 1998). O'Brien, Relyea, and Taerum (1996) obtained reports of nausea for 7 days from 161 women in the first trimester of pregnancy. The women were randomly placed in one of the following three groups: P6 acupressure band, acupressure band placed in an inappropriate place, and no-band control group. All three groups reported a significant decrease in nausea, but there were no differences between groups.

Acupressure was applied with a wristband with a button placed over the P6 point in 60 women with NVP. The placebo wrist bands had a button that applied pressure at an inappropriate site on the wrist. A nontreatment group received no acupressure in any area. The bands were worn for two weeks and a questionnaire was completed before treatment and on day 1, 3, 6, and 14 of treatment. Visual analog scales for nausea (with 0 indicating no nausea and 100 indicating severe nausea) were used. Relief from nausea appeared one day after starting the acupressure at P6 and continued for the 14 days of therapy. In contrast, patients with no treatment at all had no change in the level of nausea. Placebo-treatment patients initially improved but by day 6, their nausea symptoms were no different than the no treatment group (Werntoft & Dykes, 2001).

In a study of 97 women with first trimester nausea of pregnancy Norheim et al. (2001) applied acupressure at P6 with a wrist band with a protruding button. The placebo wristband had a felt patch rather than a protruding button. The study lasted 12 days with a 4-day run-in, 4-day treatment, and 4-day follow-up. Visual analog scales were used to record symptoms. The acupressure treatment was applied to both wrists. Results showed that 71% of the women had reduced morning sickness and reduced duration of symptoms. Of the women with placebo treatment 59% had relief of symptoms. The treatments were not statistically different except the P6 acupressure treatment subjects had reduced duration of symptoms.

Acustimulation

The P6 acupuncture point was stimulated electrically with a wristwatch-sized device in forty-one women with NVP (Evans et al., 1993). Nausea was scored on a scale of 1–5. Neonates were evaluated for congenital abnormalities. The pretreatment nausea scores averaged 4.2. On a scale of 1–5, the device was considered effective with an overall rating of 4.2, with 5 indicating significant or complete relief of nausea. No congenital abnormalities were found in the newborns. In another open-label study of NVP with an afferent nerve stimulation device, improvement in nausea symptoms and no serious adverse outcomes in the newborns were reported (Slotnick, 2001).

Acupuncture

Traditional acupuncture was used by Knight et al. (2001) on 55 women with NVP who were treated on three or four visits over a 3-week period of time. The main outcome measure was nausea as reported in a visual analog scale. Anxiety and depression were also assessed. Nausea scores decreased from 85.5 to 47.5 in the acupuncture group and from 87.0 to 48.0 in the sham treatment group, but differences were not significant.

Drug Therapies for NVP

Drug therapies for NVP are empiric, since the precise mechanisms of NVP are unknown. As mentioned above, when a specific disorder is diagnosed, such as gastroesophageal reflux or peptic ulcer disease, then specific therapy can be prescribed. Treatments range from suppressing acid with antacids to systemic drugs such as H_2 receptor antagonists or proton pump inhibitors (PPIs). For a review of the diagnosis and treatment of peptic disorders during pregnancy see Winbery and Blaho (2001).

Bendectin

Until 1983, Bendectin was used commonly for the treatment of NVP. Then the drug was alleged to cause birth defects. The manufacturer withdrew Bendectin from the market. Analyses subsequently showed no association between Bendectin use and birth defects. A meta-analysis (McKeigue et al., 1994) of cohort and case control studies again showed no association between birth defects and the use of Bendectin during pregnancy. The incidence of birth defects did not change after Bendectin was withdrawn from the market; but if Bendectin was a factor in birth defects, then the incidence of birth defects should have decreased (Lamm, 2000). The rate of hospitalizations for women with NVP doubled in the United States during the eight years after withdrawal of Bendectin from the market. The well-publicized alleged link between Bendectin use during pregnancy and birth defects sensitized women's fear or suspicion of medical therapy for their nausea and vomiting. Pharmaceutical companies were also sensitized so that drug development for these very debilitating symptoms was abandoned.

Systemic Drug Treatments for Nausea and Vomiting of Pregnancy

Before considering systemic therapy, the risk of the drug to the mother and fetus must be considered. A study by Pole et al. (2000) showed both parents and health professionals frequently rated drugs as not safe despite evidence of no association with congenital malformations. Perceptions of undue risks also sensitize and affect opinions and the advice physicians give pregnant women. These perceptions also affect receptivity toward drug treatment by pregnant women. However, fewer than 30 drugs have been proven to have teratogenic potential and many of these 30 drugs are no longer in clinical use (Koren, Pastuszak & Ito, 1998). This review by Koren, Pastuszak, and Ito (1998) provides a list of drugs that can be used during pregnancy according to a variety of common symptom conditions(Table 12.1). A comprehensive reference textbook for drugs and their risk to fetal development is available (Briggs, Freeman & Yaffe, 2008), as are reviews (Magee, Mazzotta & Koren, 2002; Jewell & Young, 2003). For a comprehensive summary of medications see Mahadevan and Kane (2006).

Vitamin Therapy

Pyridoxine hydrochloride (vitamin B6) was one of the active ingredients in Bendectin. Sahakian et al. (1991) studied 59 women treated with vitamin B6 (25 mg tablets, PO, Q 8 hrs. for 3 days) versus 28 patients who received placebo in the same format. Patients with severe nausea had a significant benefit from the B6 therapy with mean nausea scores decreasing from 4.3 to 1.8. In patients with mild to moderate nausea, no significant difference in treatment or placebo was observed. The symptomatic patients as a whole had

Table 12.1 Selected Drugs that Can Be Used Safely During Pregnancy

Condition	Drugs of Choice
Acne	Topical: erythromycin, clindamycin, benzoyl peroxide
Allergic Rhinitis	Topical: glucocorticoids, cromolyn, decongestants, xylometazoline, oxymetazoline, naphazoline, phenylephrine; Systemic: diphenhydramine, tripelennamine, astemizole
Constipation	Docusate sodium, calcium, glycerine, sorbitol, lactulose, mineral oil, magnesium hydroxide
Cough	Diphenhydramine, codeine, dextromethorphan
Depression	Tricyclic antidepressant drugs, fluoxetine
Diabetes	Insulin (human)
Headache—Tension	Acetaminophen
Migraine	Acetaminophen, codeine, dimenhydrinate
Hypertension	Labetalol, methyldopa
Mania (and bipolar affective disorder)	Lithium, chlorpromazine, haloperidol
Nausea, vomiting, motion sickness	Diclectin (doxylamine plus pyridoxine)
Peptic ulcer disease	Antacids, magnesium hydroxide, aluminum hydroxide, calcium carbonate, ranitidine
Pruritus	Topical: moisturizing creams or lotions, aluminum acetate, zinc oxide cream or ointment, calamine lotion, glucocorticoids; Systemic: hydroxyzine, diphenhydramine, glucocorticoids, astemizole
Thrombophlebitis, deep-vein thrombosis	Heparin, antifibrinolytic drugs, streptokinase

Reprinted with permission from Koch and Frissora, 2003.

significantly less vomiting episodes during B6 treatment compared with placebo. Thus, patients with severe nausea and vomiting benefited from the B6 therapy.

Ginger

Several studies have examined the effectiveness of ginger as a treatment for nausea of pregnancy, from which the following three recent examples are selected. (In this volume, see Chapter 14 for efficacy of ginger for the nausea of chemotherapy and Chapter 15 for motion sickness.) Chittumma, Kaewkiattikun, and Wiriyasiriwach (2007) compared the effectiveness of ginger and vitamin B6 for treatment of nausea and vomiting in early pregnancy. One hundred twenty-six pregnant women with nausea and vomiting were randomly allocated to receive either 650 mg of ginger or 25 mg of vitamin B6 3 times per day for 4 days. The degree of nausea and vomiting was assessed by three physical symptoms of Rhodes's score, episodes of nausea, duration of nausea, and number of vomits. Ginger and vitamin B6 significantly reduced nausea and vomiting scores. The mean score change after ginger was significantly greater than with vitamin B6.

Ensiyeh and Sakineh (2009) compared the effectiveness of ginger and vitamin B6. Seventy pregnant women were randomly assigned to receive either 1 g/day of ginger or 40 mg/day of vitamin B6 for 4 days. Subjects graded the severity of their nausea using an analog scale, and recorded the number of episodes of vomiting in the 24 hours before and 4 days during treatment. The decrease in the visual analog scores of nausea in the ginger group was significantly greater than for the vitamin B6 group. The number of vomiting episodes in both groups decreased, and there was no significant difference between the groups. Sakineh concluded that ginger is more effective than vitamin B6 for relieving the nausea of pregnancy and is equally effective for decreasing the episodes of vomiting in early pregnancy.

A study of the efficacy of ginger in comparison with dimenhydrinate in the treatment of nausea and vomiting in pregnancy was conducted by Pongrojpaw, Somprasit, and Chanthasenanont (2007). In a double-blind, randomized controlled study, 170 pregnant women with the symptoms of nausea and vomiting were randomly treated with one capsule of 0.5 g ginger twice per day or an identical capsule of 50 mg dimenhydrinate twice daily. There was no significant difference in visual analog nausea scores between the two groups in days 1–7 of treatment. No difference between groups in vomiting episodes during days 3–7 of treatment was found. There was a significantly greater side effect of drowsiness after treatment in the dimenhydrinate group. The authors concluded that from the presented data, ginger is as effective as dimenhydrinate in the treatment of nausea and vomiting during pregnancy and has fewer side effects.

To examine the effectiveness and safety of ginger in the treatment of pregnancy-induced nausea and vomiting, Borelli et al. (2005) systematically searched the literature through three computerized databases (MEDLINE, EMBASE, and Cochrane Library) and reviewed six randomized controlled trials that showed that ginger was superior to a placebo or equal in efficacy to vitamin B6 in relieving the severity of nausea and vomiting episodes. There were no spontaneous or case reports of adverse effects on pregnancy outcomes during ginger treatment in pregnancy.

Doxylamine-Pyridoxine (Diclectin®)

In the United States, there are no specific drugs labeled for the treatment of NVP. In Canada, doxylamine-pyridoxine (Diclectin®), a compound of doxylamine and vitamin B6, is a delayed-release preparation approved for NVP. The drug is typically taken in the evening to treat nausea in the morning. An additional tablet is taken in the morning and in the late afternoon to treat nausea during the day. In an observational study of 225 women with NVP, the recommended dose and higher doses of Diclectin® were prescribed. Higher doses of the drug were associated with no increase in congenital malformations, but no specific symptom assessment was reported in this study. Doses range from 5 to 12 tablets/day and were not associated with any increased incidence of sleepiness or fatigue (Atanackovic et al., 2001). A meta-analysis of controlled studies with over 170,000 first-trimester exposures to Diclectin revealed no increased risk of congenital malformations (McKeigue et al., 1994). The results of a more recent study (Shrim et al., 2006) showed no negative pregnancy outcomes when women consumed large doses of vitamin B6 during the first trimester of pregnancy.

Antihistamines

A histamine$_1$ antagonist was the other active ingredient in Bendectin. Doxylamine is the antihistamine in Diclectin®. Antihistamines are frequently used to treat the nausea of motion sickness. Meclizine (Antivert) is a widely used antihistamine for motion sickness and there is no evidence of teratogenic activity. In addition, dimenhydrinate (Dramamine) and diphenhydramine (Benadryl) are other antihistamine agents, but they have conflicting results on safety and efficacy. As early as 1949, Carliner, Radman, and Gay treated 43 women with NVP with Dramamine and obtained promising results, but no data were presented concerning safety.

Phenothiazines

The phenothiazines are also used in a nonspecific manner to control nausea and vomiting from a wide variety of causes. Promethazine (Phenergan) had no teratogenic effects as determined in one case-controlled study, but in another study a relationship with congenital hip dislocation was noted. Promethazine and prochlorperazine (Compazine), chlorpromazine (Thorazine), and trimethoben-zamide (Tigan) are other phenothiazines that have clinical efficacy, but safety in pregnancy is not established.

Agents with Gastrointestinal Actions

Metoclopramide is a drug that acts as a dopamine$_2$ receptor antagonist, a partial 5-HT$_3$ receptor antagonist, and a 5-HT$_4$ receptor agonist. Metoclopramide improves gastric emptying and corrects gastric dysrhythmias in nonpregnant patients. Metoclopramide is the antiemetic of choice for NVP in Europe (Einarson, Koren & Bergman, 1998). A recent brief report indicated that metoclopramide treatment for NVP was not associated with fetal malforma-tions (Berkovitch et al., 2000). Other prokinetic agents such as domperidone (a peripheral dopamine$_2$ antagonist), bethanechol (a muscarinic receptor agonist), and erythromycin (a motilin receptor agonist) have not been studied in NVP.

Other Drugs for Nausea and Vomiting

Droperidol (Inapsine) is a butyrophenone that has dopamine antagonist activity. This drug is an effective antiemetic and is used for postoperative nausea and vomiting and during endoscopic procedures. It is usually given by intravenous route and should be reserved for severe nausea and vomiting. A recent box warning concerning QT prolongation and cardiac dysrhythmias was issued.

The 5-HT$_3$ receptor antagonist ondansetron is commonly used for nausea and vomiting related to cancer chemotherapy agents and postoperative situations. Case reports with this drug have been limited to treating hyperemesis gravidarum and there are no double-blind, placebo-controlled trials.

In summary, according to Mazzotta and Magee (2000), there are scant evidence-based data to guide therapy for mild, moderate, or severe NVP. If nutritional counseling or acupressure or acustimulation devices are not helpful, then systemic drug therapy should be offered with Diclectin® (where available) or pyridoxine. Metoclopramide (10 mg TID), dimenhydrinate (50–100 mg PO, or by suppository) would appear to be a safe next step in systemic therapy. Some experts recommend metoclopramide only after week 10 gestation. If NVP continues, then phenothiazines would be the next step, as there are no data to indicate increased teratogenicity. Ondansetron may be considered if these other medications are not successful. Treatment approaches for hyperemesis gravidarum are described below.

HYPEREMESIS GRAVIDARUM

When pregnant women develop severe nausea and vomiting to the point of dehydration, electrolyte abnormalities, or weight loss, then the disorder is referred to as hyperemesis gravidarum (HG). The incidence of HG is between 3 and 20 per 1,000 pregnancies, with 5 per 1,000 being the most commonly accepted figure (Fairweather, 1968; Chin & Lao, 1988). A more recent study gave a higher figure of 12.8/1000 (Chin, 2000). If untreated, HG can lead to significant morbidity including maternal and fetal death. HG can coexist with gestational diseases and life-threatening pregnancy-associated diseases of the liver, which require accurate diagnosis upon initial presentation.

Pathophysiology

The underlying pathophysiology in HG is complex and poorly understood. The pathophysiology of the clinical syndrome of hyperemesis involves: (1) the hormonal changes of early pregnancy; (2) the emetic center in the brainstem; and (3) altered function in the enteric nervous system and smooth muscle function resulting in altered gastrointestinal motility.

HG has been linked to elevated levels of estrogen. Depue et al. (1987) demonstrated that estrogen, and not progesterone, levels are increased in patients with HG. The hormonal changes affect the function of neuropeptides and neurons in the central nervous system as well as the enteric nervous system. For example, estrogen stimulates nitric oxide synthetase and nitric oxide, that relaxes smooth muscle. Thus, estrogen may be one of the factors that alters gastrointestinal smooth muscle contraction or the pacemaker function of the stomach, gastric factors that may contribute to hyperemesis.

Vomiting results from activation of the so-called "emetic center" in the brain stem. This center receives afferent stimuli from the gastrointestinal tract and from the area postrema in the medulla, which is directly stimulated by toxic substances and by increased blood levels of urea and ketones (Biggs, 1975). In a perpetuating cycle, dehydration will cause further vomiting in some patients.

Altered gastric myoelectrical rhythms may be part of the pathophysiology of HG. The stomach contracts at a rate of 3 cpm for normal emptying. In three patients with HG the normal 3-cpm EGG pattern was absent and "flatline" EGG recordings were recorded (Koch, K. L., personal communications). It is known that hCG can cause gestational hyperthyroidism through cross-reaction with the TSH receptor (Glinoer, 1998). Gestational hyperthyroidism is frequently associated with HG, but the effect on gastrointestinal neuromuscular function has not been studied. Additional, unidentified mechanisms may be involved.

In the past, psychosocial factors were thought to be involved in HG. However, according to Fairweather (1968), these studies were conducted in an unblinded and biased manner, and findings have not been duplicated by more carefully performed studies. Simpson et al. (2001) found no support for the theory that HG is a psychosomatic disorder. At this time psychological factors have an unproven role in HG.

HG is more likely to occur with multiple gestation, gestational trophoblastic disease, and certain fetal abnormalities such as triploidy (partial mole), trisomy 21, and hydrops fetalis. These conditions must be excluded before attributing the symptoms to nonobstetrical causes. Basso and Olsen (2001) reviewed 9401 births from women who were hospitalized for HG from 1980 to 1996 in Denmark. Twins were twice as common in pregnancies with HG. The male to female sex ratio was 0.87 (95% CI = 0.82–0.91).

The three principle trophoblastic diseases of pregnancy are: hydatidiform mole, invasive mole, and choriocarcinoma. The risk for hyperemesis is increased in all of these disorders. Hydatidiform moles or "molar pregnancy" occur in 1 in 1500 pregnancies in the United States. Hydatidiform mole develops 10 times more often in women over the age of 45 than in those who are younger. Hydatidiform mole is a neoplastic proliferation of the trophoblast in which the terminal villi are transformed into vesicles full of clear fluid. Hydatidiform mole is usually benign but at times precedes the development of choriocarcinoma. Patients with molar pregnancy present with amenorrhea, during which time the patient considers herself to be pregnant. Nausea and vomiting are more severe and pregnancy induced hypertension is more common in trophoblastic disease. A positive diagnosis is made by sonography showing cystic lesions; also hCG levels are higher than for normal pregnancy. The uterus should be evacuated as soon as the diagnosis is made.

Differential Diagnosis

Patients with hyperemesis may have other underlying diseases that are unrelated to obstetrical causes of nausea and vomiting. HG typically begins in the first trimester. Thus, severe vomiting that develops after the first trimester is more likely to have other causes. The potentially lethal disorders to consider are: preeclampsia/eclampsia, HELLP syndrome (hemolysis, elevated liver enzymes, and low platelets), and acute fatty liver of pregnancy (AFLP).

Maternal-Fetal Complications of Hyperemesis

In mothers with HG who experienced weight loss, there is a 23% chance of the fetal weight being less than the 10th percentile (Gross, Librach & Cecutti, 1989). Fetal death rarely occurs in mothers with hyperemesis, but maternal morbidity can be significant. The most common serious disorder reported is Wernicke's encephalopathy which results from thiamine (Vitamin B1) deficiency. Wernicke's encephalopathy is sometimes associated with central pontine myelinolysis (Peeters et al., 1993). Serious injury rarely occurs as a result of severe vomiting. Yamamoto et al. (2001) reported a patient who developed esophageal rupture and presented with pneumomediastinum as a result of hyperemesis.

Clinical Presentation

HG typically presents in the first trimester of pregnancy. It is the very severe form of NVP. Predisposing factors include adolescent pregnancy, multiple gestation, and hydatidiform mole. In addition to nausea and vomiting, dry mouth, sialorrhea, hyperolfaction, dysgeusia (altered or metallic taste), and decreased gustatory discernment are reported. Clinical signs of HG include persistent vomiting beyond the first trimester and weight loss greater than 5% of prepregnancy weight. Physical exam may reveal dry mucous membranes, poor skin turgor, and hypotension. Laboratory data reveal electrolyte abnormalities and ketonuria. With hyponatremia, mental status changes can also occur. Liver transaminases and renal function are normal unless dehydration is pronounced. Abnormal liver tests should prompt a thorough investigation for HELLP syndrome and AFLP. Poor dietary intake can lead to nutritional deficits such as vitamin B1 (thiamine), iron, calcium, and folate deficiency.

Treatment

Intravenous and Oral Hydration

The initial treatment of HG is hydration. Prolonged vomiting of gastric contents results in hypochloremic metabolic alkalosis. Intravenous hydration is needed early in the course to replete intravascular volume and to restore electrolytes. Thiamine (Vitamin B1) 100 mg intravenously is administered prior to any dextrose to avoid Wernicke's encephalopathy. Ringers lactate is given intravenously through a 16 Fr IV catheter at 350 cc/hour. After 2 liters is infused, the volume can usually be decreased. After 24 hours of hydration, the intravenous fluid rate is adjusted to maintain urine output. Many patients improve promptly after rehydration and can be maintained by IV hydration as an outpatient as needed. Sodium, potassium, and magnesium levels must be frequently monitored and replaced as needed. When checking the calcium levels, it is essential to correct for the low albumin, which is common in pregnancy due to fluid shifts.

When oral hydration is tolerated it is best to begin with small, frequent volumes of salty fluids such as homemade chicken soup or pedialyte. Once oral hydration is tolerated patients can be advanced to step 2 of the gastroparesis diet (see above) which is crackers, noodles, and peanut butter.

Ginger

Fischer-Rasmussen et al. (1991) investigated the use of ginger for HG. Thirty women participated in a double-blind randomized cross-over trial of a natural product, the powdered root of ginger (Zingiber officinale) 250 mg po QID vs. placebo. The ginger was taken for 4 days with a 2-day washout in between placebo and ginger. Patients reported significantly greater relief after ginger compared to placebo (p = 0.035). The relief seemed to be achieved by reducing the degree of nausea and the number of attacks of vomiting. The preference for the ginger treatment period was statistically significant (p = 0.003). No side effects were observed. One spontaneous abortion occurred in 27 pregnancies, which was not a high rate of miscarriage. One drawback is that the study period was only 4 days, but overall the treatment appears safe and may help some patients.

Methylprednisolone

Several studies have investigated methylprednisolone treatment in HG. A double-blind study of 40 patients evaluated oral methylprednisolone (16 mg po TID) or oral promethazine (25 mg 3 TID) (Taylor, 1996). The methylprednisolone was tapered over 2 weeks whereas the promethazine dose was stable over 2 weeks. Those patients who continued to vomit for 2 days were excluded from the study. No patient from the methylprednisolone group, but five of the seven patients in the promethazine group were readmitted for hyperemesis within 2 weeks of discharge (p = 0.0001). There were no adverse effects noted for either drug. However, long-term use of steroids throughout pregnancy may be associated with adverse outcomes for the fetus (Safari et al., 1998; Taylor, 1996).

Erythromycin

El Younis, Abulafia, and Sherer (1998) reported that HG in two cases responded to oral erythromycin (250 mg QID for 5 days). Erythromycin acts as a gastric prokinetic by binding the motilin receptor in the stomach. Whether erythromycin treatment will reduce symptoms in larger groups of patients remains to be demonstrated.

Nutritional Support

In HG the absorptive function of the intestine is normal. If nutritional support is needed, an 8 Fr nasojejunal feeding tube with a weighted tip may be used.

Tube feeding can begin at 20 cc/hr and be increased as tolerated to 60–120 cc/hr for 12–24 hours depending on the amount of desired calories. Most enteral nutrition solutions have 1 calorie per cc. Therefore, a rate of 80 cc/hr would supply 1920 Kcal per day if given continuously (Hsu et al., 1996). An 8 Fr Dobbhoff nasojejunal tube with infusion rates to 110 ml. hour was tolerated in all 7 patients. In the most severe cases of hyperemesis, total parenteral nutrition (TPN) has been used to provide nutrition. TPN carries many risks including pneumothorax upon placement of the central line, line infection and sepsis, hyperglycemia, diabetes, and cholelithiasis (Levine & Esser, 1988).

Pregnancy Outcome

No significant differences in spontaneous miscarriage or birth weights have been found in women who have HG. A low risk of central nervous system and skeletal malformations in children born of women with hyperemesis was noted. Depue et al. (1987) have reported that HG may also be a risk factor for testicular cancer in male offspring.

In summary, HG is a multifactorial neurohormonal disorder of pregnancy resulting in severe and prolonged nausea and vomiting. Electrolyte abnormalities and dehydration always ensue. HG must not be confused with preeclampsia, HELLP syndrome, or AFLP, which are potentially life-threatening if unrecognized. Treatment of HG focuses on rehydration, nutritional support, and prevention of recurrence. Nondrug therapies such as ginger and acustimulation may benefit some patients. Since medications are of limited value, hydration, diet, and nutrition are the mainstay of treatment.

CONCLUSIONS

Nausea and vomiting of pregnancy and hyperemesis gravidarum reflect the broad spectrum of pregnancy-related disturbances in hormonal and gastrointestinal function. The pathophysiology of these debilitating symptoms is poorly understood. Entirely new hypotheses are needed.

An understanding of the relationships between pregnancy-related hormonal events and neuromuscular dysfunction of the gastrointestinal tract may lead to new efficacious therapies for NVP. In the meantime, the burden of the symptoms of nausea and vomiting are beginning to be appreciated and additional attempts to treat these symptoms are evolving. Blum (2000) described nausea as "irremediable suffering" which is, at the least, "an uncomfortable, disruptive, and preoccupying experience." There is much work to be done in understanding and relieving the irremediable suffering of the nausea and vomiting of pregnancy.

Chapter 13

Postoperative Nausea

Nausea frequently accompanies and/or follows surgery. In this chapter we will often discuss postoperative nausea and vomiting (PONV) because many studies in this area do not differentiate between nausea and vomiting. Nausea and vomiting are collectively often referred to as the "big little problem" (Kapur, 1991) in anesthesiology practices.

PONV is a potential problem for all patients undergoing surgical operation. PONV is a common problem for ambulatory surgery patients and occurs in an estimated 35% of all patients and 70% of high-risk patients. Complications of postoperative vomiting (POV) include wound disruption, esophageal tears and rupture, rib fracture, gastric herniation, muscular fatigue, rupture of cutaneous vessels in the upper body, dehydration, and electrolyte imbalance (Andrews, 1992). There is also the risk of aspiration of vomitus and pneumonia. Postoperative nausea (PON) can be very distressing for patients and result in anxiety about and even avoidance of future surgical operations. The prevalence of PON and PONV varies depending on the several risk factors listed below. For additional discussion of the risk factors for postoperative nausea and vomiting see Andrews (1999), Gan (2006), and Apfel (2010).

RISK FACTORS FOR PONV

Patient Risk Factors

Certain patient groups are at higher risk for PONV than others and this is important information when a decision is made whether or not to give preoperative prophylactic antiemetics, and which agents to administer. (See "Treatment" section below.)

> *Gender*—The prevalence of PONV is higher in women than men (Camilleri et al., 2005), but this difference is not evident for children or the elderly. As Andrews (1992) has pointed out, women are more sensitive than men to virtually all emetic stimuli.
>
> *Age*—Rub, Andrews, and Whitehead (1992) reported a decrease in prevalence of nausea with increasing age. The prevalence of PONV is low in very young children, increases up to age 5, and peaks in children 6–16 years old. This is similar to the effect of age on susceptibility to motion sickness (Reason & Brand, 1975). Overall, children are two times more likely to develop PONV than adults.

Motion Sickness—Patients with a history of motion sickness are more likely to develop PONV (Epstein, 1993; Thomas et al., 2007).

Obesity—Following surgery, some obese patients may experience prolonged PONV possibly because fat-soluble anesthetics may accumulate in adipose tissue and continue to be released over an extended period of time.

Migraine Headaches—Patients with a history of migraine headaches are more likely to experience PONV.

History of PONV—Such patients may have a lower threshold for nausea and/or vomiting, and anxiety due to previous experience of PONV, which may increase the risk.

Gastroparesis–Patients with delayed gastric emptying may be at greater risk of developing PONV.

Risk Factors as a Function of Type of Surgery

Longer surgical procedures are more likely to lead to PONV; and the following surgical procedures result in higher incidence of PONV including gynecological; gastrointestinal; laparoscopic; ear, nose, and throat; and strabismus and other ophthalmic procedures (Andrews, 1992).

Risk Factors as a Function of Anesthetic

The following anesthetic agents can increase the risk of PONV:

- Opioid analgesics
- Nitrous oxide
- Some inhalation agents
- Longer procedures and greater depth of anesthesia

Postoperative Risk Factors

Several postoperative factors may influence the risk of PONV. Some of the established factors are as follows:

Pain—The relationship of pain and nausea is complex. Sometimes the relief of pain relieves nausea. But if opioid analgesics are used to relieve the pain, nausea will usually increase.

Use of opioids—The use of opioids will usually increase the risk of PONV because of their known emetic potential.

Dizziness—PONV is increased in patients who experience dizziness.

Movement—Early or sudden movement following surgery can increase the risk of PONV.

Hypotension—Postoperative hypotension is common and can trigger PONV.

Premature eating or drinking—Following surgery oral intake should be limited to small sips of water, ginger ale, or electrolyte-containing sports drinks to minimize the risk of PONV.

According to Gan (2006), current risk-scoring systems have approximately 55%–80% accuracy in predicting which patient groups will suffer PONV. Apfel et al. (2002) compared the ability of different models to predict postoperative nausea and vomiting based on several different combinations of risk factors. Some models had as many as 12 factors, but Apfel et al. found that their model based on the following four risk factors had the greatest predictive value: female gender, history of motion sickness and/or PONV, no history of smoking, and use of opioids for analgesia. More recently, Peng et al. (2007) described the use of artificial neural networks to predict postoperative nausea and vomiting.

Stadler et al. (2003) conducted a somewhat unique study in this area in that they examined differences in risk factors for postoperative nausea (PON) and postoperative vomiting (POV) separately rather than combining risk factors for PONV. The study included 671 consecutive surgical patients undergoing various procedures. Nausea measures were obtained using a visual analog scale every four hours after completion of the surgical procedure. Some risk factors predicted both nausea and vomiting: female gender, history of no smoking, use of general anesthetic. But other risk factors were mainly related to nausea; for example, history of migraine, type of surgery. The authors concluded that these differences in risk factors for nausea and vomiting may be explained by considering differences in the pathophysiology of the two symptoms.

POSSIBLE CAUSES OF PON

Many articles appear in the medical literature comparing the efficacy of various pharmacological agents in preventing or reducing PONV, but few deal with the causes of PONV, and those that do (Wilhelm, Dehoorne-Smith & Kale-Pradhan, 2007) discuss possible CNS pathways involved in stimulating the chemoreceptor trigger zone (CTZ), which is located in the area postrema (see Chapter 4 in this volume) and/or the responses of this pathway to commonly used emetic anesthetic and analgesic agents. No articles have been found that deal solely with the causes of PON; therefore, the following four factors should be considered.

First, the emetic qualities of several anesthetic and analgesic agents suggest that they might also provoke nausea, but the mechanisms underlying the nausea symptoms are not known. However, the CNS-depressing effects of anesthetics and analgesics, which may be detected in gut and/or brain, are similar to those of some toxins, and, therefore, nausea may be provoked as a protective mechanism (see Chapter 1, in this volume).The other three factors that are thought to contribute to PON are ileus, lack of oral feeding, and fluid loss. In an editorial in the *New England Journal of Medicine* it was pointed out that "Postoperative ileus, a temporary impairment of gastrointestinal motility, occurs universally after major abdominal surgery. This condition exacerbates nausea and vomiting, delays oral feeding, increases postoperative pain, and prolongs hospitalization" (Steinbrook, 2001). Ileus can also occur following nonabdominal surgery (Carter, 2006). In a review article about postoperative nausea and vomiting, Kreis (2006) concludes that PONV can be secondary to the effects of ileus. Several studies have shown (e.g., Uijtdehaage, Stern & Koch, 1992) that lack of feeding leads to a loss of normal 3-cpm gastric myo-electric activity, an increase of abnormal tachygastric activity, and reports of nausea. Fluid loss that occurs during surgery together with the limited fluid intake permitted postoperatively will result in an increase in vasopressin levels in many postoperative patients, and several studies (e.g. Koch et al., 1990b) have shown that increased vasopressin is accompanied by reports of nausea. For a more complete discussion of the relationship of vasopressin levels to nausea see Chapters 6 and 7 in this volume.

TREATMENT

Drug Therapy

Patients who are at a moderate to high risk of developing PONV are treated with a combination of antiemetic drugs prior to surgery. Prophylactic treat-ment, rather than waiting until nausea and vomiting appear after surgery, is preferred by patients (White & Watcha, 1999) and is more cost-effective (Watcha & Smith, 1994).

No single drug or class of drugs is usually fully effective in controlling PONV, presumably because none block all of the receptor types implicated in nausea and vomiting. Classes of anti-emetic drugs include the 5-HT$_3$ receptor antagonists (e.g., ondansetron), corticosteroids (e.g., dexamethasone), buty-rophenones (e.g., droperidol), antihistamines (e.g., dimenhydrinate), anticho-linergics (e.g., scopolamine), mu opioid receptor antagonists (e.g., naloxone), and neurokinin-1 receptor antagonist (e.g., aprepitant) (Gan et al., 2007). Combinations of anti-emetic drugs from different classes may be used as dis-cussed below.

As mentioned at the beginning of this chapter, many investigators working on issues related to PONV fail to differentiate between *symptoms* of nausea and the act of vomiting, and this is also true for studies of treatments. However, an exception appears in an article by Gan (2002) in which he points out that it is important to distinguish between the symptoms of nausea and the act of vomiting because some drugs are more effective against nausea (e.g., droperi-dol), while others are more effective against vomiting (e.g., 5-HT$_3$ serotonin receptor antagonists). On the other hand, a retrospective study showed ondansetron (a 5-HT$_3$ receptor antagonist) provided a 26% relative risk reduc-tion in PON and a 33% relative risk reduction in POV (Jokela et al., 2009). Moreover, a post hoc analysis of a multicenter PONV drug trial showed that droperidol reduced nausea and vomiting equally in the early (0-2 hr) postop-erative period (Apfel et al., 2009).

The antiemetic drugs used as prophylaxic agents prior to surgery and their receptor site affinity are summarized by Scuderi (2003) (see Table 13.1). The reader interested in the pharmacology of antiemetics is referred to Scuderi (2003). Clearly much more investigation is needed regarding the mechanisms and treatments of PON and POV.

The system used by Gan (2002) making use of patient and surgical risk factors to determine optimal prophylactic antiemetic treatment is shown in Figure 13.1. The percentage denotes risk of developing PONV. For example,

Table 13.1 Receptor Site Affinity of Antiemetic Drugs*

Pharmacologic Group	Dopamine (D₂)	Muscarinic Cholinergic	Histamine	Serotonin
Anticholinergics				
Scopolamine	+	++++	+	-
Antihistamines				
Cyclizine	+	+++	++++	-
Dimenhydrinate	+	++	++++	-
Diphenhydramine	+	++	++++	-
Hydroxyzine	+	++	++++	-
Medizine	+	+++	++++	-
Promethazine	++	++	++++	-
Antiserotonins				
Dolasetron	-	-	-	++++
Granisetron	-	-	-	++++
Ondansetron	-	-	-	++++
Ramosetron	-	-	-	++++
Benzamides				
Domperidone	++++	-	-	+
Metoclopramide	+++	-	-	++
Butyrophenones				
Droperidol	++++	-	+	+
Haloperidol	++++	-	+	-
Phenothiazines				
Chlorpromazine	++++	++	++++	+
Fluphenazine	++++	+	++	-
Perphenazine	++++	+	++	+
Prochlorperazine	++++	++	++	+
Steroids				
Betamethasone	-	-	-	-
Dexamethasone	-	-	-	-

*Modified from Peroutka and Snyder (1982) and Watcha and White (1992).

Reproduced with permission from Scuderi, 2003.

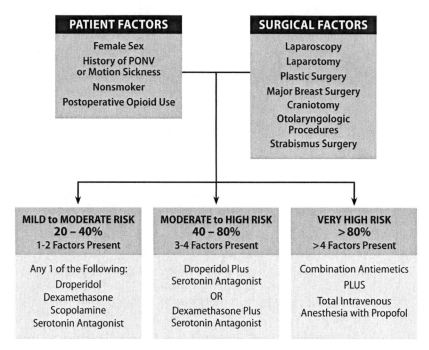

Figure 13.1 Risk factors for PONV and guidelines for prophylactic antiemetic therapy
Reproduced with permission from Gan, 2002.

a patient classified as very high risk would have at least four risk factors, and would be treated with combination antiemetics (drugs that antagonize at least two different receptors), plus total IV anesthesia (no inhaled agents), plus propofol.

   As mentioned above, many studies have been done comparing the efficacy of different drugs to prevent or reduce PONV. An example is a multicenter European study (Apfel, et al., 2004) that compared six interventions, including a comparison of three commonly used antiemetics—droperidol, dexamethasone, and ondansetron. The investigators found that the three drugs yielded similar results. White (2004), commenting on the results of the Apfel et al. study, pointed out that the low cost and excellent safety profile of both droperidol and dexamethasone make the combination of these two drugs a highly cost-effective strategy for preventing PONV. The addition of ondansetron resulted in only a small incremental benefit when administered to high-risk patients undergoing ambulatory surgery. Gan et al. (2007) in a comparison of the NK-1 antagonist, aprepitant, versus ondansetron for the prevention of PONV found aprepitant was superior to ondansetron for prevention of vomiting in the first 24 and 48 h, but no significant differences were observed between aprepitant and ondansetron for nausea control, use of rescue, or complete response. Similarly, Apfel, Malhotra, and Leslie (2008) reported that aprepitant was superior to ondansetron for reducing POV; however, its efficacy against nausea alone was not found to be superior to other antiemetics.

Gan et al. (2003) presents consensus guidelines for managing PONV based on the recommendations of a multidisciplinary panel of 12 experts in this field. What follows is a brief summary of the recommendations. The interested reader is referred to the original publication.

> *Guideline 1*—Identify adults at high risk for PONV.
>
> *Guideline 2*—Identify children at high risk for postoperative vomiting. Because of the difficulty in diagnosing nausea in young children, only vomiting is studied and treated in this population.
>
> *Guideline 3*—Reduce baseline risk factors for PONV. See Table 13.2 for suggestions as to how to accomplish this guideline.
>
> *Guideline 4*—Use specific antiemetic therapy for PONV prophylaxis in adults. See Table 13.3 for prophylactic doses and timing for the administration of antiemetics in adults.
>
> *Guideline 5*—Use specific antiemetic therapy for POV prophylaxis in children. See Table 13.4 for antiemetic doses for children.
>
> *Guideline 6*—Use prophylaxis for high risk and moderate risk patients. Patients at low risk are usually not given PONV prophylaxis unless they are at risk for medical sequelae from vomiting.
>
> *Guideline 7*—Provide antiemetic treatment to patients with PONV who did not receive prophylaxis or in whom prophylaxis failed. See Table 13.5 for recommended treatment regimens for such patients.

The conclusion of the consensus guidelines follows:

> Drugs for PONV prophylaxis for adults should be considered for use as monotherapy or in combination for patients at moderate risk for PONV. There is increasing evidence that the combination of several potentially beneficial factors (multimodal approach) may lead to an improved outcome. Double and triple antiemetic combinations are recommended for patients at high risk for PONV. All prophylaxis in children at moderate or high risk for POV should be with combination therapy using a 5-HT$_3$ antagonist and a

Table 13.2 Strategies to Reduce Baseline Risk

Use of regional anesthesia (IIIA) (16)
Use of propofol for induction and maintenance of anesthesia (IA) (29)
Use of intraoperative supplemental oxygen (IIIB) (30,31)
Use of hydration (IIIA) (32)
Avoidance of nitrous oxide (IIA) (19,33)
Avoidance of volatile anesthetics (IA) (18,20)
Minimization of intraoperative (IIA) and postoperative (IVA) opioids (7,18,21–23)
Minimization of neostigmine (IIA) (34)

Reproduced with permission from Gan et al., 2003.

second drug. Antiemetic rescue therapy should be administered to patients
who have an emetic episode after surgery. If PONV occurs within 6 h after
surgery, patients should not receive a repeat dose of the prophylactic
antiemetic. An emetic episode more than 6 h after surgery can be treated
with any of the drugs used for prophylaxis except dexamethasone and
transdermal scopolamine. (Gan et al., 2003)

Table 13.3 Antiemetic Doses and Timing for Administration in Adults

Drug	Dose	Evidence	Timing	Evidence
Ondansetron	4–8 mg IV (37)	IA	At end of surgery (38)	IIIA
Dolasetron	12.5 mg IV (39)	IA	At end of surgery (39)	IIIA
Granisetron	0.35–1 mg IV (40–42)	IA	At end of surgery (40, 42)	IIIA
Tropisetron	5 mg IV (43)	IA	At end of surgery	VA
Dexamethasone	5–10 mg IV (44)	IIA	Before induction (47)	IIIA
Droperidol	0.625–1.25 mg IV (48, 49)	IA	At end of surgery (50)	IIA
Dimenhydrinate	1–2 mg/kg IV (51)	IIA		
Ephedrine	0.5 mg/kg IM (52)	IIIB		
Prochlorperazine	5–10 mg IV (53)	IIIA	At end of surgery (53)	IIIB
Promethazine	12.5-25 mg IV (54)	IIIB	At end of surgery (54)	IIIB
Scopolamine	Transdermal patch (55, 56)	IIB	Applied prior evening or 4h before end of surgery (56)	IIB

When a dose range is presented, the smallest dose is recommended.

Reproduced with permission from Gan et al., 2003.

Table 13.4 Antiemetic Doses for Children

Drug	Dose	Evidence
Ondansetron	50–100 ug/kg up to 4 mg (37	IIA
Dolasetron	350 ug/kg up to 12.5 mg (71)	V
Dexamethasone	150 ug/kg up to 8 mg (44)	IIA
Droperidol	50–75 ug/kg up to 1.25 mg (50)	IIA
Dimenhydrinate	0.5 mg/kg (51)	IIA
Perphenazine	70 ug/kg (72,73)	IA

Reproduced with permission from Gan et al., 2003.

Table 13.5 Antiemetic Treatment for Patients with Postoperative Nausea and Vomiting (PONV) Who Did Not Receive Prophylaxis or in Whom Prophylaxis Failed—Exclude Inciting Medication or Mechanical Causes of PONV (V)

Initial Therapy	Failed Prophylaxis
No prophylaxis or dexamethasone	Administer small-dose 5-HT$_3$ antagonist[a] (IIA)
5-HT$_3$ antagonist[a] plus second agent[b]	Use drug from different class (V)
Triple therapy with 5-HT$_3$ antagonist[a] plus two other agents[b] when PONV occurs < 6 h after surgery (V)	Do not repeat initial therapy (IIIA) Use drug from different class (V) or propofol, 20 mg as needed in postanesthesia care unit (adults) (IIIB)
Triple therapy with 5-HT$_3$ antagonist[a] plus two other agents[b] when PONV occurs > 6 h after surgery (V)	Repeat with 5-HT$_3$ antagonist[a] and droperidol (not dexamethasone or transdermal scopolamine) Use drug from different class (V)

5-HT$_3$ = serotonin.

[a] Small-dose 5-HT antagonist dosing: ondansetron 1.0 mg, dolasetron 12.5 mg, granisetron 0.1 mg, and tropisetron 0.5 mg.

[b] Alternative therapies for rescue: droperiodol 0.625 mg IV, dexamethasone (2–4 mg IV), and promethazine 12.5 mg IV.

Reproduced with permission from Gan et al., 2003.

ALTERNATIVE/COMPLEMENTARY THERAPY FOR PONV

During the past few years, several studies have appeared in the literature describing attempts to use nondrug prophylaxics, alternative or complementary medicine, to reduce or prevent PONV. In the following section, examples of studies that have used ginger, acupuncture, acustimulation, and acupressure are described.

Chaiyakunapruk et al. (2006) reported the results of a meta-analysis of five studies including 363 patients in which the effects of 1 gm of dried ginger root were compared to a placebo as prophylaxis for PONV. The authors concluded that ginger was significantly better than placebo for the prevention of PONV. They stated that ginger can reduce the likelihood of having PONV by 36%. Abdominal discomfort was the only negative side effect reported.

Ezzo, Streiberger, and Schneider (2006) summarized the results of 26 trials, over 3000 patients, in which acupuncture at P6 was compared to sham acupuncture for the prevention of PONV. The P6 point is on the under side of the wrist and, according to traditional Chinese medicine, controls nausea. According to Ezzo et al., the pooled data showed that acupuncture at P6 was superior to sham acupuncture in preventing PONV in both adults and children, and was superior to several antiemetic drugs.

Electrical stimulation, rather than acupuncture, at P6 was used by Kabalak et al, (2005) and compared with the ability of ondansetron to relieve PONV in children who had tonsillectomies. There were 30 children randomly assigned to each group plus a third no-treatment group. The results showed that there was significantly less PONV in both treatment groups compared to the no-treatment group, and the parents' satisfaction score was also significantly higher for children who were in the treatment groups. However it was noted that children in the ondansetron group had more side effects than children in the two other groups. The authors concluded that acustimulation at P6 is an easy, painless, reliable, and effective means of relieving PONV in children. However, the study lacked a control for the possible placebo effect of the acustimulation. In another study using acustimulation, Habib et al. (2006b) examined the efficacy of the Reliefband, a commercial device that stimulates P6, to relieve nausea and vomiting during and after caesarean delivery under spinal anesthetic. Patients were randomly assigned to an active Reliefband group or a control Reliefband group that wore the device on the dorsal side of their wrist. The authors reported finding no differences between groups in nausea, vomiting, or patient satisfaction.

In a more recent study, Turgut et al. (2007) reported success using acupressure to relieve postoperative nausea and vomiting following gynecological surgery in women receiving patient controlled morphine. All women received a general anesthetic and following surgery 50 were randomly assigned to a group that received acupressure; a band with an attached bead that applied pressure to the P6 point was placed around both wrists. Another 50 women were assigned to a control group and had the band and bead applied to a nonacupoint site. The results showed that only 33% of the women in the acupressure group experienced nausea compared with 63% in the control group. And in the acupressure group only 25% reported vomiting, whereas 61% of the control group vomited. These results are among the strongest demonstrating the benefits of using acuprocedures to reduce postoperative nausea and vomiting. The study is also mentioned in this chapter because it is one of the few studies in the PONV literature that reports effects for nausea apart from PONV. But in general, these alternative and complementary procedures are considered promising areas of research and application about which much remains to be learned.

CONCLUSIONS

Postoperative nausea continues to be a major clinical problem for moderate- and high-risk patients. The risk for a given individual depends on the interaction of patient risks, surgery risks, and anesthetic/analgesic risks. Prophylactic treatment prior to surgery rather than treating symptoms postoperatively is preferred by patients and more cost-effective for hospitals. Some factors that are thought to contribute to postoperative nausea are the emetic characteristics of many anesthetics and analgesics, ileus, lack of feeding, and loss of fluids.

Chapter 14

Nausea Resulting from Cancer and Its Treatment

Nausea associated with radiation therapy and chemotherapy is one of the most distressing side effects of cancer treatment. Several studies have shown that incidence and/or severity of cancer chemotherapy-induced nausea is often underestimated by physicians and nurses (Wickham, 1999; Coates et al., 1983; Craig & Powell, 1987; Passik et al., 2001; Grunberg et al., 2004). This chapter discusses nausea caused by the malignancies themselves and nausea caused by radiotherapy and chemotherapy. Because some authors fail to differentiate between nausea and vomiting, the large literature in this area is difficult to summarize and conclusions are difficult to draw. And studies of chemotherapy-induced nausea sometimes do not make clear whether or not acute or delayed nausea is assessed.

NAUSEA CAUSED BY MALIGNANCIES

Although the nausea associated with cancer is usually caused by the anticancer treatment, in some cases nausea is caused by the particular malignancy. Examples include but are not limited to primary and metastatic gastrointestinal (GI), liver, or bowel obstruction caused by primary or metastatic cancers, and brain cancers.

According to Teng (2000), "The formation of a tumor impinging extrinsically on the GI tract may cause NV as a result of nerve impulses sent from the upper GI tract to the Vomiting Center or network by the way of vagal and parasympathetic nerves (p. 437)." Nausea is commonly reported by patients with infiltrating stomach cancer termed linitus plastica. Nausea is also associated with gastric or small bowel obstruction from advanced or recurrent cancers. Nausea is common in duodenal and proximal jejunal cancers. Twenty-five percent of patients with colon cancer report nausea and vomiting, but those with right colon cancer tend to report nausea but not vomiting. Nausea is reported by 19%–40% of patients with liver cancer. Twenty-four percent of patients with brain tumors report nausea; 67% of those patients who also have increased cranial pressure experience nausea (Teng, 2000).

NAUSEA CAUSED BY RADIOTHERAPY

According to Feyer et al. (2005), as many as 40%–80% of patients undergoing radiotherapy (RT) experience nausea depending on the site of irradiation. However, the nausea is usually not as severe as that experienced by chemotherapy patients (see below). Patients receiving RT to the brain or GI system have the greatest probability of experiencing nausea (Teng, 2000). The latency to reports of nausea is approximately one hour, and it tends to continue for two to three hours. Since RT often involves treatments that continue for six to eight weeks, repeated experiences of nausea sometimes cause patients to delay or refuse further RT. Incidence of RT-induced nausea depends on RT-related factors such as single and total dose fractionation, radiated volume, and RT special techniques. Patient-related factors that have been found to contribute to nausea include gender, general health, age, concurrency or recent chemotherapy, and psychological state. For a description of treatments for the nausea of RT see treatments for the nausea of chemotherapy below.

NAUSEA CAUSED BY CHEMOTHERAPY

Nausea associated with chemotherapy is usually classified as follows:

Acute Nausea—Nausea experienced during approximately the first 18–24 hours following administration of chemotherapy.

Delayed Nausea—Nausea that occurs more than 24 hours following chemotherapy.

Anticipatory Nausea—Nausea that occurs prior to administration of a chemotherapy treatment and usually after previous chemotherapy sessions that provoked nausea.

ACUTE AND DELAYED NAUSEA

The incidence of acute and delayed nausea associated with highly and moderately emetogenic chemotherapy drugs has been studied by several investigators (e.g., Grunberg et al., 2004). In their study, patients were recruited from 14 oncology clinics in six countries. Overall, more than 35% of patients reported acute nausea and 60% reported delayed nausea. For additional information about the prevalence of nausea associated with chemotherapy see Chapter 2 in this volume.

The incidence and severity of chemotherapy-induced nausea and vomiting varies according to many factors including the particular cytotoxic drug, dose, schedule of administration, and route. Individual patient variables are also relevant. Risk factors for acute and/or delayed nausea include nausea with prior chemotherapy, female gender (Aapro, Kirchner & Terrey, 1994), nausea during pregnancy (Roscoe et al., 2004), susceptibility to motion sickness (Morrow, 1985), and younger age (McMillan, 1989). Several studies of the effects of heightened anxiety prior to a chemotherapy treatment and/or expectation of nausea have found increased nausea during or after the chemotherapy session (Jacobsen et al., 1988; Haut et al., 1991; Roscoe, Hickok & Morrow, 2000; Hickok, Roscoe & Morrow, 2001; Roscoe et al., 2004). The mechanism by which risk factors such as nausea during previous chemotherapy, or provocative motion, or pregnancy influence the degree of nausea during or following chemotherapy is not known. Two possibilities are (1) prior experiences with nausea together with knowledge that nausea is commonly associated with chemotherapy may increase one's expectation, which, as mentioned above, may increase the nausea of chemotherapy (Roscoe et al., 2004); or (2), the degree of nausea experienced by an individual, no matter what the cause, may be a function of the nausea threshold of that person and, therefore, a person who experienced high levels of nausea during, for example, pregnancy, would be predicted to experience high levels of nausea during chemotherapy (see Chapter 3, in this volume).

A rating system for classifying the acute/delayed emetic potential of chemotherapy drugs developed by the American Society of Clinical Oncology (ASCO) was updated by Kris et al. (2006). The report appears online (NCI, 2009).

Physiological Mechanisms

Many questions remain with regard to the detailed mechanisms responsible for the emesis that is associated with chemotherapy, but preclinical physiological and pharmacological studies predominantly in the ferret have identified the major pathways involved in the acute and delayed emetic responses using cisplatin as an exemplar. The acute phase is predominantly due to activation of the abdominal (intestinal) vagal afferents by 5-hydroxytryptamine released from enterochromaffin cells and which acts locally on 5-HT$_3$ receptors located on the peripheral afferent terminals (see Chapters 5 and 6, in this volume). This proposed mechanism is supported by studies in humans showing the efficacy of the 5-HT$_3$ receptor antagonists primarily in the acute phase (Hesketh et al., 2003a) and elevated levels of the urinary metabolite of 5-hydroxytryptamine, 5-hydroxyindoleacetic acid (5-HIAA). The delayed phase is less well understood and there may not be a single mechanism, but ablation of the area postrema ("CTZ"-chemoreceptor trigger zone for emesis) can abolish the delayed phase of the emetic response to cisplatin in the ferret (Percie du Sert et al., 2009). It is proposed that endogenous mediators released from the gut are responsible for activation of the area postrema, but their identity is not known. It must be noted that the preclinical studies investigate the mechanisms by which a chemotherapeutic agent induces emesis and are not models of chemotherapy as, for example, the animals do not have cancer, have not had surgery, do not have concomitant medication, and do not receive multiple cycles of cytotoxic drug administration. Studies in patients undergoing chemotherapy have shown some benefit from prokinetic and antisecretory drugs in the delayed phase, suggesting that disturbances of secretion and motility may also contribute to the delayed phase. For a detailed discussion of the physiology of emesis and nausea see Chapters 4–7 in this volume. The reader interested in the physiological mechanisms thought to be associated with the vomiting resulting specifically from chemotherapy is referred to Rudd and Andrews (2005), Hesketh (2008), and Darmani et al. (2009).

Less is known about the mechanisms involved in chemotherapy-induced acute or delayed nausea than is known about emesis primarily because of the difficulties of studying nausea in animal models (Chapter 8, in this volume). However, it is likely that the pathways described above are also the ones by which the central pathways leading to induction of nausea are also activated (Chapter 4, in this volume). However, it is difficult to envisage how mechanistic studies to investigate the pathways directly can ever be performed in patients undergoing chemotherapy. It is known that cisplatin, a commonly used chemotherapy drug, induces nausea in >90% of patients and in approximately 50% of patients who receive potent antiemetic medications. We also know that nausea is far less effectively treated than vomiting in both the acute and delayed phases. The mechanisms underlying the relative incidence and intensity of nausea evoked by the various chemotherapeutic agents is at present unknown.

Some investigators look to the physiology of the emesis of chemotherapy as a model of the physiology of the nausea of chemotherapy. Two possible reasons for this approach are the common observation that nausea frequently is followed by emesis, and the finding that nausea can sometimes be induced by less intense stimulation by the same stimulus that induces vomiting. But Rudd and Andrews (2005) point out the limits of this approach. "if nausea is due to low-level activation of the [emesis] input pathways, then it might be expected that nausea would be easier to block than vomiting, but this is not the case" (p. 23).

It has been suggested by different investigators that more may be learned about the nausea of chemotherapy by examining changes in autonomic nervous system (ANS) activity, gastric motility, and vasopressin. According to the National Cancer Institute (NCI, 2009), nausea is mediated by the ANS. Chapter 5 (in this volume) provides a discussion of the relationship of ANS to nausea in general, but only a few studies appear in the literature documenting the role of ANS in the nausea of chemotherapy. Morrow, Angel, and DuBeshter (1992) recorded several ANS measures from five female cancer patients at baseline, during peak nausea, and during vomiting. The authors reported that skin temperature and pallor increased from baseline to nausea to vomiting, and that heart rate and blood volume pulse decreased from baseline to nausea and increased from nausea to emesis. In a follow-up article from Morrow's lab, Belig et al., (1995) described the ANS measures that they found to be related to reports of nausea by chemotherapy patients. In a subsequent study, Morrow et al. (1999) reported changes in clinical measures of ANS in 20 cancer patients who developed chemotherapy-induced nausea. Eight ANS measures were obtained from the patients before chemotherapy, 2 hours after, and 24 hours after. The results showed that 2 hours after chemotherapy and before any nausea was reported, the 9 patients who subsequently developed high levels of nausea had a significantly greater percentage of abnormal clinical ANS tests than the 11 patients who subsequently developed low levels of nausea. After 24 hours the results were similar, but the differences were not significant. Morrow et al. (2000) measured vagal efferent activity, as a function of heart rate variability, in 24 female cancer patients with chemotherapy-induced nausea. Data were obtained prior to chemotherapy and during the nausea that followed chemotherapy. The results showed an increase in vagal activity immediately following infusion of the cytotoxic drug, but a decrease in vagal activity when nausea was reported. In the last of this series of reports from Morrow's lab, Gianaros et al. (2001) used a within-subject design and compared vagal activity prior to chemotherapy for sessions during which the patients subsequently developed nausea and for sessions when they did not. No differences were found in vagal activity prior to chemotherapy sessions when patients developed nausea and when they did not, but the degree of abnormal gastric activity prior to chemotherapy was found to predict subsequent nausea. In all the above studies it must be noted that changes in vagal efferent activity to the heart are not necessarily reflected in the similar directional changes in either the vagal efferent supplying the GI tract or the parasympathetic innervation of other viscera.

Riezzo et al. (2005) reported finding significant increased tachygastria following chemotherapy in patients who reported nausea and other dyspeptic symptoms. The degree of tachygastria was found to be significantly associated with the severity of nausea. As was discussed in Chapter 7 in this volume, several studies using a rotating optokinetic drum as a provocative stimulus have demonstrated a strong relationship between gastric dysrhythmias, usually tachygastria, and reports of nausea (e.g., Koch et al., 1987). And some studies, such as Gianaros et al. (2001), have shown that gastric dysrhythmias prior to chemotherapy predict subsequent nausea. The authors recorded EGGs from 25 cancer patients prior to and after chemotherapy. Thirteen of the patients experienced nausea and they showed a significant reduction in normal 3-cpm gastric activity and a significant increase in tachygastria. However, others have not found a relationship between gastric dysrhythmias and nausea induced by chemotherapy (Lindberg, Nordesjö & Hellström-Lindberg, 1996; DiBaise et al., 2001).

Brand et al. (1999) suggested that gastroparesis may be the cause of the nausea of chemotherapy, and it is important to note that during tachygastria, gastric motility decreases or even completely shuts down (Koch & Stern, 2004). Wolf (1943) showed many years ago that nauseogenic situations, i.e., putting cold water in one ear, swinging, and rotation of the head inhibited gastric contractile activity AND provoked nausea. To quote from Wolf:

> These experiments show that the same bodily changes were induced by swinging as by caloric stimulation. Decreased gastric motility was a constant occurrence, but further gastric changes and the more widespread autonomic effects occurred only when nausea or discomfort was induced. (p. 880)

Vasopressin, an antidiuretic hormone released from the posterior pituitary, increases in the blood of individuals who report nausea following vection-induced motion sickness (Koch et al., 1990b), after injection of apomorphine (Feldman, Samson & O'Dorisio, 1988), after morphine (Koch et al., 1993), after the stimulation of sitting in a rotating chair (Eversmann et al., 1978), and after cancer chemotherapy agents (Fisher et al., 1982; Edwards et al., 1989). It is not clear in these situations whether plasma vasopressin increases immediately before or immediately after the experience of nausea. Several authors (e.g., Robertson, 1977) have stated that nausea causes an increase in vasopressin release. Verbalis, Richardson, and Stricker (1987) state, "Nausea, with or without emesis, is one of the most potent stimuli to arginine vasopressin (AVP) secretion known in humans." In the typical experiment (e.g., Grant et al., 1986), vasopressin levels were found to increase from baseline to the poststimulus point at which subjects reported nausea. In those few experiments in which several vasopressin measurements were made over time rather than just one prestimulus and one poststimulus measurement (Koch et al., 1990b; Xu et al., 1993), reports of nausea covaried with vasopressin levels (see Chapter 6 in this volume). It is conceivable that through classical conditioning, the sensation of nausea has come to stimulate an increase in vasopressin release, but this is thought to be a relatively weak effect since the conditioned stimulus (nausea) and the unconditioned stimulus (vomiting) often don't follow one another, and even when they do, the nausea-vomiting interval is quite long.

To summarize, much remains to be learned about the physiological mechanisms involved in the acute and delayed nausea of chemotherapy. This explains why, as outlined in the next section, about 50% of cancer patients given cytotoxic drugs such as cisplatin and the latest antiemetic drugs still report nausea.

Treatments

A large number of treatments to prevent or reduce acute and delayed nausea and vomiting associated with chemotherapy has been described in the literature. As of January 2010, Medline listed 14,488 abstracts in response to a search for TREATMENT-NAUSEA-VOMITING-CHEMOTHERAPY. In this section the use of pharmacological agents and nonpharmacological therapies are discussed. The reader is referred to the recommendations of the National Cancer Institute (NCI, 2009). For a further discussion of antiemetic therapies see Hesketh (2008).

Pharmacological Treatments

Prior to the development of serotonin receptor antagonists (5-HT$_3$ receptor antagonists), metoclopramide was considered the most effective single antiemetic agent against highly emetogenic chemotherapy drugs such as cisplatin. However, the current recommendation of the National Cancer Institute (2009) of drugs to use either singularly or in combination to prevent and/or reduce the nausea frequently associated with chemotherapy includes a corticosteroid, a 5-HT$_3$ receptor antagonist, and an NK$_1$ receptor antagonist. Schwartzberg (2007), in an article in which he discusses the use of several antiemetic agents for chemotherapy patients, mentions that other classes of drugs such as benzodiazepines and cannabinoids offer the potential for additional protection.

Dexamethasone is the corticosteroid most commonly used to prevent and/or decrease the nausea of chemotherapy. It is sometimes used as a single agent against mildly nauseogenic cytotoxic drugs, but is more commonly used in combination with other agents. Numerous studies have shown that dexamethasone potentiates the antiemetic properties of the 5-HT$_3$ receptor antagonists (e.g., Smyth et al., 1991).

There are four 5-HT$_3$ receptor antagonists currently available in the United States: ondansetron (Zofran), granisetron (Kytril), dolasetron (Anzemet), and a second-generation agent, palonosetron (Aloxi). Numerous studies have been conducted comparing the efficacy of these drugs, but the National Cancer Institute (NCI, 2009) has concluded that there is no major difference in the effectiveness of the three first-generation agents in the prevention of chemotherapy-induced acute nausea and vomiting when used in appropriate doses (e.g., Hesketh, 2000; Navari et al., 1995a; Hesketh et al., 1996; Dua et al., 2004). Although all three first-generation 5-HT$_3$ receptor antagonists have been found to reduce acute vomiting following chemotherapy, they have not been shown to be effective during the delayed stage following chemotherapy (Hickok et al., 2003; Navari, 2003; Kris, 2003). And as mentioned in Chapter 1 in this volume, Roscoe et al. (2000) studied the effectiveness of 5-HT$_3$ receptor antagonists in preventing the nausea and vomiting of 1413 cancer patients who received chemotherapy. The patients were divided into six cohorts depending on the year in which they entered the study. No patients in the first group (1987–1990) received treatment with 5-HT$_3$ receptor antagonists, and the percentage of patients who did receive such treatment increased with each successive group. In the last group (1995), 89% of the patients received a 5-HT$_3$ receptor antagonist to prevent the nausea and vomiting of chemotherapy.

Figure 14.1a shows the division of the 1413 patients into cohort groups increasing in percentage who received 5-HT$_3$ antiemetics. Figure 14.1b shows that there was a significant reduction in vomiting with successive cohort groups; i.e., the drugs acted as effective antiemetics. But in contrast, Figure 14.1c shows that there was not a reduction in the incidence of nausea, and Figure 14.1d shows that there was a significant increase in the duration of nausea following chemotherapy as a higher percentage of patients in the groups that received antiemetic treatments.

Palonosetron has been approved by the U.S. FDA for the control of acute and prevention of delayed nausea and vomiting (Eisenberg et al., 2003; Gralla et al., 2003), but acute and delayed nausea remain as serious problems for many patients.

In 2003, the U.S. FDA approved the use of the NK$_1$ receptor antagonist aprepitant (Emend) for the prevention of the nausea and vomiting that

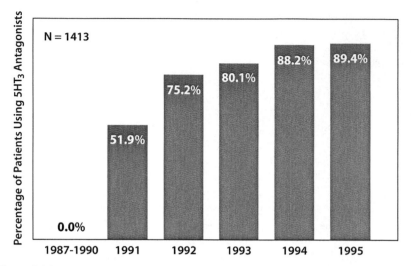

Figure 14.1 A Proportion of patients receiving 5-HT₃ receptor antagonists. Reproduced with permission from Roscoe et al., 2000.

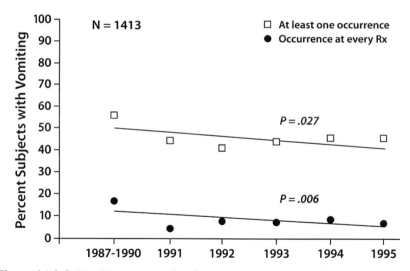

Figure 14.1 B Vomiting measured at four treatment cycles. Symbols represent proportion of patients reporting symptom. Reproduced with permission from Roscoe et al., 2000.

frequently accompany chemotherapy. Two studies were conducted, each with over 500 cancer patients receiving cisplatin, to determine the extent to which standard antiemetic therapy (dexamethasone plus ondansetron) plus aprepitant would prevent chemotherapy-induced nausea and vomiting better than standard therapy alone (Hesketh et al., 2003a; Poli-Bigelli et al., 2003).

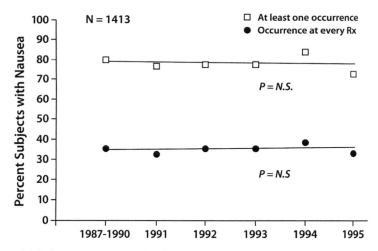

Figure 14.1 C Nausea measured at four treatment cycles. Symbols represent proportion of patients reporting nausea. Reproduced with permission from Roscoe et al., 2000.

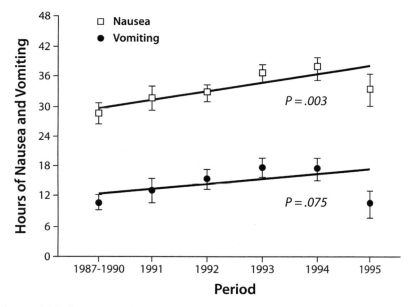

Figure 14.1 D Average duration per incident. Reproduced with permission from Roscoe et al., 2000.

In both studies the group that received standard therapy plus aprepitant experienced significantly less acute and delayed emesis than the group that only received standard therapy. However, the results for the effects on nausea were not as positive. In both studies, the addition of aprepitant did not significantly reduce either "nausea" or "significant nausea" (Merck, 2010).

In conclusion, much still remains to be learned about the causes and treatment of the nausea that is experienced by many cancer patients receiving nauseogenic cytotoxic drugs such as cisplatin. While two studies did report a significant reduction in nausea for some cancer patients using 5-HT$_3$ (Navari et al., 1995b) or NK$_1$ (Van Belle et al., 2002) receptor antagonists, differences in methodology, including the outcome measure of nausea (complete protection or partial protection) and in the subgroups of cancer patients who participated in various studies make comparative assessments difficult. In general, the majority of studies have reported that while these drugs are effective in reducing emesis, they did little to relieve either acute or delayed nausea. Progress has been made in the development of combinations of agents that decrease or prevent emesis, but treatment of nausea is still suboptimal.

Nonpharmacological Treatments

Nonpharmacological procedures and products are also being used to prevent or decrease the nausea associated with chemotherapy. Included in these treatments are acustimulation procedures, diet, and various forms of relaxation training. The last treatment has been used mostly to treat anticipatory nausea and will be discussed below.

Acustimulation   Ezzo et al. (2005) conducted a meta-analysis based on 11 studies and 1247 patients to determine the effects of various types of acustimulation (i.e., acupuncture, acupressure, and electroacustimulation) on acute and delayed nausea induced by chemotherapy. Pooling all types of acustimulation, the authors reported that stimulation reduced acute vomiting but not the severity of acute or delayed nausea. Results were similar from studies that just used needles (acupuncture); that is, the procedure did not reduce nausea. Acupressure did reduce acute nausea severity, but not acute vomiting or delayed nausea. Noninvasive electrostimulation (i.e., electroacustimulation using surface electrodes) failed to reduce nausea or vomiting. To summarize, acupressure was the only acustimulation procedure that reduced the severity of nausea induced by chemotherapy, and none reduced the severity of delayed nausea.

Dibble et al. (2007) reported the results of a multicenter study of the effects of acupressure on chemotherapy-induced nausea and vomiting. The subjects were 160 women with breast cancer receiving their second or third chemotherapy treatment. They all had experienced moderate nausea during previous treatments. The participants were randomly assigned to one of the following three groups: acupressure to P6 point (active), acupressure to S13 (placebo point), or no acustimulation. All patients received normal antiemetic drug therapy. The authors reported finding no differences among groups for acute nausea or vomiting; however, for delayed responses, the active acupressure group, compared to the other two groups, showed a significant reduction in the amount of vomiting and in the severity of nausea.

Roscoe et al. (2009) conducted a three-arm randomized clinical trial to investigate the effectiveness of acupressure bands in controlling radiation therapy-induced nausea and to test whether an informational manipulation designed to increase expectation of efficacy would enhance the effectiveness of the acupressure bands among 88 patients who experienced nausea at prior treatments. The results showed a significant reduction in nausea among those using the acupressure bands; however, the addition of information promoting the potential efficacy of the treatments did not add further to the relief of nausea.

Acupressure, together with drug therapy, appears to be a promising treatment for chemotherapy-induced nausea.

Neutraceuticals   As mentioned in several other chapters, the dried root of ginger (*Zingiber officinale*) has been shown to reduce nausea. Little is known about the optimal timing and dosage of ginger for relief of chemotherapy-induced nausea (CIN). For example, Zick et al. (2009), in a study of 162 patients who had experienced nausea and vomiting during a prior round of chemotherapy, found that neither 1.0 g or 2.0 g ginger capsule daily for three days following treatment relieved CINV significantly more than placebo. All patients were also receiving standard antiemetic therapy (5-HT$_3$ receptor antagonists and/or aprepitant).

However, Ryan et al. (2009) administered ginger in various dosages for 6 days beginning 3 days prior to treatment to 644 patients who had previously experienced CINV following chemotherapy. "All patients received 5-HT$_3$ receptor antagonist antiemetics on Day 1 of all cycles and took three 250 mg capsules of ginger or placebo twice daily for six days starting three days before the first day of the next two cycles." Their results showed a significant reduction in nausea, as measured on a semantic scale, for all dosages, with the greatest reduction found with 0.5 g and 1.0 g.

Levine et al. (2008) studied the use of ginger and protein for the treatment of chemotherapy-induced delayed nausea. Ginger capsules have been shown to decrease nausea in provocative motion situations (Lien et al., 2003), and protein has been shown to decrease nausea in the first trimester of pregnancy (Jednak et al., 1999) and in response to motion (Levine et al., 2004). In the Levine et al. (2008) study, 28 cancer patients receiving chemotherapy for the first time and standard antiemetic medication were assigned to one of three groups: Control Group patients continued with their normal diet, Protein Group patients consumed a drink with 15g of protein and 1g of ginger twice daily, and High Protein Group patients consumed a drink with 31g of protein and 1g of ginger twice daily. Patients recorded in a diary for 3 days whether they had experienced nausea, whether their nausea had been frequent, whether their nausea had been bothersome, and whether they had used any antiemetic medication. As can be seen in Figure 14.2, reports of nausea were significantly less common in the High Protein than Control and Protein Groups. Furthermore, significantly fewer patients in the High Protein Group used antiemetic medication during the 3 days following chemotherapy. The authors concluded that a randomized, placebo-controlled study is necessary before the extent to which protein with ginger can be recommended as a novel, nutritionally based treatment for the delayed nausea of chemotherapy.

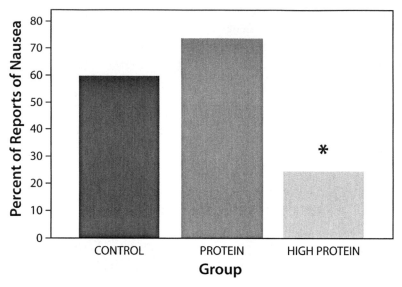

Figure 14.2 The percent of reports of nausea from the high protein, protein, and control groups of cancer patients following their first chemotherapy session. The nausea reported by the high protein group was significantly less than that reported by the other two groups. Reproduced with permission from Levine et al., 2008.

ANTICIPATORY NAUSEA

Approximately 25%–50% of cancer patients who receive chemotherapy develop anticipatory nausea and vomiting (ANV). That is, after one or more treatments with cytotoxic drugs that induce acute and or delayed nausea and/or vomiting, the patient experiences these debilitating symptoms prior to his or her next treatment. Watson, McCarron, and Law (1992) studied 95 adult cancer patients being treated with mild to moderately emetic cytotoxic drugs and determined that 23% reported anticipatory nausea. Tye et al. (1997) investigated the prevalence of anticipatory nausea among 59 pediatric cancer patients, all of whom were treated with ondansetron, and 59% indicated at least mild anticipatory nausea. As discussed in Chapter 2 in this volume, Stockhorst, Klosterhalfen, and Steingrüber (1998) published a review article summarizing what was known at that time about the prevalence of anticipatory nausea, and, unfortunately, the percentages they reported, 26%–57%, are still valid today.

Anticipatory nausea is not relieved by any drug and remains a serious negative side effect of chemotherapy. Approximately 25% to 50% of cancer patients suffering from anticipatory nausea and/or vomiting delay one or more scheduled cycles of chemotherapy, or even refuse further treatment (Laszlo, 1983). An additional negative aspect of anticipatory nausea according to Bovbjerg (2006) is that anticipatory nausea contributes to the severity of nausea experienced during or after the cancer patient's next chemotherapy session.

Morrow (1993) listed the following patient characteristics as contributing to the development of anticipatory nausea:

1. Nausea after the previous chemotherapy session
2. Severe nausea after the first chemotherapy session
3. Severe vomiting after the first chemotherapy session
4. Younger than 50 years old
5. Susceptible to motion sickness
6. Weakness following previous treatments
7. Sweating following previous treatments
8. Feeling warm or hot following previous treatments.

Morrow (1993) reported that most cancer patients who developed anticipatory nausea manifested at least four of the above characteristics. More recently, Zachariae et al. (2007) examined the role of additional individual differences in the development of anticipatory nausea in 125 women being treated with chemotherapy for breast cancer. Thirty-four percent of the women reported anticipatory nausea. Characteristics of this group were what the authors labeled as high absorption (high hypnotizability), severe delayed nausea, and pretreatment worry/anxiety.

Patient expectation is another factor that has been shown to contribute to the development of anticipatory nausea in chemotherapy patients. Hickok, Roscoe, and Morrow (2001) studied reports of nausea in 63 female cancer patients receiving chemotherapy and found that 40% of patients who expected nausea developed anticipatory nausea by their third cycle of treatment. Patients who did not expect nausea did not develop anticipatory nausea, suggesting a complex cognitive aspect to the development of anticipatory nausea. These findings also suggested the possibility that successful treatment to prevent or reduce anticipatory nausea in chemotherapy patients might involve some form of behavioral therapy (see "Treatments" below).

Anticipatory Nausea and Classical Conditioning

Anticipatory nausea is thought to be a learned response that conforms in many aspects to a classical conditioning model, or what is sometimes referred to as Pavlovian conditioning (e.g., Bovbjerg et al., 1992; Stockhorst et al., 2000; Stockhorst et al., 2006; Stockhorst, Enck & Klosterhalfen, 2007). In classical conditioning, a stimulus that initially does not provoke the response of interest (the conditioned stimulus, CS) is paired with a stimulus, the unconditioned stimulus or UCS, that does provoke the response of interest, the unconditioned response, the UCR. After these pairings, the CS begins to provoke the conditioned response (CR), a response very similar to the UCR. The sequence of events that can lead to anticipatory nausea in cancer patients receiving nauseogenic chemotherapy is as follows:

1. Patient sees the nurse who administers the chemotherapy (she/he is the CS).

2. Patient receives chemotherapy, the unconditioned stimulus (UCS) and experiences nausea, the unconditioned response (UCR).
3. After several pairings of the CS and the UCS, the patient experiences nausea, now the conditioned response (CR), at the sight of the nurse.

According to Morrow, Waight, and Black (1991), data tend to support a classical conditioning model of the development of anticipatory nausea and none refute it. For example, the more treatment cycles one has—the more pairings of the CS and UCS—the greater the probability of the cancer patient developing anticipatory nausea (Morrow & Dobkin, 1988). Other examples of observations of the mechanisms involved in the development of anticipatory nausea that fit the classical conditioning model include stimulus generalization, high-order conditioning, and the relevance of the strength of the unconditioned response.

An example of stimulus generalization commonly experienced by chemotherapy patients is their reporting nausea after several treatments not only to the sight of the nurse that administers their cytotoxic drug, but to the sight of other nurses or even the car used to travel to the cancer clinic. Higher-order conditioning refers to a situation in which a CS has been paired with a UCS a sufficient number of times so that the CS now produces a CR and acts as a UCS when paired with a new previously neutral stimulus. A hypothetical example of higher-order conditioning in a cancer treatment clinic might occur when a nurse who has been administering the cytotoxic drug (a CS that has become a UCS) calls the patient the morning of his/her next treatment to remind the patient of the appointment and the patient experiences nausea. As is apparent, higher-order conditioning can lead to many previously neutral stimuli provoking nausea in chemotherapy patients. An additional aspect of classical conditioning that is seen in the development of anticipatory nausea is the finding that the greater the intensity of the unconditioned response the greater the conditioning. To relate this relationship to the cancer clinic, the more severe the acute or delayed nausea experienced by the chemotherapy patient, the greater the probability that conditioning—anticipatory nausea—will develop. Morrow and Dobkin (1988) mention eight studies where this relationship has been found. This finding points out the importance of minimizing acute and delayed nausea during the first few chemotherapy cycles for cancer patients. It is one of the primary means of reducing or preventing the development of anticipatory nausea.

Treatment of Anticipatory Nausea

The treatment of anticipatory nausea in cancer patients undergoing chemotherapy is very difficult; there is no drug that successfully treats the condition once established. Therefore, the best treatment is prevention by decreasing acute and/or delayed nausea (e.g., Aapro, Molassiotis & Olver, 2005). When this fails, there are behavioral interventions that have achieved some success: hypnosis, progressive relaxation training, systematic desensitization, and overshadowing (Stockhorst et al., 1998).

LaBaw et al. (1975) used hypnosis with cancer patients in an effort to reduce anticipatory nausea by inducing bodily relaxation and found some success with children but not with adults. However, Marchioro et al. (2000) reported success using induction of relaxation and hypnosis to relieve 16 adult chemotherapy patients of anticipatory nausea. Following a meta-analysis of five hypnosis studies with children and one with adults, all randomized controlled trials, Richardson et al. (2007) concluded that "hypnosis could be a clinically valuable intervention for anticipatory nausea."

Yoo et al. (2005) studied the efficacy of progressive muscle relaxation training and guided imagery in reducing anticipatory nausea in breast cancer patients receiving chemotherapy. This was a randomized controlled trial with 30 patients in the muscle relaxation group and 30 in the control group. The authors reported that there was significantly less anticipatory nausea in the group that received progressive muscle relaxation plus guided imagery.

The successful use of systematic desensitization to decrease the anticipatory nausea of chemotherapy patients was demonstrated by Morrow and Morrell (1982). This technique teaches the patient how to maintain deep muscle relaxation while imagining a hierarchy of events related to anticipatory nausea. Only the subjects in the systematic desensitization group showed a significant reduction in severity, frequency, and duration of anticipatory nausea. Patients in two control groups did not show improvement.

In brief, the best method of preventing the development of anticipatory nausea in chemotherapy patients is to prevent nausea and/or vomiting during and following the first cycle of treatment. If anticipatory nausea does develop, behavioral interventions should be applied (Figueroa-Moseley et al., 2007).

CONCLUSIONS

In conclusion, nausea is still a debilitating effect of cancer in certain parts of the body, such as the brain and GI system. Unfortunately, it is also a strong negative side effect for as many as 50% of chemotherapy patients receiving nauseogenic cytotoxic drugs such as cisplatin. In some cases antiemetic medication may prolong nausea. The second generation $5\text{-}HT_3$ receptor antagonists and the NK_1 receptor antagonists have not had major impact on the treatment of nausea. Anticipatory nausea remains a very difficult symptom to treat since it does not respond to any pharmacological agent. Acute, delayed, and anticipatory nausea are more than just bothersome side effects of chemotherapy. Rather, they can have major impact on quality of life and are so unpleasant for some cancer patients that they terminate what might have been life-saving treatment. Much more needs to be learned about the mechanisms involved in the nausea of cancer and chemotherapy before successful treatments can be developed.

Chapter 15

Nausea of Motion Sickness

All individuals possessing an intact vestibular apparatus can be made motion
sick given the right quality and quantity of provocative stimulation, although
there are wide and consistent individual differences in the degree
of susceptibility
—(Reason & Brand, 1975, p. 29)

Factors that affect individual differences in susceptibility to nausea and other symptoms of motion sickness are discussed in this chapter along with treatments that have been used to prevent or reduce the nausea of motion sickness including drugs, dietary supplements, adaptation, desensitization, controlled breathing, use of acupressure, and related procedures.

In Chapter 3 (in this volume), the contribution of age, gender, and genetic factors to susceptibility to the nausea of motion sickness were discussed. In summary, infants are not susceptible, susceptibility increases in the adolescent years and then decreases with age, and, in general, women report more nausea of motion sickness than men. As the following studies showed, Asian subjects are more susceptible than European American or African American participants (Stern et al., 1996). Stern et al. (1993) reported that Chinese subjects were hypersusceptible to motion sickness provoked by a rotating optokinetic drum (see Figure 7.1 in this volume). The subjects in this first of three studies were Chinese-born women who had recently come to the United States. In a second study, Muth et al. (1994) compared the susceptibility to motion sickness of U.S.-born children of Asian parents, i.e., Asian Americans, and European Americans, and again found a significant increase in reports of nausea and other symptoms and in tachygastria among Asian subjects. In a third study of Chinese subjects, Xu et al. (1993) again found very high levels of susceptibility to motion sickness and very high levels of plasma vasopressin compared to European American subjects. More recently, Klosterhalfen et al. (2005a) reported using a rotating chair to compare the susceptibility to motion sickness of European and Chinese subjects. The average rotation time of the European subjects was significantly longer than the rotation time tolerated by the Chinese subjects. The Chinese subjects also had a significantly higher score on the Motion Sickness Susceptibility Questionnaire than the European subjects. Klosterhalfen et al. (2006) followed up on their 2005 study using a rotating optokinetic drum and reported that European subjects tolerated rotation in the drum significantly longer than Chinese subjects.

As mentioned in Chapter 3 in this volume, there is evidence of a genetic factor contributing to the racial differences found in susceptibility to the nausea of motion sickness. Individuals who are highly susceptible to motion sickness often report that their siblings and/or parents are highly susceptible (Abe, Amatomi & Kajiyama, 1970; Lentz & Collins, 1977). In addition, Bakwin (1971) reported that concordance for car sickness is significantly higher for monozygotic than dizygotic twins. Reavley et al. (2006) sent a mail questionnaire concerning susceptibility to motion sickness to 3652 monozygotic and dizygotic adult female twins. The results indicated a significant genetic contribution with heritability for a motion sickness factor score estimated as 57%. The heritability of recalled motion sickness (70%) was highest in childhood. Lockette and Farrow (1993) described the characteristics of a genetic polymorphism associated with susceptibility to motion sickness. Finley et al. (2004) have demonstrated that a genetic polymorphism of the alpha $_2$ adrenoceptor increases autonomic nervous system responses to stress and suggest that this inherited exaggerated response to stress may contribute to increased susceptibility to motion sickness. Zerbe (1985) described genetic factors involved in the secretion of vasopressin, and as described in this volume, levels of vasopressin in the blood have been linked to reports of nausea (e.g., Koch et al., 1990c).

There is sufficient evidence to indicate that susceptibility to the nausea of motion sickness is a good predictor of susceptibility to nausea in other nauseogenic situations. For example, Morrow (1985) reported finding a positive correlation between susceptibility to motion sickness and the nausea and vomiting that frequently follow chemotherapy. Morrow (1984b) and Leventhal et al. (1988) have also reported finding a positive correlation between susceptibility to motion sickness and the development of anticipatory nausea and vomiting in patients undergoing chemotherapy. Whitehead, Holden, and Andrews (1992) have reported finding a positive correlation between susceptibility to motion sickness and the nausea of pregnancy. Several investigators have reported finding a positive correlation between susceptibility to motion sickness and postoperative nausea and vomiting (e.g., Purkis, 1964; White & Shafer, 1988). Epstein (1993) considers susceptibility to motion sickness to be a risk factor for nausea and vomiting following outpatient surgery and cautions clinicians to take this into account during preoperative preparation. In summary, the correlation between the nausea of motion sickness and nausea in other situations is not only statistically significant but also clinically significant. And this finding is of importance both because it validates motion sickness as a model of nausea, and because it suggests the possibility that individuals have a threshold for nausea across different situations.

WHY ARE NAUSEA AND VOMITING SYMPTOMS OF MOTION SICKNESS?

It is not obvious why nausea and vomiting are common symptoms of motion sickness because the symptoms appear to be disadvantageous for the sufferer.

While studying sea-sickness, Claremont (1930) was the first person to our knowledge to suggest a relationship between sensory mismatch, possible toxin ingestion, and the nausea and vomiting of motion sickness.

> We are accustomed to receive certain sensations from our eyes in conjunction with others from the soles of our feet, joints, back, or other points of support. Normally the two sets "agree" with one another, or rather their occurrence in a given conjunction we are accustomed to regard as normal. This normality is disturbed on board ship. Our eyes here tell us that we are stationary, since we are moving with the room. But our sensations of support will have it that we are moving. We feel changes of pressure as the ship goes up or down. Under all known conditions, sensations of that kind would be accompanied by movements of the room about us (relative to the eye). Here there are no such movements. Some sense or other, it seems, must be misleading us. Our system concludes that we are seriously ill, poisoned probably; hence we vomit—the first precaution of nature's first aid. (p. 86)

Over 40 years after Claremont's analysis of sea-sickness, Treisman (1977) published a paper entitled "Motion Sickness: An Evolutionary Hypothesis," in which he developed more completely Claremont's hypothesized relationship between sensory mismatch, toxin ingestion, and the nausea and vomiting of motion sickness. He points out that all species have had to develop multiple levels of defense against ingested toxins (see Davis et al., 1986). As mentioned previously, Treisman suggests that sensory mismatch is a fourth level of defense against toxins, an early warning system sensitive to even minimal physiological disturbances caused by absorbed toxins:

> Even a minor degree of impairment of sensory (vestibular) input or of the coordination of eye muscles would produce mismatches between the systems. An emetic response to repeated such mismatches would be an advantageous adaptation for an unspecialized feeder which might ingest neurotoxins in vegetation or carrion. It is unfortunate that unusual or sophisticated situations, such as vehicular travel, should so often provide a stimulus of the same sort in man. (p. 494)

According to Treisman, "motion sickness is an adaptive response evoked by an inappropriate stimulus."

Money and Cheung (1983) also stated that motion sickness can be considered the result of activation, by motion, of a mechanism that normally facilitates vomiting in response to the ingestion of toxins. In their paper entitled, "Another Function of the Inner Ear: Facilitation of the Emetic Response to Poisons," they describe a study in which they surgically removed the vestibular apparatus of seven dogs and then observed their emetic response to certain poisons. Removal of the vestibular apparatus resulted in impairment of the emetic response to lobeline, levodopa, and nicotine, but had no effect on pilocarpine or apomorphine.

Money (1990) summarizes his position as follows:

> In the absence of a better explanation of how inner ear surgery can cause major defects in the responses to emetic poisons, it can be concluded that

there exists a physiological mechanism that facilitates vomiting in response to "early or minimal physiological disturbances produced by absorbed toxins" as predicted by Treisman and that the mechanism is at least partly vestibular. Parsimony would suggest that this same vestibular mechanism underlies that "vestibulo-gastric illness" called motion sickness. (p. 5)

PHYSIOLOGICAL MECHANISMS INVOLVED IN THE NAUSEA OF SUSCEPTIBLE INDIVIDUALS

A working hypothesis of the physiological changes that lead to the sensation of nausea in susceptible subjects who are exposed to the sensory mismatch created by a rotating optokinetic drum is depicted in Figure 15.1. Subjects who experience nausea in the drum show an increase in sympathetic nervous system (SNS) activity and a decrease in parasympathetic nervous system (PNS) activity, followed by a change in gastric myoelectric activity from a regular 3 cycles per minute (cpm) to dysrhythmic 4–9 cpm activity, or gastric tachygastria (e.g., Hu et al., 1991). This is usually followed by reports of nausea and an increase in vasopressin levels in blood plasma (Koch et al., 1990c).

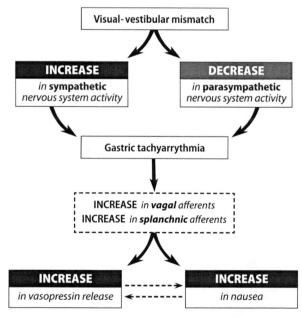

Figure 15.1 A working hypothesis of the temporal order of physiological changes that occur in susceptible subjects between exposure to a rotating optokinetic drum and reports of nausea. Solid lines indicate established relationships, dotted lines indicate hypothesized relationships. Reproduced with permission from Stern and Koch, 2006.

Vasopressin, an antidiuretic hormone that is released in the posterior pituitary, increases in the blood of individuals who report nausea after injection of apomorphine (Feldman, Samson & O'Dorisio, 1988), after cancer chemotherapy agents (e.g., Fisher et al., 1982), and after the stimulation of sitting in a rotating chair (Eversmann et al., 1978). It is not clear in these situations whether plasma vasopressin increases immediately before or immediately after the perception of nausea. Several authors (e.g., Robertson, 1977) have stated that nausea causes an increase in vasopressin release. An alternative hypothesis is that vagal afferents may stimulate both vasopressin release and the sensation of nausea. Still another possibility is that increased levels of vasopressin are experienced as nausea. The complexity of the nausea-vasopressin relationship is discussed further in Chapter 6 in this volume, and in Cheung et al. (1994).

There are several published reports showing that in animals an increase in SNS activity and decrease in PNS activity often lead to tachygastria (e.g., Kelly, 1977). We know of no study that demonstrates that tachygastria leads to a change in vagal afferent nerve activity, but we suspect that it does. And it has been demonstrated (Hawthorn et al., 1988) that vagal afferent nerve stimulation increases the release of vasopressin.

Xu et al. (1993) reported that for most subjects gastric dysrhythmias preceded the onset of nausea and vasopressin release during exposure to a rotating optokinetic drum. It is suggested that the shift to gastric dysrhythmias may alter ongoing gastric vagal afferent nerve activity, which then modulates neuronal activity in the tractus solitarius and hypothalamus, and ultimately results in vasopressin secretion. This possibility is supported by the fact that asymptomatic subjects develop neither gastric dysrhythmias nor increased vasopressin release during drum rotation. For a review of theories of the causes of motion sickness see Shupak and Gordon (2006).

TREATMENTS

Drugs

Drugs that reduce nausea and other symptoms of motion sickness are mainly antihistamines or anticholinergics. This is not surprising since both histamine H_1 receptors and muscarinic acetylcholine receptors are found in the vestibular nuclei and appear to be involved in transmission to the so-called vomiting center (de Waele, Mühlethaler & Vidal, 1995). Sympathomimetics such as amphetamine or ephedrine have some anti–motion sickness effects and, in addition, they have been used by NASA, together with scopolamine and promethazine, to reduce drowsiness (Wood, 1990).

Attempts to develop an animal model to test motion sickness drugs using cats and dogs were unsuccessful (Cheung et al., 1992). The dogs did not show any benefit from scopolamine (one of the most effective anti–motion sickness drugs for humans), and results from cats were inconclusive.

Subsequently, Cheung and other investigators reported that they were more successful using squirrel monkeys as subjects, but the difficulty of extrapolating what we think is the experience of nausea in 'lower' animals to humans must always be considered when attempting to work with animal models of nausea. For a discussion of this important issue see Chapter 8, in this volume.

The following material on the effects of antihistamines and anticholinergics is reprinted with permission from Skidgel and Erdös (2006, p. 637).

Antihistamines

The first-generation H_1 antagonists can both stimulate and depress the CNS. Stimulation occasionally is encountered in patients given conventional doses, who become restless, nervous, and unable to sleep. Central excitation also is a striking feature of overdose, which commonly results in convulsions, particularly in infants. Central depression, on the other hand, usually accompanies therapeutic doses of the older H_1 antagonists. Diminished alertness, slowed reaction times, and somnolence are common manifestations. Some of the H_1 antagonists are more likely to depress the CNS than others, and patients vary in their susceptibility and responses to individual drugs. The ethanolamines (e.g., diphenhydramine) are particularly prone to cause sedation.

The second-generation ("nonsedating") H_1 antagonists, e.g., loratadine, cetirizine, and flexofenadine, are largely excluded from the brain when given in therapeutic doses because they do not cross the blood-brain barrier appreciably. Their sedative effects are similar to those of placebo. Because of the sedation that occurs with first-generation antihistamines, these drugs cannot be tolerated or used safely by many patients unless given only at bedtime. Even then, patients may experience an antihistamine "hangover" in the morning, resulting in sedation with or without psychomotor impairment. Thus the development of nonsedating antihistamines was an important advance that allowed the general use of these agents.

The capacity to counter motion sickness was first observed with dimenhydrinate and subsequently with diphenhydramine (the active ingredient of dimenhydrinate), various piperazine derivatives, and promethazine.

Anticholinergic Agents

Many of the first-generation H_1 antagonists tend to inhibit responses to acetylcholine that are mediated by muscarinic receptors. These atropinelike actions are sufficiently prominent in some of the drugs to be manifest during clinical usage. Promethazine has perhaps the strongest muscarinic-blocking activity among these agents and is among the most effective of the H_1 antagonists in combating motion sickness. Since scopolamine is a potent preventer of motion sickness, it is possible that the anticholinergic properties of H_1 antagonists are largely responsible for this effect. Golding and Stott (1997) found that hyoscine (scopolamine) and the selective muscarinic receptor antagonist zamifenacin (UK-76654), with selective M3 and/or m5 antagonism, were equally effective in decreasing symptoms of motion sickness. The second-generation H_1 antagonists have no effect on muscarinic receptors.

Table 15.1 from the Centers for Disease Control (CDC, 2009b) shows the dosages, contraindications, and adverse effects of drugs commonly used to combat motion sickness. Note that drowsiness is an adverse side effect of all drugs used to combat motion sickness. This may not be a problem for passengers in a commercial plane, but it is a serious matter for pilots, astronauts, and anyone else who must stay alert while being subjected to provocative motion. In early Skylab flights the astronauts took scope-dex, 0.35 mg of scopolamine to prevent space motion sickness with 5 mg of d-amphetamine to prevent drowsiness. According to Graybiel (1980), this combination of drugs was not very helpful and in later Skylab flights the astronauts used a combination of 25 mg of promethazine and 50 mg of ephedrine during the first four days of the flight but remained mildly susceptible to space motion sickness. More recently, astronauts in the Space Shuttle have used IM injections of promethazine, and Bagian (1991) reported no symptoms of space motion sickness in 28 of 29 crew members.

Two recent laboratory studies have assessed the negative effects of different drugs used as countermeasures for space motion sickness on cognitive functioning and psychomotor performance (Paule et al., 2004; Paul, MacLellan & Gray, 2005). The first study concluded that at clinically useful doses, the rank order of the drugs with the least cognitive deficits were meclizine, scopolamine, promethazine, and lorazepam. The Paule et al. study concluded that only promethazine plus d-amphetamine, of drugs and drug combinations used by astronauts, was free from impact on psychomotor performance and did not increase drowsiness.

Uijtdehaage, Stern, and Koch (1993) compared the efficacy of scopolamine and methscopolamine for the prevention of nausea and other symptoms of motion sickness provoked by exposure to a rotating optokinetic drum. Sixty subjects ingested either 0.6 mg scopolamine, 2.5 mg methscopolamine, or a placebo. Heart rate (HR), respiratory sinus arrhythmia (an index of vagal tone), and electrogastrograms were measured prior to and during the exposure to a rotating optokinetic drum. Compared to the other groups, the scopolamine group reported fewer motion sickness symptoms, and displayed lower HR, higher vagal tone, enhanced normal gastric myoelectric activity, and depressed gastric dysrhythmias before and during motion sickness induction. It was concluded that scopolamine offered motion sickness protection by initiating a pattern of increased vagal tone and normal gastric myoelectric stability. Methscopolamine, which does not cross the blood-brain barrier, offered no protection.

Spinks et al. (2004) reviewed the results of 12 studies that used scopolamine for the prevention of motion sickness. The protective value of scopolamine was compared against placebos, calcium channel antagonists, antihistamines, methscopolamine, and scopolamine plus ephedrine. The authors concluded that scopolamine was superior to placebos in preventing the development of symptoms of motion sickness. However, they indicated that the results of comparisons of the effects of scopolamine versus the other drugs tested

Table 15.1 Anti–Motion Sickness Medications

Medications	Dose	Caution	Adverse Effects	Drug Interactions	Comments
Antimuscarinic Agents Scopolamine Available in transdermal patch (1.5 mg), tablets (0.4 mg), and intramuscular injection Brands: Scopace, Transderm-scop	Patch: apply to hairless area behind ear at least 4 hrs before travel. Remove or replace with new patch after 72 hrs. Do not cut patch in half. Oral: 0.4–0.8 mg every 8 hrs. Take about 1 hr before travel. IM: 0.3–0.6 mg every 6–8 hrs.	Contraindicated in glaucoma, urinary retention, gastrointestinal (GI) obstruction, ulcerative colitis, myasthenia gravis, hypersensitivity Caution in extreme heat, thyroid, cardiopulmonary, gastroesophageal reflux, liver, or kidney disease, seizure or psychotic disorder, autonomic neuropathy Should not be used in children.	Common: dry mouth/nose/throat, blurred vision, drowsiness Less common: dry skin, contact dermatitis (from patch), palpitations, urinary retention, nausea, vomiting, bloating, constipation, loss of taste, headache, confusion, memory impairment, paradoxical hyperexcitability, insomnia, acute toxic psychosis Withdrawal symptoms after patch removal: nausea, vomiting, headache, dizziness, weakness, bradycardia, hypotension	Additive effects with alcohol and other CNS depressants, anticholinergics, antihistamines, some antidepressants (e.g., tricyclic antidepressants), and other neurologic drugs. Antacids impair absorption of oral scopolamine. Scopolamine may significantly impair GI motility when used with antidiarrheal drugs. Scopolamine impairs absorption of oral medications. Scopolamine may increase risk of GI lesions related to potassium chloride use.	Caution when operating machinery, driving a car, or engaging in underwater sports. Wash hands after patch application to prevent transfer to eye. FDA Pregnancy category C

| Antihistamines | Contraindicated in hypersensitivity

Caution in glaucoma, urinary retention, GI obstruction, liver or kidney disease, chronic obstructive pulmonary disease (COPD), seizure disorder | Common: drowsiness, anticholinergic symptoms (dry mouth/nose/throat, blurred vision, urinary retention), thick respiratory secretions

Less common: dizziness, weakness, hypotension or hypertension, cardiac arrhythmia, wheezing, sweating, nausea, vomiting, bloating, diarrhea, constipation, jaundice, anorexia, headache, confusion, tinnitus, paradoxical hyperexcitability, seizures, psychosis, acute dystonic reaction, paresthesias, photosensitivity, anaphylaxis | Additive effects with alcohol and other CNS depressants, anticholinergics, some antidepressants (e.g., tricyclic antidepressants) and use of more than one antihistamine. Antihistamine effects may be potentiated by monamine oxidase inhibitors.

Antacids may impair absorption of antihistamines. | Caution when operating machinery, driving a car, or engaging in underwater sports

Take with food or milk to reduce nausea. |

(continued)

Table 15.1 (*continued*)

Medications	Dose	Caution	Adverse Effects	Drug Interactions	Comments
Dimenhydrinate Available in chewable and nonchewable tablets (50 mg), syrup (12.5 mg/ 5 mL), rectal suppositories, and intramuscular injection (50 mg/mL). Brands: Calm X, Dramamine, Triptone	Oral: Take at least 30 min before travel. Adults: 50–100 mg every 4–6 hrs, max 400 mg per day Children (6–12 yrs): 25–50 mg every 6–8 hrs, max 150 mg per day Children (2–6 yrs): 12.5–25 mg every 6–8 hrs, max 75 mg per day Rectal: Children (8–12 yrs): 25–50 mg every 8–12 hrs Children (6–8 yrs): 12.5–25 mg every 8–12 hrs IM: Adults: same as oral dose Children <12 yrs: 1.25 mg/kg every 6 hrs, max 300 mg per day	Should not be used in children < 2 yr		May block effectiveness of apomorphine	FDA Pregnancy category B

Drug	Dosing	Contraindications/Cautions	Side Effects	Interactions	FDA Pregnancy Category
Diphenhydramine Available in oral capsules and tablets (25 mg, 50 mg), elixir (12.5 mg/5 mL), and intramuscular injection (10 or 50 mg/mL) Multiple brands available	Oral: Take at least 30 min before travel. Adults: 10–50 mg every 4–6 hrs Children (6–12 yrs): 12.5–25 mg every 4–6 hrs Children (<6 yrs): 6.25–12.5 mg every 4–6 hrs IM: Adults: start 10 mg, may increase up to 50 mg, every 2–3 hrs, max 400 mg per day Children: 1–1.5 mg/kg every 6 hrs, max 300 mg per day	Not recommended in infants or neonates			FDA Pregnancy category B
Promethazine Available in oral tablets (12.5 mg, 25 mg, 50 mg), syrup (6.25 mg/5 mL, 25 mg/5 mL), rectal suppositories, and intramuscular injection. Brands: Phenergan, Promacot	Oral: Take at least 30 min before travel Adults: 25 mg every 8–12 hrs Contraindicated in children under 2 and not recommended for children <16 yrs (12)	Also caution in sulfa allergy (some formulations contain sulfite), cardiovascular disease, peptic ulcer disease	Pronounced sedation, postural hypotension, skin rash, body temperature dysregulation, extrapyramidal symptoms, delirium, neuroleptic malignant syndrome	May interact with other neurologic drugs. Epinephrine may worsen hypotension when used with antihistamine.	FDA Pregnancy category C

(continued)

Table 15.1 (*continued*)

Medications	Dose	Caution	Adverse Effects	Drug Interactions	Comments
Meclizine	Oral: Take 1 hour before travel.			May block effectiveness of apomorphine.	
Available in chewable and nonchewable tablets (12.5 mg, 25 mg, 50 mg)	Adults: 25–50 mg every 24 hrs				
Brands: Antivert (Rx), Bonine (OTC), Dramamine II (OTC), Meclicot (Rx), Medivert (Rx)	Not recommended for children <12 yrs				
Cyclizine	Oral: Take 30 min before travel	Caution in heart failure			
Available in oral tablets (50 mg)	Adults: 50 mg every 4–6 hrs, max 200 mg per day				
Brands: Marezine (OTC)	Not recommended for children <12 yrs				
	IM: Adults: same as oral dose				

were equivocal. Possible reasons given include different modes of administration of scopolamine and the comparison drugs, small number of subjects in most studies, and different dosages from study to study. The authors also concluded that scopolamine was no more likely to induce drowsiness, blurred vision, or dizziness compared to the other drugs tested. However, dry mouth was a more likely side effect with scopolamine than the other agents tested.

Gil et al. (2005) examined the effects of plasma concentration of scopolamine, not just dosage, on symptom reports. A transdermal scopolamine patch was applied to 61 naval crewmembers. Blood samples and symptom reports were obtained 8 hours after the patch was applied. Subjects were divided by symptom reports into Responders, who reported fewer symptoms of seasickness with the patch compared to other days at sea without the patch, and Non-Responders, who reported no benefit from the patch. The mean concentration of scopolamine in the blood of the 37 Responders was 156.77 pg/ml, which was significantly higher than that found in the blood of the 24 Non-Responders (97.03 pg/ml). The authors conclude that an attempt should be made to increase the plasma levels of scopolamine in individuals exposed to provocative motion either by increasing the dosage or improving transdermal absorption.

In conclusion, the nausea of motion sickness can be reduced or even prevented by the use of scopolamine or several over-the-counter antihistamines, but there are side effects such as drowsiness and dry mouth and large individual differences in responses. Neither the 5-HT$_3$ nor the NK$_1$ receptor antagonists used to treat the nausea and vomiting that often follows chemotherapy prevent nausea and other symptoms of motion sickness (Levine et al., 2000; Reid et al., 2000).

Dietary Supplements

It has been shown that factors that increased peripheral parasympathetic nervous system activity, such as eating, strengthens the normal 3 cpm rhythm of the stomach (e.g., Jones & Jones, 1985; Koch, Stewart & Stern, 1987) and reduces nausea. Uijtdehaage, Stern, and Koch (1992) demonstrated that the ingestion of a small meal significantly reduced nausea and other symptoms of motion sickness. The results also showed that the meal increased normal 3 cpm stomach activity compared to a no-meal control group, and inhibited the development of gastric dysrhythmias during exposure to provocative motion.

Jednak et al. (1999) compared the use of both liquid and solid protein, carbohydrate, and fat meals to reduce the nausea of women in the first trimester of pregnancy. Their major finding was that protein-predominant meals reduced nausea and dysrhythmic stomach activity significantly more than equicaloric carbohydrate and fat meals.

Levine et al. (2004) followed up on this research demonstrating that both liquid protein and carbohydrate meals reduced dysrhythmic gastric activity during exposure to provocative motion, but only the group receiving the protein meal showed significantly lower motion sickness scores when compared to the no-meal control condition. Williamson, Levine, and Stern (2005) investigated the efficacy of drink palatability and nutritional composition in preventing nausea and other subjective symptoms of motion sickness, decreased normal gastric activity, and withdrawal of vagal tone in response to optokinetic motion. Participants received a liquid, high protein/low carbohydrate, moderate protein/high carbohydrate, low protein/high carbohydrate, or water meal 30 minutes prior to exposure to a rotating optokinetic drum. The results showed that palatability and high protein content appear to be important factors in attenuating the nausea associated with exposure to optokinetic motion.

Protein, more so than other kinds of nutrients, has been shown to provide amino acids to the stomach that specifically stimulate the gastric hormone, gastrin (Richardson et al., 1976; Taylor et al., 1982). Gastrin, in turn, binds to receptors on the smooth muscle of the stomach, thereby increasing gastric contractility and normal electrical activity that accompanies these contractions (Elwin, 1974; Baur & Bacon, 1976; Szurszewski, 1975). And as has been mentioned previously, treatments that enhance normal 3 cpm gastric activity reduce nausea.

There are many anecdotal reports of the use of foods, herbs, etc. to treat the nausea of motion sickness, but the one most often mentioned in publications is ginger. Dried ginger root (*Zingiber officinale*) has a long history as an herbal remedy for upset stomach, loss of appetite, and motion sickness. For many centuries, Chinese sailors have taken ginger to avoid seasickness. Mowrey and Clayson (1982) reported that ginger was superior to a placebo and dimenhydrinate in reducing motion sickness provoked by exposure to a rotating chair. However, Stewart et al. (1991) subsequently reported that ginger failed to prevent the development of symptoms of motion sickness in subjects who were required to move their head forward and back while sitting in a rotating chair. There were many differences in the procedures used in these two studies and therefore it is difficult to account for the different findings, but one possibility is that the head movements required in the Stewart et al. study were a much more provocative stimulus, and one that could not be prevented by the dosage of ginger used and/or the time from ingestion of the ginger to motion exposure.

Lien et al. (2003) tested the efficacy of 1 gram of ginger in preventing the nausea and accompanying physiological changes that usually results from exposure to a rotating optokinetic drum. They reported that ginger reduced nausea, gastric dysrhythmia, and plasma vasopressin, a hormone that usually increases along with nausea. They also found that ginger prolonged latency before nausea onset and shortened recovery time after rotation. Two grams of ginger were no better than one. In an additional study that looked at possible mechanisms by which ginger reduces nausea, Gonlachanvit et al. (2003a) reported that 1 gram of ginger reduced the gastric dysrhythmia and nausea reported by a placebo group following infusion of dextrose to produce hyperglycemia in healthy human subjects. It should be noted that gastric dysrhythmia and nausea are commonly seen in patients with advanced diabetes mellitus. Gonlachanvit et al. hypothesized that the ability of ginger to prevent hyperglycemia-evoked dysrhythmia and nausea stems from inhibition of the action of endogenous prostaglandins.

In conclusion, it appears that both high-protein meals and ginger inhibit the development of the nausea of motion sickness probably as the result of reducing tachygastria, the abnormal gastric activity that has been shown to accompany nausea. It should be noted that the studies cited above that used ginger, used tablets of dried ginger root usually available in health food stores in 250 mg tablets. Some ginger drinks are artificially flavored and contain no ginger.

Additional Treatments for the Nausea of Motion Sickness

In this section the use of the following treatments for the nausea of motion sickness are described: adaptation, desensitization, controlled breathing, use of acuprocedures, and others. This list is not exhaustive, and there is considerable overlap among some of the treatments.

Adaptation to Provocative Motion

As mentioned in Chapter 3 in this volume, an early attempt to reduce symptoms of motion sickness by subjecting susceptible individuals to repeated exposure to provocative motion, such as occurs in gymnastic procedures and other movement, on a schedule of approximately every 48 hours until symptoms abated was described by Popov (1943). Stern et al. (1989), using a rotating optokinetic drum, demonstrated the importance of the time between repeated exposure to provocative motion for adaptation to occur. In the first of two studies, healthy participants were exposed to the rotating drum with intersession intervals of 4 to 24 days, and few showed adaptation to the nausea and other symptoms of motion sickness after three sessions. Several participants reported that with the long intersession interval, "re-exposure was like starting all over." However, the results of a second study, in which the intersession interval was shortened to 48 hours, revealed significant adaptation of subjective symptoms of motion sickness from session to session. Group means for subjective symptoms were 12.1, 6.9, and 3.9. Tachygastria, the abnormal gastric activity that usually accompanies nausea, also showed adaptation with the shortened intersession interval: 46.9, 15.9, and 5.8.

Hu et al. (1991) exposed participants to the same rotating drum used in the previous study for three sessions with a 48-hour intersession interval and again reported significant adaptation of both the subjective symptoms of motion sickness and tachygastria. In addition, the authors reported finding less change in measures of both sympathetic and parasympathetic nervous system activity with repeated exposure to the rotating drum and concluded that adaptation to motion sickness is accompanied by recovery of autonomic nervous system balance.

In the next study in this series, Hu, Stern, and Koch (1991) investigated the effects of two different preexposure procedures on adaptation to the symptoms of motion sickness in the same rotating drum. The control group had no preexposure rotation procedure, only a standard 16-min exposure to the rotating drum at 60 degrees/s. The incremental exposure group had two 4-min preexposure periods, one at 15 degrees/s and another at 30 degrees/s, in the rotating drum immediately prior to the standard 16-min exposure period at 60 degrees/s. The abrupt exposure group also had two 4-min preexposure periods, but both were at 60 degrees/s. The results showed that the subjects in the incremental exposure group reported significantly fewer subjective symptoms of motion sickness and less tachygastria during the standard 16-min rotation period at 60 degrees/s compared to the other two groups. The authors concluded that incremental exposure to motion stimuli may be a useful method for training resistance to the nausea and other symptoms of visually induced motion sickness.

Hu and Hui (1997) asked the question, Is it necessary for individuals who are susceptible to motion sickness to experience nausea during repeated exposure to a rotating drum in order to adapt? All subjects were exposed to a rotating optokinetic drum for 16 min per session with a 48-hour intersession interval, and participants in one group, the Nausea group, continued to be exposed even if they reported nausea. The mean number of sessions to reach adaptation for the Nausea group was 3.9, and for the other group 3.2 sessions. It was concluded that subjects susceptible to motion sickness can adapt to a nauseogenic optokinetic drum by repeated exposure without experiencing nausea and/or vomiting during adaptation. Recent research by Klosterhalfen et al. (2005b) took these findings one step further and tested adaptation to a rotating chair when subjects were repeatedly exposed to the stationary chair for 4 days prior to exposure to the rotating chair on day 5. The authors reported that the preexposure, labeled by them as latent inhibition, reduced anticipatory but not postrotational nausea.

An important applied issue for individuals who make use of laboratory motion sickness adaptation training to aid in the adaptation of, for example, astronauts in zero gravity, is how long will the adaptation last? Hu and Stern (1999) compared the retention of adaptation to a rotating optokinetic drum after one month and after one year. Participants who developed symptoms of motion sickness during a preliminary session in the drum were reexposed to the drum repeatedly with a 48-hour intersession interval until they reported no feeling of nausea. Subjects were reexposed to the drum after either one month or one year. The mean rating of nausea after one month was 0.94, almost no nausea, compared to the initial rating of 9.23. The mean nausea rating after one year was 6.88, compared to the group initial rating of 8.94. In summary, the results indicate that adaptation of the nausea of motion sickness was almost completely retained after one month and partially retained after one year.

Another important applied issue is the extent to which adaptation of nausea and other symptoms of motion sickness in a motion situation will transfer to other situations involving provocative motion. Cheung and Hofer (2005) exposed three groups of subjects to 4 days of adaptation to one of the following conditions: cross-coupled motion, torso rotation, or simulated aircraft motion. On the fifth day, all three groups were exposed to the simulated aircraft motion. Within each group, the participants showed adaptation during the 4 days. Cross-coupled motion was found to be the most provocative stimulus, but there was no significant difference in reports of motion sickness on the fifth day regardless of the adapted stimuli. Cheung and Hofer suggest, based on their results, that desensitization, or adaptation, to one provocative motion may transfer to a less severe motion stimulus.

Williamson, Higgins, and Stern (2003) recruited a group of participants who suffered from severe carsickness. The subjects were adapted in a rotating optokinetic drum using repeated exposures with a 48-hour intersession interval. Each session was terminated as soon as the participant reported any nausea or other discomfort. The mean number of sessions required to adapt this special group of subjects was five. The subjects kept a diary of their symptoms and behavior related to riding in cars and other forms of motion, and most reported dramatic improvement. As can be seen in Figure 15.2, the group showed a significant decrease in self-reports of car sickness after adaptation in the rotating drum, and the benefit lasted for at least 7 months. Some reported that for the first time in their lives they could ride in the passenger seat of a car without experiencing motion sickness. Others reported being symptom free while going on carnival rides, fishing boats, etc. It should be noted that even though the results of this unique study are very promising, there was no placebo control condition. However, these were individuals who had not obtained relief from other forms of motion sickness therapy.

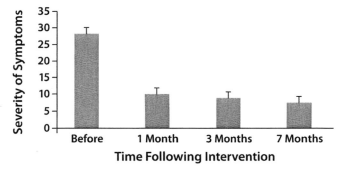

Figure 15.2 Mean severity of reports of car sickness before adaptation in a rotating optokinetic drum and symptom reports 1 month, 3 months, and 7 months after adaptation. Symptoms were significantly less than pretreatment for the three delayed periods tested. Reproduced with permission from Williamson, Higgins, and Stern, 2003.

Adaptation to the sensory rearrangement of microgravity is a major concern for NASA. According to Reschke et al. (1994), most astronauts show signs of adaptation to the sensory rearrangement of space flights usually within the first 48 hours of orbital flight. For example, gastrointestinal symptoms often appear shortly after launch but usually resolve after 30 to 48 hours (Thornton et al., 1987). A second indication that adaptation to space flight occurs can be seen in the difference in incidence of space motion sickness manifested by first-time astronauts and repeat flyers. Of first-time flyers in the Space Shuttle, 83% experienced motion sickness, but only 61% of repeat flyers reported space motion sickness (Reschke et al., 1994). NASA continues to develop various training devices, including virtual environments, to preadapt astronauts to the sensory rearrangement of microgravity.

In conclusion, most healthy individuals adapt to the illusion of motion produced by a rotating optokinetic drum in about three trials if the intersession interval is 48 hours or less. With adaptation the subjective reports of nausea and other symptoms decrease accompanied by a decrease in tachygastria and a return to autonomic nervous system balance. Adaptation is retained for 6 months and may transfer to outside forms of provocative motion, e.g., cars, boats, etc. There is evidence that adaptation to one motion situation may transfer to other situations involving provocative motion.

Desensitization

"Adaptation" and "desensitization" are often used interchangeably in the literature. In this chapter, desensitization is conceptualized as adaptation plus an effort to reduce anxiety and/or expectation. Most desensitization treatment programs expose the individual to situations involving gradually increasing nauseogenic stimuli and aim to decrease anxiety and expectation of the pilot in training, naval recruit, etc.

There are several studies in the literature documenting the role of anxiety and expectation in nausea (e.g., Marten et al., 1993; Levine, Stern & Koch, 2006). Research has also shown that anxious individuals are hyperalert to any type of threat and, therefore, extreme anxiety would be expected to lower one's threshold for the detection of toxins, among other things, resulting in loss of appetite and/or nausea. Several studies (e.g., Morrow & Rosenthal, 1996) have found that expectations about nausea prior to initial chemotherapy treatment can lower that individual's nausea threshold and in so doing affect appraisal of the procedure and one's bodily responses. This would be predicted by response expectancy theories such as that proposed by Kirsch (1999). Specifically, Kirsch states that if an individual is presented with information that indicates that sickness may result due to exposure to some new stimulus situation, and the stimulus exposure itself supports that prediction, then the nausea response to the stimulus is likely to be augmented more so than if either the response expectation or the stimulus were not present together. The results of a recent study (Levine, Stern & Koch, 2006) demonstrated the importance of the strength of the expectation and the strength of the nauseogenic stimulus in determining the response. Prior to being exposed to a rotating optokinetic drum, three groups of subjects were given placebos. One group was told that the pills would reduce nausea, a second group was told that the pills would increase nausea, and a third group was told that the pills were a placebo. The first group reported the same degree of nausea as the placebo-control group. *The surprise finding was that the group that was told that the pills would increase their nausea reported significantly less nausea than the other two groups* and significantly less gastric dysrthymia than usually accompanies nausea. A tentative explanation is that these subjects had a strong negative expectation that was not supported by the actual stimulus. Thus, when their bodily reaction was not very great, this observation caused an increase in their nausea threshold, as the stimulus was appraised as not very noxious, and consequently they reported little nausea.

Several programs designed to reduce motion sickness of pilots in training have been reported. As mentioned previously, an early training procedure was successful in reducing symptoms in 78% of susceptible pilots (Popov, 1943). Various air forces have developed programs subsequently to desensitize flight personnel who suffer from airsickness. One such program was developed by the U.S. Air Force School of Aviation Medicine (Levy, Jones & Carlson, 1981). Aircrew who were affected by severe airsickness were repeatedly exposed to a rotating and tilting chair while being taught to control their autonomic nervous system responses using biofeedback. The authors reported that 16 of 19 participants were returned to full flying duty. Cowings and Toscano (2000) compared the effectiveness of autogenic-feedback training and intramuscular injections of promethazine for control of motion sickness. Autogenic feedback training makes use of biofeedback to help an individual learn to control his/her autonomic nervous system responses. Promethazine is the drug currently used to control space motion sickness. The dependent measure of interest was motion sickness tolerance in a rotating chair. After four sessions of autogenic-feedback training, subjects reported significantly fewer symptoms of motion sickness in the rotating chair compared to subjects who received promethazine. More recently the desensitization program of the Italian Air Force was described by Lucertini and Lugli (2004). In brief, this desensitization program involves 2 weeks of exposure to increasingly more intense nauseogenic stimuli plus autogenic training and cognitive-behavioral therapy. They reported a success rate of 88%.

Controlled Breathing

There are many anecdotal reports of slow deep breathing being used to relieve nausea and other symptoms of motion sickness. In a controlled laboratory study, Jokerst et al. (1999b) compared physiological responses and reports of symptoms of motion sickness of three groups of subjects all of whom were exposed to a rotating optokinetic drum. The group that did slow deep breathing showed significantly less tachygastria during rotation than a group that counted their breaths and a second control group that breathed normally.

The slow deep breathing group also reported significantly fewer symptoms than the group that counted their breaths. It was concluded that slow deep breathing prevented the development of gastric dysrhythmias and decreased symptoms of motion sickness.

Yen Pik Sang, Golding, and Gresty (2003) conducted a study similar to the Jokerst et al. (1999b) study, but motion sickness was induced by whole body pitch oscillations while subjects viewed a video image of the environment oscillating in 180 degrees counter-phase rather than a rotating optokinetic drum. The subjects in the controlled breathing group took significantly longer to reach the endpoint of mild nausea. It was also reported that controlled breathing prolonged time tolerated with nausea and reduced the recovery time after motion cessation. Yen Pik Sang et al. (2005) examined the effects of controlled breathing on an accelerated motion sickness desensitization training program. A controlled breathing group and a control group, matched for susceptibility to motion sickness, were exposed to four trials in an off-vertical axis rotation device within 1 hour. Both groups showed an increased tolerance for motion and a reduction in symptoms with stimulus repetition. The authors reported a tendency for greater habituation in the controlled breathing group.

The results of these three studies suggest that controlled breathing may be effective for reducing motion-induced nausea, although the physiological basis is not known. Ziavra et al. (2003) determined that breathing supplementary oxygen did not reduce the nausea of motion sickness.

Acupuncture, Acustimulation, and Acupressure

Acupuncture and related procedures (referred to here collectively as acuprocedures) have been used to treat GI symptoms in China and other Asian countries for centuries. One of the most commonly used points for acuprocedures is P6, the Neiguan point on the pericardinal meridian, the underside of the wrist. Attempts to study the efficacy of acuprocedures to reduce or prevent nausea and other symptoms of motion sickness in the laboratory have produced mixed results.

In one of the first such studies, Warwick-Evans, Masters, and Redstone (1991) compared the effects of acupressure and a placebo on symptoms provoked by rotation about two orthogonal axes. They reported that acupressure provided no protection for subjects who were either high or low susceptible to motion sickness. On the other hand, Hu, Stern, and Koch (1992) reported obtaining positive results from two studies that tested the effects of electrical acustimulation on symptoms and gastric activity of participants exposed to a rotating optokinetic drum. In the first study, 16 Chinese subjects familiar with acustimulation were each tested twice in counterbalanced order, once with acustimulation and once without. With acustimulation the subjects showed significantly less tachygastria and reported significantly fewer symptoms of motion sickness. With acustimulation five reported nausea;

without, 11 reported nausea. A second study was conducted to determine if the results of the first study were influenced by a placebo effect or the fact that all subjects were Chinese. In the second study 45 European American subjects not familiar with acuprocedures were divided into the following three independent groups: acustimulation, sham acustimulation, and no acustimulation. The results indicated that the acustimulation group had significantly fewer motion sickness symptoms than either of the other two groups and significantly less tachygastria than the no acustimulation group. In a similar study that used a rotating optokinetic drum to provoke symptoms of motion sickness, Hu et al. (1995) compared symptom reports and gastric activity of the following four groups: P6 acupressure, dummy-point acupressure, sham P6 acupressure, and no acupressure control. Subjects in the P6 acupressure group reported significantly less nausea and less tachygastria than the other groups during drum rotation.

The complexity of selecting appropriate placebo control groups in this area of research and drawing valid conclusions about the effects of acuprocedures on nausea and other symptoms of motion sickness can be seen in a study by Stern et al. (2001b). Using a within-subject design, the authors exposed participants to a rotating optokinetic drum on three days with the following three counterbalanced conditions: acupressure at P6, acupressure on the upper arm, and no acupressure. Acupressure on the upper arm was selected as a placebo condition because, according to traditional Chinese medicine, it is not a point with a connection to nausea. But the results revealed that subjects had fewer motion sickness symptoms and less tachygastria during rotation while receiving acupressure at P6 and on the upper arm compared to the no acupressure condition. These results suggest a placebo effect, but there is also the possibility that acupressure at P6 stimulated the meridian nerve and acupressure on the upper arm may have stimulated the same nerve. Alkaissi et al. (2005) conducted a similar study and obtained similar results. Women were divided into three groups: acupressure at P6, placebo acupressure on the forearm, and a no acupressure control group. All subjects were exposed to eccentric rotation in a chair with head movement. Both acupressure groups reported significantly less nausea than the control group, but the acupressure group did only marginally better than the placebo acupressure group. Miller and Muth (2004) compared the efficacy of acupressure and acustimulation for the prevention of nausea and other symptoms of motion sickness. They exposed subjects to a rotating optokinetic drum and reported that neither treatment prevented the development of symptoms, but participants provided with acustimulation had a longer delay until symptom onset.

Based on the laboratory studies reported in the literature to date, it is not possible to draw valid conclusions about the efficacy of the acuprocedures for preventing the development of nausea and other symptoms of motion sickness. Some of the relevant factors that have varied from study to study and made it impossible to draw valid conclusions include, subject knowledge of and expectation about acuprocedures, placebo control group, intensity and quality of stimulation across procedures, nature of provocative motion, and measure of nausea and/or other symptoms of motion sickness.

Other Procedures for Reducing the Nausea of Motion Sickness

In addition to the treatments described above that have been used to reduce the nausea of motion sickness, a few unique procedures have been described in the literature. Stern et al. (1990) investigated the effects on nausea and other symptoms of motion sickness of having a fixation point between the subject and the inside of a rotating optokinetic drum, and in a second group, the effects of wearing glasses that restricted the visual field to 15 degrees. Fixation greatly reduced nystagmus and slightly reduced vection. The restricted visual field slightly reduced nystagmus and greatly reduced vection. Both of the conditions significantly reduced nausea and other symptoms of motion sickness and tachygastria compared to a control group.

Jeng-Weei Lin et al. (2005) exposed subjects to complex visual motion through a cartoon-like simulated environment in a driving simulator. The variable manipulated was the level of cue salience for the upcoming simulated vehicle motion. The results showed that subjects experienced significantly greater simulator sickness in the no-cue condition.

Reschke, Somers, and Ford (2006) have suggested the use of stroboscopic illumination to combat space motion sickness. Promising results were obtained from a laboratory study in which participants read text and made horizontal head movements while wearing left-right reversing prisms. During the condition with the strobe light, motion sickness scores were significantly lower than in the control condition with normal light. Similar results were obtained using liquid crystal display shutter glasses.

In a correlational study using 1829 students, Caillet et al. (2006) examined the effect of involvement in sports and susceptibility to motion sickness. The first finding reported was that subjects who practiced a sport before the age of 18 were less susceptible to motion sickness than were the other subjects. The second finding was that subjects who practiced sports involving greater proprioception experienced less motion sickness than other subjects. The authors concluded that by practicing sports that make much use of proprioceptive cues, individuals become less dependent on visual input and use vestibular cues more effectively, and this enables them to manage better conflicting sensory inputs thereby reducing susceptibility to motion sickness.

CONCLUSIONS

The nausea of motion sickness can be prevented by the use of scopolamine and several over-the-counter antihistamines, but there are side effects such as drowsiness and dry mouth and large individual differences in responses. High protein meals and dried ginger root have shown promise as prophylactics for the nausea of motion sickness, but more research is needed with these products. Adaptation has been shown to reduce the nausea of motion sickness when subjects are reexposed to provocative motion within 48 hours in the laboratory, and there is some evidence of retention of adaptation for at least six months and of transfer from laboratory provocative motion to "real world" motion. Several government organizations including NASA and military groups have reported the successful use of exposure to increasingly provocative motion to desensitize pilots in training, astronauts, etc., to motion sickness. There is some evidence that controlled breathing can be used to reduce the nausea of motion sickness, but support for the use of acupressure and related procedures is weak. To summarize, there is no successful treatment for the nausea of motion sickness that is efficacious for everyone and free of negative side effects. The development of such a treatment must await the results of basic research on the mechanisms of motion sickness.

Chapter 16

Future Research: Management and Mechanisms

This final chapter describes research in progress and research that the authors believe is necessary for a greater understanding of the psychology, gastroenterology, and physiology underlying nausea and for the development of new, more effective treatments.

THREE NOVEL TREATMENTS FOR NAUSEA: BIOFEEDBACK, NUTRACEUTICALS, AND ADAPTATION

The three preliminary studies described below may lead to the development of novel treatments for nausea. The first study involved the use of biofeedback (Stern et al., 2004). The rationale for this study was that since nausea is usually accompanied by tachygastria and the loss of normal 3-cpm EGG activity, an effort could be made to use biofeedback to increase the normal 3-cpm activity in terms of amplitude and consistency of the signal. An initial study was done with healthy subjects. Thirteen participants were provided with biofeedback of their EGG activity as projected on a computer screen in real time. They were instructed to try to relax and increase their 3-cpm activity by making their own EGG match a 3-cpm signal that was always present on the computer screen. Thirteen different participants formed a control group that received the same instructions to relax and try to increase their 3-cpm activity, but they received no biofeedback. All participants reported to the lab after a 3-hour fast and agreed to return for four sessions with a 7-day intersession interval. EGG electrodes were applied during a 10-minute baseline period. During the following 10 minutes participants tried to increase their 3-cpm activity either with or without biofeedback with the ideal 3-cpm signal projected beside their own EGG recording. Neither group received biofeedback during the final 10 minutes. The subjects who received biofeedback increased their normal 3-cpm EGG activity significantly from session 1 to sessions 3 and 4. In contrast, the control subjects failed to increase their normal 3-cpm activity. In conclusion, this first biofeedback study of EGG with healthy subjects with normal gastric activity demonstrated that with biofeedback of their EGG they could increase their 3-cpm activity. Note that this initial study was done with healthy subjects who had a considerable amount of normal

3-cpm activity at baseline, but they were still able to increase it significantly by the third biofeedback session. We hope to develop this procedure as a treatment for chronic nausea, for patients who show very little normal 3-cpm activity at baseline.

The second study, which was described fully in Chapter 14 in this volume, used nutraceuticals to reduce the delayed nausea of chemotherapy (Levine et al., 2008). The results were very encouraging even though the number of subjects was small. As can be seen in Figure 14.2 (p. 326), the percentage of patients in the high protein group who reported nausea was significantly less compared with the patients in the other two groups. Patients in the high protein group also used significantly less antiemetic medication during the study period after their chemotherapy. A limitation of this first study of its type was the lack of sufficient control groups to distinguish the effects of the high protein drink from the effects of ginger. We look forward to seeing future studies with larger numbers of patients, sufficient control groups, and nauseogenic conditions other than chemotherapy.

The third study, which was described in Chapter 15 in this volume, used the transfer of adaptation to drum rotation to treat car motion sickness (Williamson, Higgins & Stern, 2003). As discussed in Chapter 7 in this volume, exposure to a rotating drum induces nausea and gastric dysrhythmias in susceptible subjects. And in Chapter 3, we discussed the role of adaptation to provocative motion. The question that was asked in this study was if adaptation to a rotating drum would decrease drum-induced nausea in the laboratory, and would that adaptation transfer to a real-world situation, namely car sickness? As seen in Figure 15.2 (p. 347), transfer of adaptation from the rotating drum to the moving car did take place for most subjects. This figure shows the magnitude of self-reported symptoms of car sickness before and after adaptation sessions (treatment) in the rotating drum. We are eager to see the results of a similar study that includes a control group to make sure that the results obtained were not simply a function of attention being focused on the subjects. This study demonstrated that adaptation to a rotating optokinetic drum shows significant transfer to the real-world problem of car sickness and further studies may show to other nauseogenic conditions, such as chemotherapy, as well.

It is our hope to see this procedure of adapting people to a rotating drum being used to help cancer patients deal with the nausea that they frequently experience after chemotherapy or for patients at high risk of postoperative nausea and vomiting. For example, a group of cancer patients could be adapted in a rotating drum prior to their first chemotherapy treatment. A control group would also visit the drum rotation lab the same number of times as the subjects in the experimental group, but the control patients would not be adapted to the rotating drum. It would be exciting to find that these non-pharmacological treatment approaches might prevent or at least reduce the nausea induced by chemotherapy and/or other nauseogenic stimuli.

DRUGS, DEVICES, AND REGENERATION: A FUTURE FOCUSED
ON GASTRIC NEUROMUSCULAR DISORDERS AND NAUSEA

To make advances in the treatment of nausea, the specific details of the pathophysiology of nausea must be understood. As reviewed in Chapters 4–7 in this volume, there are multiple CNS and peripheral neurohormonal mechanisms that mediate nausea. Nevertheless, many causes of nausea are ultimately associated with disturbances in gastric electrical rhythm, the gastric dysrhythmias (see Chapter 7, in this volume), although their involvement in the genesis of the sensation of nausea is still unclear (see Chapter 5, in this volume). Thus, in the diverse situations where gastric dysrhythmias occur associated with nausea (e.g., mesenteric ischemia, gastric cancer, postsurgery, diabetic gastroparesis, pregnancy, motion sickness, chronic renal failure, functional dyspepsia), therapies targeted at their correction may provide an approach to the treatment of nausea (Owyang & Hasler, 2002). Specific antiarrhythmic drugs may have different cellular targets: central nervous system, abdominal vagal afferent or efferent neurons, gastric interstitial cells of Cajal (ICC), enteric nervous system, or gastric smooth muscle. For example, it is known that dopamine D_2 receptor antagonists, such as domperidone, correct gastric dysrhythmias (Koch et al., 1989) in humans; but, there are numerous other peripherally targeted receptors including motilin and $5\text{-}HT_4$ receptor agonists, vasopressin, $5\text{-}HT_3$ and NK_1 receptor antagonists, and inhibitors of prostaglandin synthesis that require systematic investigation. Modulation of the CNS autonomic outflows to the stomach such as selective muscarinic receptor antagonists provide another approach to maintenance of normal gastric rhythm (Owyang & Hasler, 2002). However, rational approaches rely on a more detailed understanding of the physiological processes underlying the EGG changes and the relationships among the EGG signal, gastric electromechanical coupling, gastric motility, and afferent signaling of these peripheral stomach changes to relevant CNS centers.

Drugs need to be developed that regulate the interstitial cells of Cajal (ICC), the pacemaker cells of the stomach, since abnormal ICC function and numbers contribute to the onset of gastric dysrhythmias. Such drugs may also help correct gastric dysrhythmias and control nausea. Thus, the future of gastric antiarrhythmia therapies will mirror the past successes in cardiology where the development of antiarrhythmic drugs for cardiac dysrhythmias has been successful. In view of similarities between ion channels in many excitable tissues, it is possible that knowledge of the ion channels regulating ICCs may identify antiarrhythmic drugs with efficacy in the stomach. Tissue engineering approaches that repopulate the stomach with normal ICCs, enteric nerves, or even smooth muscle may also be developed to restore function where these key elements are damaged or destroyed.

Advanced instrumentation to help diagnose gastric dysrhythmias will include expanded use of electrogastrography methods to record EGGs during various provocative test meals and to evoke gastric dysrhythmias in patients with unexplained nausea (Koch & Stern, 2004). Mapping of the gastric pacesetter potentials in the antrum and corpus with fixed electrodes or special catheters that are passed through endoscopes will help to localize gastric dysrhythmias and direct therapies that will correct the dysrhythmic foci. Recordings of gastric contractile activity and pH levels with an ingestible capsule will reveal new patterns of disordered gastric motility that will stimulate new ideas for treatments. Ambulatory EGG recording equipment is available to expand such recordings from the laboratory and clinic into real life situations.

Gastric electrical stimulation therapies will continue to be developed for the treatment of severe gastroparesis, nausea, and vomiting (Abell et al., 2003; McCallum et al., 2005; Lin et al., 2006). Application of various electrical currents to the stomach via electrodes placed in the muscular wall is still in its infancy (Hasler, 2009). These electrical stimulation approaches will become more precise and more sophisticated in the future. Improved patient selection criteria for electrical stimulation also will help to make these therapies more successful in reducing nausea and vomiting. More sophisticated placement of the electrodes in the corpus or antrum to achieve maximum efficacy is still under development. Variable stimulation characteristics, from frequency to duration to current amplitude, need further refinement for optimal reduction of nausea and vomiting and to improve gastric neuromuscular function. These gastric electrical stimulation techniques will also be used to treat other forms of nausea that may be temporary, but severe (e.g., severe nausea after cancer chemotherapy and prolonged postoperative nausea). For a comprehensive review of the use of gastric electrical stimulation see Hasler (2009).

Another treatment approach for patients with severe nausea and vomiting is to identify the focus of tachygastria and then to ablate that area using radiofrequency, laser, or other modalities. In the future the dysrhythmia focus in the corpus or antrum will be localized with electrical mapping techniques and then endoscopic technologies will be used to apply the ablation therapies.

The discipline of regenerative medicine offers hope for the future when end-stage gastroparesis will be treated by replacing the failed stomach with a regenerated stomach. The regenerated stomach will be formed by gastric smooth muscle that grows over specialized scaffolds in the presence of specific growth factors to form a functional sphere of smooth muscle. The regenerated stomach will replace key portions of the failed stomach (e.g., antrum or fundus). The regenerated portions of the fundus, corpus, or antrum of the stomach will be sutured into position between the esophagus and the duodenum during surgery. Many hurdles face regeneration of the stomach or intestine: formation of the mucosal/smooth muscle wall, stimulation of peristalsis, production of organs of sufficient size, regulatory approval, and commercialization (Dunn, 2008). Urinary bladders have been regenerated using these techniques and successfully implanted in animals and humans (Atala et al., 2006). The bladders provide physiologic function where none existed.

Targeting the Central Nervous System

The focus of the above sections has been on correcting the EGG dysrhythmias, as this is probably currently the most objective signal to target therapy. However, elevated plasma vasopressin has been equally widely but not universally implicated in the pathogenesis of nausea. Studies have shown that ginger treatment during vection, which blunted the secretion of vasopressin, reduced the sensation of nausea (Lien et al., 2003). Studies of selective vasopressin receptor antagonists have not been very promising (see Chapter 6, in this volume), although it must be emphasized that the development of selective vasopressin receptor antagonists lags behind other areas of relevance to nausea. Approaches to modulate the pituitary secretion of vasopressin driven by stimuli evoking nausea may prove more tractable as the neuropharmacology of the hypothalamic-pituitary axis is relatively well studied.

Irrespective of the stimuli inducing nausea and to whatever extent either vasopressin or gastric dysrhythmias are involved, it is of concern to patients when it becomes an unpleasant conscious sensation. Ultimately it will only be possible to treat nausea in all situations by identification of the central pathways and their neurotransmitters so that the central processing of the signals giving rise to the sensation can be modified. Approaches and barriers to the study of the central pathways were reviewed in Chapter 4 (in this volume).

CONCLUSIONS

Nausea is a very common unpleasant sensation, a queasy feeling usually in the stomach that is sometimes followed by emesis. Nausea is a component of a complex protective mechanism that signals us not to eat, and from which we learn to avoid certain substances. When nausea becomes persistent or occurs after meals (in the absence of poison), then nausea is a noxious and debilitating symptom. Individual differences in the experience of nausea are in part a function of one's "nausea threshold" at a certain point in time, but we do not completely understand differences in the individual experience of nausea. Psychological factors such as anxiety, expectation, and anticipation are thought to lower the threshold, and adaptation to raise it. We hypothesize that changes in the "nausea threshold" affect cognitive appraisal of the nauseogenic stimulus and/or the bodily changes (e.g., gastric dysrhythmias) that follow exposure.

A difficult problem facing health care providers is how to reduce selectively this very effective protective mechanism, nausea, when it is not needed or wanted; e.g., following chemotherapy, postoperatively, during threats such as speech preparation, during provocative motion stimuli, or after a meal. In the clinical setting, persistent, chronic nausea can cause "irremediable suffering." This suffering will only be reduced after we gain a greater understanding of the complex interaction of the inherent and psychological factors and their accompanying gastrointestinal, autonomic, central nervous system, and endocrine changes that contribute to the experience of nausea.

At this time we conclude that nausea is usually accompanied by gastric dysrhythmia, characteristic changes in the autonomic outflow, and increased release of vasopressin. A giant step forward in our understanding of nausea will take place when future research progresses from the "accompanied" variety to conclusions about cause and effect.

References

Aapro, M. S., Kirchner, V., & Terrey, J. P. (1994). The incidence of anticipatory nausea and vomiting after repeat cycle chemotherapy: the effect of granisetron. *Br J Cancer, 69,* 957–960.

Aapro, M. S., Molassiotis, A., & Olver, I. (2005). Anticipatory nausea and vomiting. *Support Care Cancer, 13,* 117–121.

Abe, K., Amatomi, M., & Kajiyama, S. (1970). Genetic and developmental aspects of susceptibility to motion sickness and frost-bite. *Human Heredity, 20,* 507–516.

Abell, T. L., Bernstein, V. K., Cutts, T., Farrugia, G., Forster, J., Hasler, W. L., McCallum, R. W., Olden, K. W., Parkman, H. P., Parrish, C. R., Pasricha, P. J., Prather, C. M., Soffer, E. E., Twillman, R., & Vinik, A. I. (2006). Treatment of gastroparesis: A multidisciplinary clinical review. *Neurogastroenterol Motil, 18,* 263–283.

Abell, T. L., & Malagelada, J.-R. (1985). Glucagon-evoked gastric dysrhythmias in humans shown by an improved electrogastrographic technique. *Gastroenterology, 88,* 1932–1940.

Abell, T., McCallum, R., Hocking, M., Koch, K., Abrahamsson, H., LeBlanc, I., Lindberg, G., Konturek, J., Nowak, T., Quigley, E. M. M., Tougas, G., & Starkebaum, W. (2003). Gastric electrical stimulation for medically refractory gastroparesis. *Gastroenterology, 125,* 421–428.

Abrahamsson, H. (1973). Studies on the inhibitory nervous control of gastric motility. *Acta Physiol Scand Suppl, 390,* 1–38.

Abrahamsson, H., & Jansson, G. (1969). Elicitation of reflex vagal relaxation of the stomach from pharynx and esophagus in the cat. *Acta Physiol Scand, 77,* 172–178.

Abrahamsson, H., & Thoren, P. (1973). Vomiting and reflex vagal relaxation of the stomach elicited from heart receptors in the cat. *Acta Physiol Scand, 88,* 433–439.

Ader, R. (1976). Conditioned adrenocortical steroid elevations in the rat. *J Comp Physiol Psychol, 90,* 1156–1163.

AGA (2001). American Gastroenterological Association. Medical position statement: Nausea and vomiting. *Gastroenterology, 120,* 261–263.

Aggarwal, S. K., San Antonio, J. D., Sokhansanj, A., & Miller, C. (1994). Cisplatin-induced peptic ulcers, vagotomy, adrenal and calcium modulation. *Anticancer Drugs, 5,* 177–193.

Aikins Murphy, P. (1998). Alternative therapies for the nausea and vomiting of pregnancy. *Obstet Gynecol, 91,* 149–155.

Aldrich, C. G., Rhodes, M. T., Miner, J. L., Kerley, M. S., & Paterson, J. A. (1993). The effects of endophyte-infected tall fescue consumption and use of a dopamine antagonist on intake, digestibility, body temperature, and blood constituents in sheep. *J Anim Sci, 71,* 158–163.

Alexander, S. P., Mathie, A., & Peters, J. A. (2008). Guide to Receptors and Channels (GRAC), 3rd. *Br J Pharmacol, 153*(Suppl. 2), S1–209.

Ali, F., Guglin, M., Vaitkevicius, P., & Ghali, J. K. (2007). Therapeutic potential of vasopressin receptor antagonists. *Drugs, 67,* 847–858.

Alkaissi, A., Ledin, T., Odkvist, L. M., & Kalman, S. (2005). P6 acupressure increases tolerance to nauseogenic motion stimulation in women at high risk for PONV. *Can J Anaesth, 52,* 703–709.

Allen, M. E., McKay, C., Eaves, D. M., & Hamilton, D. (1986). Naloxone enhances motion sickness: Endorphins implicated. *Aviat Space Environ Med, 57,* 647–653.

Alvarez, W. C. (1922). New methods of studying gastric peristalsis. *J Am Med Assoc, 22,* 1281–1284.

Alvarez, W. C. (1925). Reverse peristalsis in the bowel, a precursor of vomiting. *JAMA, 85,* 1051–1054.

Alvarez, W. C. (1940). *An introduction to gastroenterology: The mechanics of the digestive tract* (3rd ed.). New York: Hoeber.

Amber, E. I., Henderson, R. A., Adeyanju, J. B., & Gyang, E. O. (1990). Single-drug chemotherapy of canine transmissible venereal tumor with cyclophosphamide, methotrexate, or vincristine. *J Vet Intern Med, 4,* 144–147.

Andersen, R., & Krohg, K. (1976). Pain as a major cause of postoperative nausea. *Can Anaesth Soc J, 23,* 366–369.

Andersson, B., & Larsson, S. (1954). Inhibitory effect of emesis on water diuresis in the dog. *Acta Physiol Scand, 32,* 19–27.

Andersson, B., & Persson, N. (1958). Intravenous assay of antidiuretic hormone using the goat. *Acta Physiol Scand, 42,* 257–261.

Andresen, M. C., & Kunze, D. L. (1994). Nucleus tractus solitarius: Gateway to neural circulatory control. *Ann Rev Physiol, 56,* 93–116.

Andrew, B. L. (1956). The nervous control of the cervical oesophagus of the rat during swallowing. *J Physiol, 134,* 729–740.

Andrews, P. L. R. (1986). Vagal afferent innervation of the gastrointestinal tract. *Prog Brain Res, 67,* 65–86.

Andrews, P. L. R. (1992). Physiology of nausea and vomiting. *Br J Anaesthesia, 69* (Suppl. 1), 2S–19S.

Andrews, P. L. R. (1999). Postoperative nausea and vomiting. In M. K. Herbert, P. Holzer, & N. Roewer (Eds.), *Problems of the gastrointestinal tract in anesthesia, the perioperative period, and intensive care* (pp. 267–288). Berlin and Heidelberg: Springer-Verlag.

Andrews, P. L., Axelsson, M., Franklin, C., & Holmgren, S. (2000). The emetic reflex in a reptile (Crocodylus porosus). *J Exp Biol, 203,* 1625–1632.

Andrews, P. L., & Bhandari, P. (1993). The 5-hydroxytryptamine receptor antagonists as antiemetics: preclinical evaluation and mechanism of action. *Eur J Cancer, 29A*(Suppl. 1), S11–16.

Andrews, P. L. R., Bhandari, P., & Davis, C. J. (1992). Plasticity and modulation of the emetic reflex. In A. L. Bianchi, L. Grelot, A. D. Miller, & G. L. King (Eds.), *Mechanisms and Control of Emesis* (pp. 275–284). Montrouge, France: Coloque INSERM/John Libbey Eurotext.

Andrews, P. L. R., Bhandari, P., Garland, S., Bingham, S., Davis, C. J., Hawthorn, J., Davidson, H. I. M., Rolance, R., & Lane, S. (1990a). Does retching have a function? An experimental study in the ferret. *Life Sce Adv: Pharmacodyn and Therapeut, 9,* 135–152.

Andrews, P. L. R., Davis, C. J., Bingham, S., Davidson, H. I., Hawthorn, J., & Maskell, L. (1990b). The abdominal visceral innervation and the emetic reflex: Pathways, pharmacology, and plasticity. *Can J Physiol Pharmacol, 68,* 325–345.

Andrews, P. L. R., Friedman, M. I., Liu, Y. L., Smith, J. E., & Sims, D. W. (2005). Potential energetic implications of emesis in the house musk shrew (Suncus murinus). *Physiol Behav, 84,* 519–524.

Andrews, P. L. R., Grundy, D., & Scratcherd, T. (1980). Vagal afferent discharge from mechanoreceptors in different regions of the ferret stomach. *J Physiol, 298,* 513–524.

Andrews, P. L. R., & Hawthorn, J. (1988). The neurophysiology of vomiting. *Clin Gastroenterol, 2,* 141–168.

Andrews, P. L. R., & Horn, C. C. (2006). Signals for nausea and emesis: Implications for models of upper gastrointestinal diseases. *Auton Neurosci, 125,* 100–115.

Andrews, P. L. R., Rapeport, W. G., & Sanger, G. J. (1988). Neuropharmacology of emesis induced by anti-cancer therapy. *Trends Pharmacol Sci, 9,* 334–341.

Andrews, P. L. R., & Rudd, J. A. (2004). The role of tachykinins and the tachykinin NK1 receptor in nausea and emesis. In P. Holzer (Ed.), *Tachykinins, handbook of experimental pharmacology* (Vol. 164, pp. 359–440). Berlin: Springer Verlag.

Andrews, P. L. R., Sims, D. W., & Young, J. Z. (1998). Induction of emesis by the sodium channel activator veratrine in the lesser spotted dogfish, Scyliorhinus canicula (Chondrichthyes: Elasmobranchii). *J Mar Biol Ass U.K., 78,* 1269–1279.

Andrews, P. L. R., Torii, Y., Saito, H., & Matsuki, N. (1996). The pharmacology of the emetic response to upper gastrointestinal tract stimulation in Suncus murinus. *Eur J Pharmacol, 307,* 305–313.

Andrews, P. L. R., & Wood, K. L. (1988). Vagally mediated gastric motor and emetic reflexes evoked by stimulation of the antral mucosa in anaesthetized ferrets. *J Physiol, 395,* 1–16.

Andrews, P. L. R., & Young, J. Z. (1993). Gastric-motility patterns for digestion and vomiting evoked by sympathetic-nerve stimulation and 5-hydroxytriptamine in the dogfish Scyliorhinus canicula. *Philosophical Transactions of the Royal Society of London, 342,* 363–380.

Andrykowski, M. A. (1990). The role of anxiety in the development of anticipatory nausea in cancer chemotherapy: A review and synthesis. *Psychosom Med, 52,* 458–475.

Annese, V., Bassotti, G., Caruso, N., De Cosmo, S., Gabbrielli, A., Modoni, S., Frusciante, V., & Andriulli, A. (1999). Gastrointestinal motor dysfunction, symptoms, and neuropathy in noninsulin-dependent (type 2) diabetes mellitus. *J Clin Gastroenterol, 29,* 171–177.

Apfel, C. C. (2010). Postoperative nausea and vomiting. In R. D. Miller et al. (Eds.), *Miller's Anesthesia* (7th ed., pp. 2729–2755). New York: Churchill Livingstone Elsevier.

Apfel, C. C., Cakmakkaya, O. S., Frings, G., Kranke, P., Malhotra, A., Stader, A., Turan, A., Biedler, A., & Kolodzie, K. (2009). Droperidol has comparable clinical efficacy against both nausea and vomiting. *Brit J Anaesthesia, 103,* 359–363.

Apfel, C. C., Kortilla, K., Abdalla, M., Kerger, H., Turan, A., Vedder, I., Zernak, C., Danner, K., Jokela, R., Pocock, S. J., Trenkler, S., Kredel, M., Biedler, A., Sessler, D. I., Roewer, N., & IMPACT Investigators (2004). A factorial trial of six interventions for the prevention of postoperative nausea and vomiting. *N Engl J Med, 350*, 2441–2451.

Apfel, C. C., Kranke, P., Eberhart, L. H., Roos, A., & Roewer, N. (2002) Comparison of predictive models for postoperative nausea and vomiting. *Br J Anaesthesiol, 89*, 339–340.

Apfel, C. C., Malhotra, A., & Leslie, J. B. (2008). The role of neurokinin-1 receptor antagonists for the management of postoperative nausea and vomiting. *Curr Opinion in Anesth, 21*, 427–432.

Appenzeller, O., & Oribe, E. (1997). *The autonomic nervous system, an introduction to basic and clinical concepts.* Amsterdam: Elsevier.

Araya, M., McGoldrick, M. C., Klevay, L. M., Strain, J. J., Robson, P., Nielsen, F., Olivares, M., Pizarro, F., Johnson, L., & Poirer, K. A. (2001). Determination of an acute no-observed-adverse-effect level (NOAEL) for copper in water. *Reg Toxicol Pharmacol, 34*, 137–145.

Arwas, S., Rolnick, A., & Lubow, R. E. (1989). Conditioned taste aversion in humans using motion-induced sickness as the US. *Behav Res Ther, 27*, 295–301.

Asakawa, H., Hayashi, I., Fukui, T., & Tokunaga, K. (2003). Effect of mosapride on glycemic control and gastric emptying in type 2 diabetes mellitus patients with gas-tropathy. *Diabetes Res Clin Pract, 61*, 175–182.

Atala, A., Bauer, S. B., Soker, S., Yoo, J. J., & Retik, A. B. (2006). Tissue-engineered autologous bladders for patients needing cystoplasty. *Lancet, 367*, 1241–1426.

Atanackovic, G., Navioz, Y., Moretti, M. E., & Koren, G. (2001). The safety of higher than standard dose of doxylamine-pyridoxine (Diclectin®) for nausea and vomiting of pregnancy. *J Clin Pharmacol, 41*, 842–845.

Atanackovic, G., Wolpin, J., & Koren, G. (2001). Determinants of the need for hospital care among women with NVP. *Clin Invest Med, 24*, 90–93.

Atkinson, A. J., & Ivy, A. C. (1938). Studies on the control of gastic secretions. *Am J Dig Dis, 4*, 811–816.

Attenborough, D. (2002). *The life of mammals.* London: BBC Wordwide Ltd.

Aung, H. H., Dey, L., Mehendale, S., Xie, J. T., Wu, J. A., & Yuan, C. S. (2003). Scutellaria baicalensis extract decreases cisplatin-induced pica in rats. *Cancer Chemother Pharmacol, 52*, 453–458.

Aung, H. H., Mehendale, S. R., Xie, J. T., Moss, J., & Yuan, C. S. (2004). Methylnaltrexone prevents morphine-induced kaolin intake in the rat. *Life Sci, 74*, 2685–2691.

Avanzino, G. L., Bradley, P. B., & Wolstencroft, J. H. (1966). Actions of prostaglandins E1, E2, and F2-alpha on brain stem neurones. *Br J Pharmacol Chemother, 27*, 157–163.

Axelrod, F. B. (1999). Familial Dysautonomia. In C. J. Mathias and R. Bannister (Eds.), *Autonomic failure, a textbook of clinical disorders of the autonomic nervous system* (4th ed., pp. 402–409). New York: Oxford University Press.

Aylett, P. (1962). Gastric emptying and change of blood glucose level, as affected by glucagon and insulin. *Clin Sci, 22*, 171–178.

Aziz, Q., Thompson, D. G., Ng, V. W., Hamdy, S., Sarkar, S., Brammer, M. J., Bullmore, E. T., Hobson, A., Tracey, I., Gregory, L., Simmons, A., & Williams, S. C. (2000). Cortical processing of human somatic and visceral sensation. *J Neurosci, 20*, 2657–2663.

Azziz, R., Marin, C., Hoq, L., Badamgarav, E., & Song, P. (2005). Health care–related economic burden of the polycystic ovary syndrome during the reproductive life span. *J Clin Endocrinol Metab, 90,* 4650–4658.

Badary, O. A., Awad, A. S., Sherief, M. A., & Hamada, F. M. (2006). In vitro and in vivo effects of ferulic acid on gastrointestinal motility: Inhibition of cisplatin-induced delay in gastric emptying in rats. *World J Gastroenterol, 12,* 5363–5367.

Badell, M. L., Ramin, S. M., & Smith, J. A. (2006). Treatment options for nausea and vomiting during pregnancy. *Pharmacotherapy, 26,* 1273–1287.

Bagian, J. P. (1991). First intramuscular administration in the U.S. space program. *J Clin Pharmacol, 31,* 920.

Bailey, P. L., Rhondeau, S., Schafer, P. G., Lu, J. K., Timmins, B. S., Foster, W., Pace, N. L., & Stanley, T. H. (1993). Dose-response pharmacology of intrathecal morphine in human volunteers. *Anesthesiology, 79,* 49–59.

Baker, P. C., & Bernat, J. L. (1985). The neuroanatomy of vomiting in man: Association of projectile vomiting with a solitary metastasis in the lateral tegmentum of the pons and the middle cerebellar peduncle. *J Neurol Neurosurg Psychiatry, 48,* 1165–1168.

Bakwin, H. (1971). Car-sickness in twins. *Dev Med Child Neurol, 13,* 310–312.

Balme, D. M. (Ed. and Trans.). (1991). *Aristotle, History of Animals* (books 7–10). Cambridge, MA: Harvard University Press.

Banks, W. A. (2006). The blood-brain barrier as a regulatory interface in the gut-brain axes. *Physiol Behav, 89,* 472–476.

Barclay, A. E. (1936). *The digestive tract.* London: Cambridge University Press.

Barcroft, H., & Swan, H. J. C. (1953). *Sympathetic control of human blood vessels.* London: Edward Arnold & Co.

Barker, L. M., Best, M. R., & Domjan, M. (1977). *Learning mechanisms in food selection.* Waco, TX: Baylor University Press.

Barnes, N. M., Bunce, K. T., Naylor, R. J., & Rudd, J. A. (1991). The actions of fentanyl to inhibit drug-induced emesis. *Neuropharmacology, 30,* 1073–1083.

Barnes, P. J. (1999). Autonomic control of the airways. In C. J. Mathias and R. Bannister (Eds.), *Autonomic failure: A textbook of clinical disorders of the autonomic nervous system* (4th ed., pp. 109–116). New York: Oxford University Press.

Barnett, J. L., & Owyang, C. (1988). Serum glucose concentration as a modulator of interdigestive gastric motility. *Gastroenterology, 94,* 739–744.

Barreca, T., Corsini, G., Cataldi, A., Garibaldi, A., Cianciosi, P., Rolandi, E., & Franceschini, R. (1996). Effect of the 5-HT3 receptor antagonist ondansetron on plasma AVP secretion: A study in cancer patients. *Biomed Pharmacother, 50,* 512–514.

Basso, O., & Olsen, J. (2001). Sex ratio and twinning in women with hyperemesis of pre-eclampsia. *Epidemiology, 12,* 747–749.

Baur, S., & Bacon, V. C. (1976). A specific gastrin receptor on plasma membranes of antral smooth muscle. *Biochem Biophys Res Commun, 73,* 928–933.

Bayley, T. M., Dye, L., Jones, S., DeBono, M., & Hill, A. J. (2002). Food cravings and aversions during pregnancy: Relationships with nausea and vomiting. *Appetite, 38,* 45–51.

Baylis, P. H. (1983). Posterior pituitary function in health and disease. *Clin Endocrinol Metab, 12,* 747–770.

Bear, M. F., Connors, B. W., & Paradiso, M. A. (1996). *Neuroscience: Exploring the brain.* Baltimore: Williams & Wilkins.

Beattie, D. T., Beresford, I. J., Connor, H. E., Marshall, F. H., Hawcock, A. B., Hagan, R. M., Bowers, J., Birch, P. J., & Ward, P. (1995). The pharmacology of GR203040, a novel, potent and selective non-peptide tachykinin NK$_1$ receptor antagonist. *Br J Pharmacol, 116,* 3149–3157.

Beattie, W. S., Lindblad, T., Buckley, D. N., & Forrest, J. B. (1991). Incidence of postoperative nausea and vomiting in women undergoing laparoscopy is influenced by the day of menstrual cycle. *Can J Anaesth, 38,* 298–302.

Beleslin, D. B., Krstic, S. K., Stefanovic-Denic, K., Strbac, M., & Micic, D. (1981). Inhibition by morphine and morphine-like drugs of nicotine-induced emesis in cats. *Brain Res Bull, 6,* 451–453.

Belig, A. J., Morrow, G. R., Barry, M., Angel, C., & DuBeshter, B. (1995). Autonomic measures associated with chemotherapy-related nausea: Techniques and issues. *Cancer Invest, 13,* 313–323.

Bensafi, M., Sobel, N., & Khan, R. M. (2007). Hedonic-specific activity in piriform cortex during odor imagery mimics that during odor perception. *J Neurophysiol, 98,* 3254–3262.

Bense, S., Stephan, T., Yousry, T. A., Brandt, T., & Dieterich, M. (2001). Multisensory cortical signal increases and decreases during vestibular galvanic stimulation (fMRI). *J Neurophysiol, 85,* 886–899.

Bergman, J., & Glowa, J. R. (1986). Suppression of behavior by food pellet-lithium chloride pairings in squirrel monkeys. *Pharmacol Biochem Behav, 25,* 973–978.

Berkovitch, M., Elbirt, D., Addis, A., Schuler-Faccini, L., & Ornov, A. (2000). Fetal effects of metoclopramide therapy for nausea and vomiting of pregnancy. *N Engl J Med, 343,* 445–446.

Bermudez, J., Boyle, E. A., Miner, W. D., & Sanger, G. J. (1988). The anti-emetic potential of the 5-hydroxytryptamine$_3$ receptor antagonist BRL 43694. *Br J Cancer, 58,* 644–650.

Bernard, C. (1949). *An introduction to the study of experimental medicine* (H. C. Green, Trans.). New York: Henry Schuman. (Original work published 1865)

Bernstein, I. L. (1978) Learned taste aversions in children receiving chemotherapy. *Science, 200,* 1302–1303.

Bernstein, I. L. (1999). Taste aversion learning: A contemporary perspective. *Nutrition, 15,* 229–234.

Bernstein, I. L., Chavez, M., Allen, D., & Taylor, E. M. (1992). Area postrema mediation of physiological and behavioural effects of lithium chloride in the rat. *Brain Res, 575,* 1132–1137.

Berridge, K., Grill, H. J., & Norgren, R. (1981). Regulation of consummatory responses and preabsorptive insulin release to palatability and learned taste aversions. *J Comp Physiol Psychol, 95,* 363–382.

Bersherdas, K., Leahy, A., Mason, I., Harbord, M., & Epstein, O. (1998). The effect of cisapride on dyspepsia symptoms and the electrogastrogram in patients with non-ulcer dyspepsia. *Aliment Pharmacol Ther, 12,* 755–759.

Berthoud, H. R. (2008). The vagus nerve, food intake, and obesity. *Reg Peptides, 149,* 15–25.

Berthoud, H. R., & Neuhuber, W. L. (2000). Functional and chemical anatomy of the afferent vagal system. *Auton Neurosci, 85,* 1–17.

Bertin, E., Schneider, N., Abdelli, N., Wampach, H., Cadiot, G., Loboquerrero, A., Leutenegger, M., Liehn, J. C., & Thiefin, G. (2001). Gastric emptying is accelerated in obese type 2 diabetic patients without autonomic neuropathy. *Diabetes Metab, 27,* 357–364.

Beyak, M. J., & Grundy, D. (2005). Vagal afferents innervating the gatrointestinal tract. In B. J. Undem and D. Weinreich (Eds.), *Advances in vagal afferent neurobiology* (pp. 315–350). Boca Raton, FL: Taylor & Francis/CRC Press.

Biggs, J. S. G. (1975). Vomiting in pregnancy: Causes and management. *Drugs, 9,* 299–306.

Bilgutay, A. M., Wingrove, R., Griffen, W. O., Bonnabeau, R. C., Jr., & Lillehei, C. W. (1963). Gastro-intestinal pacing: a new concept in the treatment of ileus. *Ann Surg, 158,* 338–348.

Billig, I., Yates, B. J., & Rinaman, L. (2001). Plasma hormone levels and central c-Fos expression in ferrets after systemic administration of cholecystokinin. *Am J Physiol Regul Integr Comp Physiol, 281,* R1243–1255.

Billington, C. J., Morley, J. E., Levine, A. S., Wright, F., & Seal, U. S. (1985). Naloxone induced suppression of feeding in tigers. *Physiol Behav, 34,* 641–643.

Blackburn-Munro, G. (2004). Pain-like behaviours in animals: How human are they? *Trends Pharmacol Sci, 25,* 299–305.

Blackshaw, L. A., Grundy, D., & Scratcherd, T. (1987). Involvement of gastrointestinal mechano- and chemoreceptors in vagal reflexes: An electrophysiological study. *J Autonom Nerv Syst, 18,* 225–234.

Blair, R., & Amit, Z. (1981). Morphine conditioned taste aversion reversed by periaqueductal gray lesions. *Pharmacol Biochem Behav, 15,* 651–653.

Blakemore, C., & Jennett, S. (Eds.). (2001). *Oxford companion to the body.* New York: Oxford University Press.

Blancquaert, J. P., Lefebvre, R. A., & Willems, J. L. (1982). Gastric relaxation by intravenous and intracerebroventricular administration of apomorphine, morphine, and fentanyl in the conscious dog. *Arch Int Pharmacodyn Ther, 256,* 153–154.

Bloomfield, A. L., & Polland, W. S. (1931). Experimental referred pain from the gastrointestinal tract: Part 2. Stomach, duodenum, and colon. *J Clin Invest, 10,* 453–473.

Blum, R. (2000). Pregnancy, nausea, and vomiting: Further explorations in theory. In R. H. Blum and W. L. Heinrichs (Eds.), *Nausea and vomiting: Overview, challenges, practical treatments, and new perspectives* (pp. 246–268). Philadelphia: Whurr.

Blum, R. H., Heinrichs, W. L., & Herxheimer, A. (2000). *Nausea and vomiting.* London: Whurr.

Boeckxstaens, G. E., Hirsh, D. P., van den Elzen, B. D., Heisteramp, S. H., & Tytgat, G. N. (2001). Impaired drinking capacity in patients with functional dyspepsia: Relationship with proximal stomach function. *Gastroenterology, 121,* 1054–1063.

Boneva, R. S., Moore, C. A., Botto, L., Wong, L. Y., & Erickson, J. D. (1999). Nausea during pregnancy and congenital heart defects: A population-based case-control study. *Am J Epidemiol, 149,* 717–725.

Bonham, A. C., & Chen, C-Y. (2005). Synaptic transmission in the nucleus tractus solitarius. In B. J. Undem and D. Weinreich (Eds.), *Advances in vagal afferent neurobiology* (pp. 193-208). Boca Raton, FL: Taylor & Francis/CRC Press.

Borelli, F., Capasso, R., Aviello, G., Pittler, M. H., & Isso, A. A. (2005). Effectiveness and safety of ginger in the treatment of pregnancy-induced nausea and vomiting. *Obstet Gynecol, 105,* 849–856.

Boring, E. G. (1942). *Sensation and perception in the history of experimental psychology.* New York: Appleton Century Crofts.

Borison, H. L. (1959). Effect of ablation of medullary emetic chemoreceptor trigger zone on vomiting responses to cerebral intraventricular injection of adrenalin, apomorphine, and piocarpine in the cat. *J Physiol, 147,* 172–177.

Borison, H. L. (1989). Area postrema: Chemoreceptor circumventricular organ of the medulla oblongata. *Prog Neurobiol, 32,* 351–390.

Borison, H. L., & Wang, S. C. (1953). Physiology and pharmacology of vomiting. *Pharmacol Rev, 5,* 193–230.

Borsini, F., & Rolls, E. T. (1984). Role of noradrenaline and serotonin in the basolateral region of the amygdala in food preferences and learned taste aversions in the rat. *Physiol Behav, 33,* 37–43.

Borsook, D., Becerra, L., & Hargreaves, R. (2006). A role for fMRI in optimizing CNS drug development. *Nat Rev Drug Discov, 5,* 411–424.

Bos, G. (Ed. and Trans.). (2004). *Maimonides: Medical Aphorisms, Treatises 1–5.* Provo, UT: Brigham Young University Press.

Bos, J. E., Damala, D., Lewis, C., Ganguly, A., & Taran, O. (2007). Susceptibility to seasickness. *Ergonomics, 50,* 890–901.

Bost, J., Mccarthy, L. E., Colby, E. D., & Borison, H. L. (1968). Rumination in sheep: Effects of morphine, deslanoside, and ablation of area postrema. *Physiol Behav, 3,* 877–881.

Bouchier, I. A. D. (1985) Nausea and vomiting. *Med Internat, 24,* 980.

Bovbjerg, D. H. (2006). The continuing problem of post chemotherapy nausea and vomiting: Contributions of classical conditioning. *Auton Neurosci, 129,* 92–98.

Bovbjerg, D. H., Redd, W. H., Jacobsen, P. B., Manne, S. L., Taylor, K. L., Surbone, A., Crown, J. P., Norton, L., Gilewski, T. A., Hudis, C. A. et al. (1992). An experimental analysis of classically conditioned nausea during cancer chemotherapy. *Psychosom Med, 54,* 623–637.

Bovbjerg, D. H., Redd, W. H., Maier, L. A., Holland, J. C., Lesko, L. M., Niedzwiecki, D., Rubin, S. C., & Hakes, T. B. (1990). Anticipatory immune suppression and nausea in women receiving cyclic chemotherapy for ovarian cancer. *J Consult Clin Psychol, 58,* 153–157.

Boyle, R. (1996). *A free enquiry into the vulgarly received notion of nature* (E. B. Davis and M. Hunter, Eds.). Cambridge, UK: Cambridge University Press. (Original work published 1686).

Bradner, W. T., & Schurig, J. E. (1981). Toxicology screening in small animals. *Cancer Treat Rev, 8,* 93–102.

Bradshaw, W. A., Gregory, B. C., Finley, C. R., Ross, A., Wilds, T., Still, M., & Smith, C. D. (2002). Frequency of postoperative nausea and vomiting in patients undergoing laparoscopic foregut surgery. *Surg Endosc, 16,* 777–780.

Brand, R. E., DiBaise, J. K., Quigley, E. M., Gobar, L. S., Harmon, K. S., Lynch, J. C., Bierman, P. J., Bishop, M. R., & Tarantolo, S. R. (1999). Gastroparesis as a cause of nausea and vomiting after high-dose chemotherapy and haemopoietic stem-cell transplantation. *Lancet, 353,* 846.

Brandes, J. M. (1967). First trimester nausea and vomiting as related to outcome of pregnancy. *Obstet Gynecol, 30,* 427–431.

Brandt, T., & Strupp, M. (2005). General vestibular testing. *Clin Neurophysiol, 116,* 406–426.

Braveman, N. S. (1974). Poison-based avoidance learning with flavored or colored water in guinea pigs. *Learning and Motivation, 5,* 182–194.

Braveman, N. S., & Bronstein, P. (1985). Experimental assessments and clinical applications of conditioned food aversions. *Ann N Y Acad Sci, 443,* 1–441.

Briggs, D. B., & Carpenter, D. O. (1986). Excitation of neurons in the canine area postrema by prostaglandins. *Cell Mol Neurobiol, 6,* 421–426.

Briggs, G. G., Freeman, R. K., & Yaffe, S. J. (2008). *Drugs in pregnancy and lactation: A reference guide to fetal and neonatal risk* (8th ed.). Philadelphia: Wolters Kluwer Health/Lippincott Williams & Wilkins.

Brizzee, K. R. (1956). Effect of localized brain stem lesions and supradiaphragmatic vagotomy on x-irradiation emesis in the monkey. *Am J Physiol, 187,* 567–570.

Broadley, K. J. (1996). *Autonomic pharmacology.* London: Taylor and Francis.

Brock, A. J. (Trans.). (1916). *Galen, on the natural faculties* (Loeb edition). Cambridge, MA: Harvard University Press.

Brookes, J. H., Zagorodnyuk, V. P., & Costa, M. (2005). Mechanotransduction by vagal tension receptors in the upper gut. In B. J. Undem and D. Weinreich (Eds.), *Advances in vagal afferent neurobiology* (pp. 147–166). Boca Raton, FL: Taylor & Francis/CRC Press.

Broomhead, J. A., Fairlie, D. P., & Whitehouse, M. W. (1980). cis-Platinum(II) amine complexes: Some structure-activity relationships for immunosuppressive, nephrotoxic, and gastrointestinal (side) effects in rats. *Chem Biol Interact, 31,* 113–132.

Brown, J. E., Kahn, E. S., & Hartman, T. J. (1997). Profet, profits, and proof: Do nausea and vomiting of early pregnancy protect women from "harmful" vegetables? *Am J Obstet Gynecol, 176*(part 1), 179–181.

Brunnschweiler, J. M., Andrews, P. L. R., Southall, E. J., Pickering, M., & Sims, D. W. (2005). Rapid voluntary stomach eversion in a free-living shark. *J Mar Biol Ass U.K., 85,* 1141–1144.

Bryan, C. P. (Trans.), & Smith, G. E. (Intro.). (1974). *Ancient Egyptian medicine: The Papyrus Ebers.* Chicago: Ares Publishers Inc.

Brzana, R. J., & Koch, K. L. (1997). Gastroesophageal reflux disease presenting with intractable nausea. *Ann Intern Med, 126,* 704–707.

Brzana, R. J., Koch, K. L., & Bingaman, S. (1998). Gastric myoelectrical activity in patients with gastric outlet obstruction and idiopathic gastroparesis. *Am J Gastroenterol, 93,* 1083–1089.

Buck, A. H. (1917). *The growth of medicine from the earliest times to about 1800.* New Haven, CT: Yale University Press.

Burchfield, S. R., Elich, M. S., & Woods, S. C. (1977). Geophagia in response to stress and arthritis. *Physiol Behav, 19,* 265–267.

Burdyga, G., Lal, S., Varro, A., Dimaline, R., Thompson, D. G., & Dockray, G. J. (2004). Expression of cannabinoid CB1 receptors by vagal afferent neurons is inhibited by cholecystokinin. *J Neurosci, 24,* 2708–2715.

Burguière, P., Gourevitch, D., & Malinas, Y. (2003). *Soranos d'Éphèse, maladies des femmes.* Paris: Les Belles Lettres.

Butler, A. B., & Hodos, W. (1996). *Comparative vertebrate neuroanatomy: Evolution and adaptation.* New York: Wiley-Liss.

Buysschaert, M., Moulart, M., Urbain, J. L., Pauwels, S., de Roy, L., Ketelslegers, J. M., & Lambert, A. E. (1987). Impaired gastric emptying in diabetic patients with cardiac autonomic neuropathy. *Diabetes Care, 10,* 448–452.

Bytzer, P., Talley, N. J., Hammer, J., Young, L. J., Jones, M. P., & Horowitz, M. (2002). GI symptoms in diabetes mellitus are associated with both poor glycemic control and diabetic complications. *Am J Gastroenterol, 97,* 604–611.

Bytzer, P., Talley, N. J., Leemon, M., Young, L. J., Jones, M. P., & Horowitz, M. (2001). Prevalence of gastrointestinal symptoms associated with diabetes mellitus: A population-based survey of 15,000 adults. *Arch Intern Med, 161,* 1989–1996.

Cabezos, P. A., Vera, G., Castillo, M., Fernandez-Pujol, R., Martin, M. I., & Abalo, R. (2008). Radiological study of gastrointestinal motor activity after acute cisplatin in the rat: Temporal relationship with pica. *Autonom Neurosci, 141,* 54–65.

Cahen, R. L. (1972). Emetic effect of biogenic amines. *Res Clin Stud Headache, 3,* 227–244.

Caillet, G., Bosser, G., Gauchard, G. C., Chau, N., Benamghar, L., & Perrin, P. P. (2006). Effect of sporting activity practice on susceptibility to motion sickness. *Brain Res Bull, 69,* 288–293.

Camilleri, M. (2006). New imaging in neurogastroenterology: An overview. *Neurogastroenterol Motil, 18,* 805–812.

Camilleri, M., Dubois, D., Coulie, B., Jones, M., Kahrilas, P. J., Rentz, A. M., Sonnenberg, A., Stanghellini, V., Stewart, W. F., Tack, J., Talley, N. J., Whitehead, W., & Revicki, D. A. (2005). Prevalence and socioeconomic impact of upper gastrointestinal disorders in the United States: Results of the US upper gastrointestinal study. *Clin Gastroenterol Hepat, 3,* 543–552.

Camilleri, M., Toouli, J., Herrera, M. F., Kulseng, B., Kow, L., Pantoja, J. P., Marvik, R., Johnsen, G., Billington, C. J., Moody, F. G., Knudson, M. B., Tweden, K. S., Vollmer, M., Wilson, R. R., & Anvari, M. (2008). Intra-abdominal vagal blocking (VBLOC therapy): Clinical results with a new implantable medical device. *Surgery, 143,* 723–731.

Cannon, D. S., Best, M. R., Batson, J. D., & Feldman, M. (1983). Taste familiarity and apomorphine-induced taste aversions in humans. *Behav Res Ther, 21,* 669–673.

Cannon, W. B. (1898). The movements of the stomach studies by means of Röntgen Rays. *Am J Physiol, 1,* 359–382.

Cappell, M. S., Sidhom, O., & Colon, V. (1996). Study at eight medical centers of the safety and clinical efficacy of esophagogastroduodenoscopy in 83 pregnancies with follow up fetal outcome. *Am J Gastroenterol, 91,* 348–354.

Caras, S. D., Soykan, I., Beverly, V., Lin, Z., & Mccallum, R. W. (1997). The effect of intravenous vasopressin on gastric myoelectrical activity in human subjects. *Neurogastroenterol Motil, 9,* 151–156.

Carliner, P. E., Radman, H. M., & Gay, L. N. (1949). Treatment of nausea and vomiting of pregnancy with dramamine: Preliminary report. *Science, 110,* 215–216.

Carnett, J. B. (1926). Intercostal neuralgia as a cause of abdominal pain and tenderness. *Surg Gynecol Obstet, 12,* 625–632.

Carpenter, D. O., & Briggs, D. B. (1986). Insulin excites neurons of the area postrema and causes emesis. *Neurosci Lett, 68,* 85–89.

Carpenter, D. O., Briggs, D. B., & Strominger, N. (1983). Responses of neurons of canine area postrema to neurotransmitters and peptides. *Cell Mol Neurobiol, 3,* 113–126.

Carpenter, D. O., Briggs, D. B., & Strominger, N. (1984). Peptide-induced emesis in dogs. *Behav Brain Res, 11,* 277–281.

Carrell, L. E., Cannon, D. S., Best, M. R., & Stone, M. J. (1986). Nausea and radiation-induced taste aversions in cancer patients. *Appetite, 7,* 203–208.

Carter, S. (2006). The surgical team and outcomes management: Focus on post-operative ileus. *J PeriAnesth Nurs, 21,* 52–56.

Castejon, A. M., Paez, X., Hernandez, L., & Cubeddu, L. X. (1999). Use of intravenous microdialysis to monitor changes in serotonin release and metabolism induced by cisplatin in cancer patients: Comparative effects of granisetron and ondansetron. *J Pharmacol Exp Ther, 291,* 960–966.

Castell, J. A., Gedeon, R. M., & Castell, D. O. (2002). Esophageal manometry. In M. M. Schuster, M. D. Crowell, & K. L. Koch (Eds.), *Atlas of gastrointestinal motility in health and disease* (pp. 69–85). Hamilton, Ontario, Canada: B. C. Decker.

Castillo, E. J., Delgado-Aros, S., Camilleri, M., Burton, D., Stephens, D., O'Connor-Semmes, R., Walker, A., Shachoy-Clark, A., & Zinsmeister, A. R. (2004). Effect of oral CCK-1 agonist GI181771X on fasting and postprandial gastric functions in healthy volunteers. *Am J Physiol Gastrointest Liver Physiol, 287,* G363–369.

Caul, E. O. (1994). Small round structured viruses: Airborne transmission and hospital control. *Lancet, 343,* 1240–1242.

CDC (2009a). National Diabetes Fact Sheet. Retrieved May 15, 2009, from http://www.cdc.gov/diabetes/pubs/estimates07.htm#top

CDC (2009b). Motion sickness. Retrieved March 24, 2009, from http://wwwn.cdc.gov/travel/yellowBookCh6-MotionSickness.aspx

Cechetto, D. F., & Saper, C. B. (1990). Role of the cerebral cortex in autonomic function. In A. D. Loewy & K. M. Spyer (Eds.), *Central regulation of autonomic functions* (pp. 208–233). Oxford and New York: Oxford University Press.

Cepeda, M. S., Farrar, J. T., Baumgarten, M., Boston, R., Carr, D. B., & Strom, B. L. (2003). Side effects of opioids during short-term administration: Effect of age, gender, and race. *Clin Pharmacol Ther, 74,* 102–112.

Cervero, F. (1982). Afferent activity evoked by natural stimulation of the biliary system in the ferret. *Pain, 13,* 137–151.

Cervero, F., & Janig, W. (1992). Visceral nociceptors: A new world order? *Trends Neurosci, 15,* 374–378.

Chaiyakunapruk, N., Kitikannakorn, N., Nathisuwan, S., Leeprakobboon, K., & Leelasettagool, C. (2006). The efficacy of ginger for the prevention of postoperative nausea and vomiting: A meta-analysis. *Am J Obstet Gynecol, 194,* 95–99.

Chan, M. Y. T., Cross-Melor, S. K., Kavaliers, M., & Ossenkopp, K.-P. (2009). Lipopolysaccharide (LPS) blocks the acquisition of LiCl-induced gaping in a rodent model of anticipatory nausea. *Neurosci Lett, 450,* 301–305.

Chang, C. S., Kao, C. H., Wang, Y. S., Chen, G. H., & Wang, S. J. (1996). Discrepant pattern of solid and liquid gastric emptying in Chinese patients with type II diabetes mellitus. *Nucl Med Commun, 17,* 60–65.

Chang, C. S., Lien, H. C., Yeh, H. Z., Poon, S. K., Tung, C. F., & Chen, G. H. (1998). Effect of cisapride on gastric dysrhythmia and emptying of indigestible solids in type-II diabetic patients. *Scand J Gastroenterol, 33,* 600–604.

Chaudhri, O., Small, C., & Bloom, S. (2006). Gastrointestinal hormones regulating appetite. *Philos Trans R Soc Lond B Biol Sci, 361,* 1187–1209.

Chelen, W. E., Kabrisky, M., & Rogers, S. K. (1993). Spectral analysis of the electroencephalographic response to motion sickness. *Aviat Space Environ Med, 64,* 24–29.

Chen, C. Y., & Bonham, A. C. (2005). Glutamate suppresses GABA release via presynaptic metabotropic glutamate receptors at baroreceptor neurones in rats. *J Physiol, 562,* 535–551.

Chen, J. D., & McCallum, R.W. (1993). Clinical applications of electrogastrography. *Am J Gastroenterol, 88,* 1324–1336.

Chen, J. D., Qian, L., Ouyang, H., & Yin, J. (2003). Gastric electrical stimulation with short pulses reduces vomiting but not dysrhythmias in dogs. *Gastroenterology, 124,* 401–409.

Cheung, B., & Hofer, K. (2005). Desensitization to strong vestibular stimuli improves tolerance to simulated aircraft motion. *Aviat Space Environ Med, 76,* 1099–1104.

Cheung, B. S., Kohl, R. L., Money, K. E., & Kinter, L. B. (1994). Etiologic significance of arginine vasopressin in motion sickness. *J Clin Pharmacol, 34,* 664–670.

Cheung, B. S., Money, K. E., Kohl, R. L., & Kinter, L. B. (1992). Investigation of anti-motion sickness drugs in the squirrel monkey. *J Clin Pharmacol, 32,* 163–175.

Chin, R. K. H. (2000). Antenatal complications and perinatal outcome in patients with nausea and vomiting–complicated pregnancy. In G. Koren & R. Bishai (Eds.), *Nausea and vomiting of pregnancy: State of the art 2000* (pp. 31–35). Toronto: Motherisk.

Chin, R. K. H., & Lao, T. T. (1988). Low birth weight and hyperemesis gravidarum. *Eur J Obstet Gynecol Repro Biol, 28,* 179–183.

Chinn, H. I. (1951). Motion sickness in the military service. *Military Surgery, 108,* 20–29.

Chittumma, P., Kaewkiattikun, K., & Wiriyasiriwach, B. (2007). Comparison of the effectiveness of ginger and vitamin B6 for treatment of nausea and vomiting in early pregnancy: A randomized double blind controlled study. *J Med Assoc Thai, 90,* 15–20.

Choi, K. M., Gibbons, S. J., Nguyen, T.V., Stoltz, G. J., Lurken, M. S., Ördög, T., Szurszewski, J.H., & Farrugia, G. (2008). Heme oxygenase-1 protects interstitial cells of Cajal from oxidative stress and reverses diabetic gastroparesis. *Gastroenterology, 135,* 2055–2064.

Claremont, C. A. (1930). The psychology of sea-sickness. *Psyche, 11,* 86–90.

Clark, J. A., Jr., Myers, P. H., Goelz, M. F., Thigpen, J. E., & Forsythe, D. B. (1997). Pica behavior associated with buprenorphine administration in the rat. *Lab Anim Sci, 47,* 300–303.

Clark, R. A., & Gralla, R. J. (1993). Delayed emesis: A dilemma in antiemetic control. *Support Care Cancer, 4,* 182–185.

Clouse, R. E., & Lustman, F. J. (1989). Gastrointestinal symptoms in diabetic patients: Lack of association with neuropathy. *Am J of Gastroenterol, 84,* 869–872.

Coates, A., Abraham, S., Kaye, S. B., Sowerbutts, T., Frewin, C., Fox, R. M., & Tattersall, M. H. (1983). On the receiving end: Patient perception of the side-effects of cancer chemotherapy. *Eur J Cancer Clin Oncol, 19,* 203–208.

Code, C. F., Steinbach, J. H., Schlegel, J. F., Amberg, J. R., & Hallenbeck, G. A. (1984). Pyloric and duodenal motor contributions to duodenogastric reflux. *Scand J Gastroenterol Suppl, 92,* 13–16.

Coen, S. J., Gregory, L. J., Yaguez, L., Amaro, E., Brammer, M., Williams, S. C. R., & Aziz, Q. (2007). Reproducibility of human brain activity evoked by esophageal stimulation using functional magnetic resonance imaging. *Am J Physiol Gastrointest Liver Physiol, 293,* G188–G197.

Cohen, J. M., & Cohen, M. J. (1972). *The penguin dictionary of quotations.* Middlesex, UK: Penguin Books Ltd.

Cohen, M. M., Duncan, P. G., DeBoer, D. P., & Tweed, W. A. (1994). The postoperative interview: Assessing risk factors for nausea and vomiting. *Anesth Analg, 78,* 7–16.

Coil, J. D., Hankins, W. G., Jenden, D. J., & Garcia, J. (1978). The attenuation of a specific cue-to-consequence association by anti-emetic agents. *Psychopharmacology (Berlin), 56,* 21–25.

Coleski, R., & Hasler, W. L. (2004). Directed endoscopic mucosal mapping of normal and dysrhythmic gastric slow waves in healthy humans. *Neurogastroenterol Motil, 16,* 557–565.

Coleski, R., & Hasler, W. L. (2009). Coupling and propagation of normal and dysrhythmic gastric slow waves during acute hyperglycaemia in healthy humans. *Neurogastroenterol Motil, 21,* 492–499.

Collins, K. J. (1999). Temperature regulation and the autonomic nervous system. In C. J. Mathias and R. Bannister (Eds.), *Autonomic failure: A textbook of clinical disorders of the autonomic nervous system* (4th ed., pp. 92–98). New York: Oxford University Press.

Contarino, A., & Gold, L. H. (2002). Targeted mutations of the corticotropin-releasing factor system: Effects on physiology and behavior. *Neuropeptides, 36,* 103–116.

Contreras, M., Ceric, F., & Torrealba, F. (2007). Inactivation of the interoceptive insula disrupts drug craving and malaise induced by lithium. *Science, 318,* 655–658.

Cooper, J. R., & Mattsson, J. L. (1979). Control of radiation-induced emesis with promethazine, cimetidine, thiethylperazine, or naloxone. *Am J Vet Res, 40,* 1057–1061.

Cooper, M. (1957). *Pica.* Springfield, Ill: Charles C. Thomas.

Corbett, R. W., Ryan, C., & Weinrich, S. P. (2003). Pica in pregnancy: Does it affect pregnancy outcomes? *MCN Am J Matern Child Nurs, 28,* 183–189.

Cordts, R. E., Yochmowitz, M. G., & Hardy, K. A. (1987). Evaluation of domperidone as a modifier of gamma-radiation-induced emesis. *Int J Radiat Oncol Biol Phys, 13,* 1333–1337.

Coresetti, M., Caenepeel, P., Fischler, B., Janssens, J., & Tack, J. (2004). Impact of coexisting irritable bowel syndrome on symptoms and pathophysiological mechanisms in functional dyspepsia. *Am J Gastroenterol, 99,* 1152–1159.

Costall, B., Domeney, A. M., & Naylor, R. J. (1986). A model of emesis in the common marmoset. *Br J Pharmacol, 30,* 375P.

Costello, D. J., & Borison, H. L. (1977). Naloxone antagonizes narcotic self blockade of emesis in the cat. *J Pharmacol Exp Ther, 203,* 222–230.

Cowings, P. S., & Toscano, W. B. (2000). Autogenic-feedback training exercise is superior to promethazine for control of motion sickness symptoms. *J Clin Pharmacol, 40,* 1154–1165.

Craig, A. D. (2002). How do you feel? Interoception: The sense of the physiological condition of the body. *Nat Rev Neurosci, 3,* 655–666.

Craig, A. D. (2003). Interoception: The sense of the physiological condition of the body. *Curr Opinion Neurobiol, 13,* 500–505.

Craig, A. D. (2009a). A rat is not a monkey is not a human [comment on Mogil, (2009), *Nature Rev Neurosci, 10,* 283–294]. *Nat Rev Neurosci, 10,* 466.

Craig, A. D. (2009b). How do you feel-now? The anterior insula and human awareness. *Nat Rev Neurosci, 10,* 59–70.

Craig, J. B., & Powell, B. L. (1987). The management of nausea and vomiting in clinical oncology. *Am J Med Sci, 293,* 34–44.

Crampton, G. H., & Daunton, N. G. (1983). Systemic naloxone increases the incidence of motion sickness in the cat. *Pharmacol Biochem Behav, 19,* 827–829.

Cubeddu, L. X., & Hoffmann, I. S. (1993). Participation of serotonin on early and delayed emesis induced by initial and subsequent cycles of cisplatinum-based chemotherapy: Effects of antiemetics. *J Clin Pharmacol, 33,* 691–697.

Cubeddu, L. X., Lindley, C. M., Wetsel, W., Carl, P. L., & Negro-Vilar, A. (1990). Role of angiotensin II and vasopressin in cisplatin-induced emesis. *Life Sci, 46,* 699–705.

Cubeddu, L. X., O'Connor, D. T., Hoffmann, I., & Parmer, R. J. (1995). Plasma chromogranin A marks emesis and serotonin release associated with dacarbazine and nitrogen mustard but not with cyclophosphamide-based chemotherapies. *Br J Cancer, 72,* 1033–1038.

Cucchiara, S., Minella, R., Riezzo, G., Vallone, G., Vallone, P., Castellone, F., & Auricchio, S. (1992). Reversal of gastric electrical dysrhythmias by cisapride in children with functional dyspepsia: Report of three cases. *Dig Dis Sci, 37,* 1136–1140.

Cummins, A. J. (1958). The physiology of symptoms: 3. Nausea and vomiting. *Am J Dig Dis, 3,* 710.

Curry, S. L., Rine, J., Whitney, C. W., Nahhas, W. A., Mortel, R., & Demers, L. M. (1981). The role of prostaglandins in the excessive nausea and vomiting after intravascular cis-platinum therapy. *Gynecol Oncol, 12,* 89–91.

Curtis, K. S., Sved, A. F., Verbalis, J. G., & Stricker, E. M. (1994). Lithium chloride-induced anorexia, but not conditioned taste aversions, in rats with area postrema lesions. *Brain Res, 663,* 30–37.

Dantzer, R., & Kelley, K. W. (2007). Twenty years of research on cytokine-induced sickness behavior. *Brain Behav Immun, 21,* 153–160.

Darmaillacq, A. S., Chichery, R., Poirier, R., & Dickel, L. (2004). Effect of early feeding experience on subsequent prey preference by cuttlefish, Sepia officinalis. *Dev Psychobiol, 45,* 239–244.

Darmani, N. A. (2001). Delta-9-tetrahydrocannabinol differentially suppresses cisplatin-induced emesis and indices of motor function via cannabinoid CB(1) receptors in the least shrew. *Pharmacol Biochem Behav, 69,* 239–249.

Darmani, N. A., & Crim, J. L. (2005). Delta-9-tetrahydrocannabinol differentially suppresses emesis versus enhanced locomotor activity produced by chemically diverse dopamine D2/D3 receptor agonists in the least shrew (Cryptotis parva). *Pharmacol Biochem Behav, 80,* 35–44.

Darmani, N. A., Crim, J. L., Janoyan, J. J., Abad, J., & Ramirez, J. (2009). A re-evaluation of the transmitter basis of chemotherapy-induced immediate and delayed vomiting: Evidence from the least shrew. *Brain Res, 1248,* 40–58.

Darmani, N. A., Janoyan, J. J., Kumar, N., & Crim, J. L. (2003a). Behaviorally active doses of the CB1 receptor antagonist SR 141716A increase brain serotonin and dopamine levels and turnover. *Pharmacol Biochem Behav, 75,* 777–787.

Darmani, N. A., & Johnson, J. C. (2004). Central and peripheral mechanisms contribute to the antiemetic actions of delta-9-tetrahydrocannabinol against 5-hydroxytryptophan-induced emesis. *Eur J Pharmacol, 488,* 201–212.

Darmani, N. A., Sim-Selley, L. J., Martin, B. R., Janoyan, J. J., Crim, J. L., Parekh, B., & Breivogel, C. S. (2003b). Antiemetic and motor-depressive actions of CP55,940: Cannabinoid CB1 receptor characterization, distribution, and G-protein activation. *Eur J Pharmacol, 459,* 83–95.

Darolova, A. (1991). Food composition in the eagle-owl (Bubo bubo Linnaeus, 1758) in Small Carpathians. *Biologia* (Bratislava), *45,* 831–840.

Darwin, C. (1872). *The expression of the emotions in man and animals.* London: John Murray.

Datta, S., Alper, M. H., Ostheimer, G. W., & Weiss, J. B. (1982). Method of ephedrine administration and nausea and hypotension during spinal anesthesia for cesarean section. *Anesthesiology, 56,* 68–70.

Davey, V. A., & Biederman, G. B. (1998). Conditioned antisickness: Indirect evidence from rats and direct evidence from ferrets that conditioning alleviates drug-induced nausea and emesis. *J Exp Psychol Anim Behav Process, 24,* 483–491.

Davidoff, R. A. (1995). *Migraine: Manifestations, pathogenesis, and management.* Philadelphia: F. A. Davis Company.

Davidson, A. (1999). *The Oxford companion to food.* Oxford: Oxford University Press.

Davidson, H. I. M., & Pilot, M.-A. (1993). Changes in gastro-intestinal motility associated with vomiting and nausea. In P. L. R. Andrews & G. J. Sanger (Eds.), *Emesis in anti-cancer therapy* (pp. 71–89). London: Chapman & Hall.

Davis, C. J., Harding, R. K., Leslie, R. A., & Andrews, P. L. R. (1986). The organisation of vomiting as a protective reflex: A commentary on the first day's discussions. In C. J. Davis, G. V. Lake-Bakaar, & D. G. Grahame-Smith (Eds.), *Nausea and vomiting: Mechanisms and treatment* (pp. 65–75). Berlin: Springer-Verlag.

Davis, J. R., Vanderploeg, J. M., Santy, P. A., Jennings, R. T., & Stewart, D. F. (1988). Space motion sickness during 24 flights of the Space Shuttle. *Aviat Space Environ Med, 59,* 1185–1189.

Davis, T. G., Peterson, J. J., Kou, J-Y., Capper-Spudich, E. A., Ball, D., Nials, A. T., Wiseman, J., Solanke, Y. E., Lucas, F. S., Williamson, R. A., Ferrari, L., Wren, P., Knowles, R. G., Barnette, M. S., & Podolin, P.L. (2009). The identification of a novel phophodiesterase 4 inhibitor, 1-ethyl-5-{5-[(4-methyl-1-piperazinyl)methyl]-1,3,4-oxadiazol-2-yl}-N-(tetrahydro-2*H*-pyran-4-yl)-1*H*-pyrazolo[3,4-*b*]pyridin-4-amine (EPPA-1), with improved therapeutic index using pica feeding in rats as a measure of emetogenicity. *J Pharmacol Exp Ther, 330,* 922–931.

Davison, J. M., Gilmore, E. A., Dürr, J., Robertson, G. L., & Lindheimer, M. D. (1984). Altered osmotic thresholds for vasopressin secretion and thirst in human pregnancy. *Am J Physiol, 246,* F105–F109.

Davison, J. M., Shiells, E. A., Phillips, P. R., & Lindheimer, M. D. (1988). Serial evaluations of vasopressin release and thirst in human pregnancy: Role of human chorionic gonadotropin in the osmoregulatory changes of gestation. *J Clin Invest, 81,* 798–806.

Day, T. A., & Sibbald, J. R. (1988). Solitary nucleus excitation of supraoptic vasopressin cells via adrenergic afferents. *Am J Physiol Regul Integr Comp Physiol, 254,* R711–716.

DeGabriel, J.L., Moore, B.D., Marsh, K.J., & Foley, W.J. (2010). The effect of plant secondary metabolites on the interplay between the internal and external environments of marsupial folivores. *Chemoecology, 20,* 97-108.

De Jonghe, B. C., & Horn, C. C. (2008). Chemotherapy-induced pica and anorexia are reduced by common hepatic branch vagotomy in the rat. *Am J Physiol Regul Integr Comp Physiol, 294,* R756–765.

De Jonghe, B. C., & Horn, C. C. (2009). Chemotherapy agent cisplatin induces 48-h Fos expression in the brain of a vomiting species, the house musk shrew (Suncus murinus). *Am J Physiol Integr Comp Physiol, 296,* R902–911.

De Jonghe, B. C., Lawler, M. P., Horn, C. C., & Tordoff, M. G. (2009). Pica as an adaptive response: Kaolin consumption helps rats recover from chemotherapy-induced illness. *Physiol Behav, 97,* 87–90.

de Lartigue, G., Dimaline, R., Varro, A., & Dockray, G. J. (2007). Cocaine- and amphetamine-regulated transcript: Stimulation of expression in rat vagal afferent neurons by cholecystokinin and suppression by ghrelin. *J Neurosci, 27,* 2876–2882.

De Ponti, F., Malagelada, J.-R., Azpiroz, F., Yaksh, T. L., & Thomforde, G. M. (1990). Variations in gastric tone associated with duodenal motor events after activation of central emetic mechanisms in the dog. *J Gastroint Motil, 2,* 1–11.

de Waele, C., Muhjethaler, M., & Vidal, P. P. (1995). Neurochemistry of the central vestibular pathways. *Brain Res Rev, 20,* 24–46.

Del Favero, A., Roila, F., Basurto, C., Minotti, V., Ballatori, E., Patoia, L., Tonato, M., & Tognoni, G. (1990). Assessment of nausea. *Eur J Clin Pharmacol, 38,* 115–120.

Del Favero, A., Tonato, M., & Roila, F. (1992). Issues in the measurement of nausea. *Br J Cancer Suppl, 66,* S69–S71.

Delaney, B. C., Wilson, S., Roalfe, A., Roberts, L., Redman, V., Wearn, A., Briggs, A., & Hobbs, F. D. (2000). Cost effectiveness of initial endoscopy for dyspepsia in patients over age 50 years: A randomized controlled trial in primary care. *Lancet, 356,* 1965–1969.

Depue, R. H., Bernstein, L., Ross, R. K., Judd, H. L., & Henderson, B. E. (1987). Hyperemesis gravidarum in relation to estradiol levels, pregnancy outcome and other maternal factors: Sero-epidemiologic study. *Am J Obstet Gynecol, 156,* 1137–1141.

Derbyshire, S. W. (2003). A systematic review of neuroimaging data during visceral stimulation. *Am J Gastroenterol, 98,* 12–20.

Devinsky, O., Morrell, M. J., & Vogt, B. A. (1995). Contributions of the anterior cingulate cortex to behaviour. *Brain, 118,* 279–306.

DiBaise, J. K., Brand, R. E., Lyden, E., Tarantolo, S. R., & Quigley, E. M. (2001). Gastric myoelectric activity and its relationship to the development of nausea and vomiting after intensive chemotherapy and autologous stem cell transplantation. *Am J Gastroenterol, 96,* 2873–2881.

Dibattista, D. (1988). Conditioned taste aversion produced by 2-deoxy-D-glucose in rats and hamsters. *Physiol Behav, 44,* 189–192.

Dibble, S. L., Luce, J., Cooper, B. A., Israel, J., Cohen, M., Nussey, B., & Rugo, H. (2007). Acupressure for chemotherapy-induced nausea and vomiting: A randomized clinical trial. *Oncol Nurs Forum, 34,* 813–820.

Dietrich, S., Smith, J., Scherzinger, C., Hofmann-Preiss, K., Freitag, T., Eisenkolb, A., & Ringler, R. (2008). [A novel transcutaneous vagus nerve stimulation leads to brainstem and cerebral activations measured by functional MRI]. *Biomed Tech (Berlin), 53,* 104–111.

DiIorio, C. (1985). First trimester nausea in pregnant teenagers: Incidence, characteristics, intervention. *Nursing Research, 34,* 372–374.

Dobie, T. G., & May, J. G. (1994). Cognitive-behavioral management of motion sickness. *Aviat Space Environ Med, 65,* C1–20.

Doig, R. K., Wolf, S., & Wolff, H. G. (1953). Study of gastric function in a decorticate man with gastric fistula. *Gastroenterology, 23,* 40–44.

Dols, M. W. (1984). *Medieval Islamic medicine.* Berkeley: University of California Press.

Dorland, W. A. (2003). *Dorland's illustrated medical dictionary* (26th ed.). Philadelphia: Saunders.

Doyle, A. C. (1894). Silver blaze. In *Memoirs of Sherlock Holmes* (pp. 1–31). London: George Newnes, Ltd.

Drummer, C., Stromeyer, H., Riepl, R. L., Konig, A., Strollo, F., Lang, R. E., Maass, H., Rocker, L., & Gerzer, R. (1990). Hormonal changes after parabolic flight: Implications on the development of motion sickness. *Aviat Space Environ Med, 61,* 821–828.

Drummond, P. D. (1999). Autonomic disorders affecting cutaneous blood flow. In C. J. Mathias and R. Bannister (Eds.), *Autonomic failure: A textbook of clinical disorders of the autonomic nervous system* (4th ed., pp. 487–493). New York: Oxford University Press.

du Bois, A., Vach, W., Siebert, C., Holy, R., Ledergerber, M., Wechsel, U., & Kriesinger-Schroeder, H. (1997). The relationship between parameters of serotonin metabolism and emetogenic potential of platinum-based chemotherapy regimens. *Support Care Cancer, 5,* 212–218.

Dua, N., Bhatnagar, S., Mishra, S., & Singhal, A. K. (2004). Granisetron and ondanse-tron for prevention of nausea and vomiting in patients undergoing modified radical mastectomy. *Anaesth Intensive Care, 32,* 761–764.

Dubois, A., Dorval, E. D., Steel, L., Fiala, N. P., & Conklin, J. J. (1987). Effect of ionizing radiation on prostaglandins and gastric secretion in rhesus monkeys. *Radiat Res, 110,* 289–293.

Dunbar, R. I., & Shultz, S. (2007). Understanding primate brain evolution. *Philos Trans R Soc Lond B Biol Sci, 362,* 649–658.

Duncan, G. G. (1962). Intermittent fasts in the correction and control of intractable obesity. *Trans Am Clin Climatol Assoc, 74,* 121–129.

Dunckley, P., Wise, R. G., Fairhurst, M., Hobden, P., Aziz, Q., Chang, L., & Tracey, I. (2005). A comparison of visceral and somatic pain processing in human brainstem using functional magnetic resonance imaging. *J Neurosci, 25,* 7333–7341.

Dundee, J. W., Sourial, F. B. R., Ghaly, R. G., & Bell, P. F. (1988). P6 acupressure reduces morning sickness. *J Royal Soc Med, 81,* 456–457.

Dunn, J. C. Y. (2008). Is the tissue-engineered intestine clinically viable? *Nature Clinical Practice, 5,* 366–367.

Ebenezer, I. S., Thornton, S. N., & Parrott, R. F. (1989). Anterior and posterior pituitary hormone release induced in sheep by cholecystokinin. *Am J Physiol Regul Integr Comp Physiol, 256,* R1355–1357.

Eberhart, L. H., Morin, A. M., & Georgieff, M. (2000). The menstruation cycle in the postoperative phase: Its effect on the incidence of nausea and vomiting. *Anaesthesist, 49,* 532–535.

Ebers, G. (1875). *Papyros Ebers: Das hermetische Buch conservirt in der Universitäts-Bibliothek zu Leipzig* (fasc. ed.). Leipzig: W. Engelmann.

Eddie, L. W., Bell, R. J., Lester, A., Geier, M., Bennett, G., Johnston, P. D., & Niall, H. D. (1986). Radioimmunoassay of relaxin in pregnancy with an analog of human relaxin. *Lancet, 1*(8494), 1344–1346.

Edwards, C. M., Carmichael, J., Baylis, P. H., & Harris, A. L. (1989). Arginine vasopres-sin: A mediator of chemotherapy induced emesis? *Br J Cancer, 59,* 467–470.

Edwards, M. (1994). Risks of medical imaging. In C. Putnam & C. Ravine (Eds.), *Textbook of diagnostic imaging* (p. 83). Philadelphia: W. B. Saunders.

Eeckhout, C. (1989). Effects of prokinetics with a different mechanism of action on cisplatin-induced slowing of gastric emptying in the rat. *J Gastrointest Mot, 1,* A52.

Eeckhout, C., & Vedder, A. (1988). 5-HT3 antagonists reverse the cisplatin-induced slowing of gastric emptying in fed rats. *Gastroenterology, 94,* A111.

Einarson, A., Koren, G., & Bergman, U. (1998). Nausea and vomiting of pregnancy: A comparative European study. *Eur J Obstet Gynecol Reprod Biol, 76,* 1–3.

Einthoven, W., Flohil, A., & Battaerd, P. J. T. A. (1908). On vagus currents examined with the string galvanometer. *Q J Exp Physiol, 1,* 243–245.

Eisenberg, P., Figueroa-Vadillo, J., Zamora, R., Charu, V., Hajdenberg, J., Cartmell, A., Macciocchi, A., & Grunberg, S. (2003). Improved prevention of moderately emeto-genic chemotherapy-induced nausea and vomiting with palonosetron, a pharmaco-logically novel 5-HT_3 receptor antagonist: Results of a phase III, single-dose trial versus dolasetron. *Cancer, 98,* 2473–2482.

Ekman, P. (1999). Introduction, afterword, and commentaries. In C. Darwin, *The expression of emotion in man and animals.* London: Fontana Press.

Eldred, E., & Trowbridge, W. V. (1954). Radiation sickness in the monkey. *Radiology, 62,* 65–73.

Elke, S., Pardo, J. V., Faris, P. L., Hartman, B. K., Kim, S. W., Ivanov, E. H., Daughters, R. S., Costello, P. A., & Goodale, R. L. (2003). Functional neuroimaging of gastric distension. *J Gastrointest Surg, 7*, 740–749.

Elliott, C. J., & Susswein, A. J. (2002). Comparative neuroethology of feeding control in molluscs. *J Exp Biol, 205*, 877–896.

Elwin, C. E. (1974). Gastric acid responses to antral application of some amino acids, peptides, and isolated fractions of a protein hydrolysate. *Scand J Gastroenterol, 68*, 662–666.

El Younis, C. M., Abulafia, O., & Sherer, D. M. (1998). Rapid marked response of severe hyperemesis gravidarum to oral erythromycin. *Am J Perinatology, 15*, 533–534.

Emelianova, S., Mazzotta, P., Einarson, A., & Koren, G. (1999). Prevalence and severity of NVP and effect of vitamin supplementation. *Clin Invest Med, 22*, 106–110.

Emond, M., Schwartz, G. J., Ladenheim, E. E., & Moran, T. H. (1999). Central leptin modulates behavioral and neural responsivity to CCK. *Am J Physiol Regul Integr Comp Physiol, 276*, R1545–R1549.

Enck, P., Rathmann, W., Spiekermann, M., Czerner, D., Tschöpe, D., Ziegler, D., Strohmeyer, G., & Gries, F.A. (1994). Prevalence of gastrointestinal symptoms in diabetic patient and non-diabetic subjects. *Z Gastroenterol, 32*, 637–641.

Engel, C. (2002). *Wild health: How animals keep themselves well and what we can learn from them*. London: Weidenfeld & Nicholson.

Ensiyeh, J., & Sakineh, M.-A. C. (2009). Comparing ginger and vitamin B6 for the treatment of nausea and vomiting in pregnancy: A randomized controlled trial. *Midwifery, 25*, 649–653.

Epstein, B. S. (1993). Preventing postoperative nausea and vomiting. In M. H. Sleisenger (Ed.), *Handbook of nausea and vomiting* (pp. 94–109). New York: Parthenon.

Ervin, G. N., Mosher, J. T., Birkemo, L. S., & Johnson, M. F. (1995). Multiple, small doses of cholecystokinin octapeptide are more efficacious at inducing taste aversion conditioning than single, large doses. *Peptides, 16*, 539–545.

Etscorn, F. (1980). Sucrose aversions in mice as a result of injected nicotine or passive tobacco smoke inhalation. *Bull Psychonom Soc, 15*, 54–56.

Etscorn, F., Moore, G. A., Hagen, L. S., Caton, T. M., & Sanders, D. L. (1986). Saccharin aversions in hamsters as a result of nicotine injections. *Pharmacol Biochem Behav, 24*, 567–570.

Etscorn, F., Moore, G. A., Scott, E. P., Hagen, L. S., Caton, T. M., Sanders, D. L., & Divine, K. K. (1987). Conditioned saccharin aversions in rats as a result of cutaneous nicotine or intraperitoneal nicotine administered in divided doses. *Pharmacol Biochem Behav, 28*, 495–502.

Evans, A., Samuels, S., Marshall, C., & Bertolucci, L. E. (1993). Suppression of pregnancy-induced nausea and vomiting with sensory afferent stimulation. *J Reprod Med, 8*, 603–606.

Eversmann, T., Gottsmann, M., Uhlich, E., Ulbrecht, G., Von Werder, K., & Scriba, P. C. (1978). Increased secretion of growth hormone, prolactin, antidiuretic hormone, and cortisol induced by the stress of motion sickness. *Aviat Space Environ Med, 49*, 53–57.

Ezzo, J., Streiberger, K., & Schneider, A. (2006). Cochrane systematic reviews examine P6 acupuncture point stimulation for nausea and vomiting. *J Altern Complement Med, 12*, 489–495.

Ezzo, J., Vickers, A., Richardson, M. A., Allen, C., Dibble, S. L., Issell, B., Lao, L., Pearl, M., Ramirez, G., Roscoe, J. A., Shen, J., Shivnan, J., Streitberger, K., Treish, I., & Zhang, G. (2005). Acupuncture-point stimulation for chemotherapy-induced nausea and vomiting. *J Clin Oncol, 23,* 7188–7198.

Faas, H., Feinle, C., Enck, P., Grundy, D., & Boesiger, P. (2001). Modulation of gastric motor activity by a centrally acting stimulus, circular vection, in humans. *Am J Physiol Gastrointest Liver Physiol, 280,* G850–857.

Fairweather, D. V. (1968). Nausea and vomiting in pregnancy. *Am J Obstet Gynecol, 102,* 135–175.

Fasold, O., Von Brevern, M., Kuhberg, M., Ploner, C. J., Villringer, A., Lempert, T., & Wenzel, R. (2002). Human vestibular cortex as identified with caloric stimulation in functional magnetic resonance imaging. *Neuroimage, 17,* 1384–1393.

Feinle, C., & Read, N.W. (1996). Ondansetron reduces nausea induced by gastroduodenal stimulation without changing gastric motility. *Am J Physiol Gastrointest Liver Physiol, 271,* G591–597.

Feinle, C., Grundy, D., & Read, N. W. (1995). Fat increases vection-induced nausea independent of changes in gastric emptying. *Physiol Behav, 58,* 1159–1165.

Feinle, C., Rades, T., Otto, B., & Fried, M. (2001). Fat digestion modulates gastrointestinal sensations induced by gastric distention and duodenal lipid in humans. *Gastroenterology, 120,* 1100–1107.

Feldberg, W., & Sherwood, S. L. (1954). Injection of drugs into the lateral ventricle of the cat. *J Physiol, 123,* 148–167.

Feldman, M., Samson, W. K., & O'Dorisio, T. M. (1988). Apomorphine-induced nausea in humans: Release of vasopressin and pancreatic polypeptide. *Gastroenterology, 95,* 721–726.

Feldman, M., & Schiller, L. R. (1983). Disorders of gastrointestinal motility associated with diabetes mellitus. *Ann Intern Med, 98,* 378–384.

Felten, D. L., & Jósefowicz, R. F. (2003). *Netter's atlas of human neuroscience.* Teterboro, NJ: Icon Learning Systems.

Fetting, J. H., Grochow, L. B., Folstein, M. F., Ettinger, D. S., & Colvin, M. (1982a). The course of nausea and vomiting after high-dose cyclophosphamide. *Cancer Treat Rep, 66,* 1487–1493.

Fetting, J. H., McCarthy, L. E., Borison, H. L., & Colvin, M. (1982b). Vomiting induced by cyclophosphamide and phosphoramide mustard in cats. *Cancer Treat Rep, 66,* 1625–1629.

Fetting, J. H., Wilcox, P. M., Sheidler, V. R., Enterline, J. P., Donehower, R. C., & Grochow, L. B. (1985). Tastes associated with parenteral chemotherapy for breast cancer. *Cancer Treat Rep, 69,* 1249–1251.

Feyer, P. Ch., Maranzano, E., Molassiotis, A., Clark-Snow, R. A., Roila, F., Warr, D., & Olver, I. (2005). Radiotherapy-induced nausea and vomiting (RINV): Antiemetic guidelines. *Support Care Cancer, 13,* 122–128.

Figueroa-Moseley, C., Jean-Pierre, P., Roscoe, J. A., Ryan, J. L., Kohli, S., Palesh, O. G., Ryan, E. P., Carroll, J., & Morrow, G. R. (2007). Behavioral interventions in treating anticipatory nausea and vomiting. *J Natl Compr Canc Netw, 5,* 44–50.

Finley, J. C., O'Leary, M., Wester, D., MacKenzie, S., Shepard, N., Farrow, S., & Lockette, W. (2004). A genetic polymorphism of the alpha 2-adrenergic receptor increases autonomic responses to stress. *J Appl Physiol, 96,* 2231–2239.

Fischer-Rasmussen, W., Kjaer, S. K., Dahl, C., & Asping, U. (1991). Ginger treatment of hyperemesis gravidarum. *Europ J Obstet Gynecol Reprod Biol, 38,* 19–24.

Fisher, R. D., Rentschler, R. E., Nelson, J. C., Godfrey, T. E., & Wilbur, D. W. (1982). Elevation of plasma antidiuretic hormones (ADH) associated with chemotherapy-induced emesis in man. *Cancer Treat Rep, 66,* 25–29.

Fisher, R. S., Roberts, G. S., Grabowski, C. J., & Cohen, S. (1978). Altered lower esophageal sphincter function during early pregnancy. *Gastroenterology, 74,* 1233–1237.

FitzGerald, C. M. (1984). Nausea and vomiting in pregnancy. *Br J Med Psychol, 57,* 159–165.

Flanagan, L. M., Verbalis, J. G., & Stricker, E. M. (1989). Effects of anorexigenic treatments on gastric motility in rats. *Am J Physiol Regul Integr Comp Physiol, 256,* R955–961.

Flaxman, S. M., & Sherman, P. W. (2000). Morning sickness: A mechanism for protecting mother and embryo. *Q Rev Biol, 75,* 113–148.

Forster, E. R., & Dockray, G. J. (1990). The effect of ondansetron on gastric emptying in the conscious rat. *Eur J Pharmacol, 191,* 235–238.

Forster, J., Damjanov, I., Lin, Z., Sarosiek, I., Wetzel, P., & McCallum, R. W. (2005). Absence of the interstitial cells of Cajal in patients with gastroparesis and correlation with clinical findings. *J Gastrointest Surg, 9,* 102–108.

Foss, J. F., Bass, A. S., & Goldberg, L. I. (1993). Dose-related antagonism of the emetic effect of morphine by methylnaltrexone in dogs. *J Clin Pharmacol, 33,* 747–751.

Foss, J. F., Yuan, C. S., Roizen, M. F., & Goldberg, L. I. (1998). Prevention of apomorphine- or cisplatin-induced emesis in the dog by a combination of methylnaltrexone and morphine. *Cancer Chemother Pharmacol, 42,* 287–291.

Foubert, J., & Vaessen, G. (2005). Nausea: The neglected symptom? *Eur J Oncol Nurs, 9,* 21–32.

Fox, R. A. (1977). Poison aversion and sexual behavior in the golden hamster. *Psychol Rep, 41,* 993–994.

Fox, R. A. (1992). Current status: Animal models of nausea. In A. L. Bianchi, L. Grelot, A. D. Miller, & G. L. King (Eds.), *Mechanisms and control of emesis* (pp. 341–350). Marseille, France: John Libbey Eurotext.

Fox, R. A., Corcoran, M., & Brizzee, K. R. (1990). Conditioned taste aversion and motion sickness in cats and squirrel monkeys. *Can J Physiol Pharmacol, 68,* 269–278.

Fox, R. A., Keil, L. C., Daunton, N. G., Crampton, G. H., & Lucot, J. (1987). Vasopressin and motion sickness in cats. *Aviat Space Environ Med, 58,* A143–147.

Frank, L., Kleinman, L., Ganoczy, D., McQuaid, K., Sloan, S., Eggleston, A., Tougas, G., & Farup, C. (2000). Upper gastrointestinal symptoms in North America: Prevalence and relationship to healthcare utilization and quality of life. *Dig Dis Sci, 45,* 809–818.

Frank, J. W., Saslow, S. B., Camilleri, M., Thomforde, G. M., Dinneen, S., & Rizza, R. A. (1995). Mechanism of accelerated gastric emptying of liquids and hyperglycemia in patients with type II diabetes mellitus. *Gastroenterology, 109,* 755–765.

Fraser, R., Horowitz, M., & Dent, J. (1991). Hyperglycemia stimulates pyloric motility in normal subjects. *Gut, 32,* 475–478.

Fraser, R. J., Horowitz, M., Maddox, A. F., Harding, P. E., Chatterton, B. E., & Dent, J. (1990). Hyperglycemia slows gastric emptying in type 1 (insulin-dependent) diabetes mellitus. *Diabetologia, 33,* 675–680.

Frazer, J. G. (1922/1998). *The golden bough* (repr. of abridged edition). Harmondsworth, UK: Penguin Classic.

Freeland, W. J., & Janzen, D. J. (1974). Strategies of herbivory in mammals: The role of plant secondary compounds. *Am Naturalist, 108,* 269–289.

Frissora, C. L., & Harris, L. A. (2001). Choosing the appropriate oral contraceptive pill is part of treating functional nausea in women. *Am J Gastroenterol, 96,* S198.

Fujisaki, Y., Yamauchi, A., Shuto, H., Niizeki, M., Makino, K., Kataoka, Y., & Oishi, R. (2001). Pharmacological characterization of cyclosporine A-induced kaolin intake in rats. *Pharmacol Biochem Behav, 70,* 267–271.

Fukuda, H., Koga, T., Furukawa, N., Nakamura, E., Hatano, M., & Yanagihara, M. (2003). The site of the antiemetic action of NK1 receptor antagonists. In J. Donnerer (Ed.), *Antiemetic therapy* (pp. 33–77). Basel, Switzerland: Karger.

Fukui, H., Yamamoto, M., Sasaki, S., & Sato, S. (1993). Involvement of 5-HT3 receptors and vagal afferents in copper sulfate- and cisplatin-induced emesis in monkeys. *Eur J Pharmacol, 24,* 13–18.

Furness, J. B. (2006). The organisation of the autonomic nervous system: Peripheral connections. *Auton Neurosci, 130,* 1–5.

Furukawa, N., & Okada, H. (1994). Canine salivary secretion from the submaxillary glands before and during retching. *Am J Physiol Gastrointest Liver Physiol, 267,* G810–817.

Furukawa, N., Fukuda, H., Hatano, M., Koga, T., & Shiroshita, Y. (1998). A neurokinin-1 receptor antagonist reduced hypersalivation and gastric contractility related to emesis in dogs. *Am J Physiol Gastrointest Liver Physiol, 275,* G1193–1201.

Gadsby, R. (1994). Pregnancy sickness and symptoms: Your questions answered. *Prof Care Mother Child, 4,* 16–17.

Gadsby, R. (2000). A prospective study of nausea and vomiting in pregnancy. In G. Koren & R. Bishai (Eds.), *Nausea and vomiting of pregnancy: State of the art 2000* (pp. 27–30). Toronto: Motherisk.

Gadsby, R., Barnie-Adshead, A. M., & Jagger, C. (1993). A prospective study of nausea and vomiting during pregnancy. *Brit J Gen Pract, 43,* 245–248.

Galef, B. G., Jr., Attenborough, K. S., & Whiskin, E. E. (1990). Responses of observer rats (Rattus norvegicus) to complex, diet-related signals emitted by demonstrator rats. *J Comp Psychol, 104,* 11–19.

Galef, B. G., Jr., & Beck, M. (1985). Aversive and attractive marking of toxic and safe foods by Norway rats. *Behav Neural Biol, 43,* 298–310.

Galef, B. G., Jr., Mason, J. R., Preti, G., & Bean, N. J. (1988). Carbon disulfide: A semiochemical mediating socially-induced diet choice in rats. *Physiol Behav, 42,* 119–124.

Gan, T. J. (2002). Post-operative nausea and vomiting: Can it be eliminated? *JAMA, 287,* 1233–1236.

Gan, T. J. (2006). Risk factors for postoperative nausea and vomiting. *Anesth Analg, 102,* 1884–1898.

Gan, T. J., Apfel, C. C., Kovac, A., Philip, B. K., Singla, N., Minkowitz, H., Habib, A. S., Knighton, J., Carides, A. D., Zhang, H., Horgan, K. J., Evans, J. K., Lawson, F. C., The Aprepitant-PONV Study Group (2007). A randomized, double-blind comparison of the NK1 antagonist, aprepitant, versus ondansetron for the prevention of postoperative nausea and vomiting. *Anesth Analg, 104,* 1082–1089.

Gan, T. J., Jiao, K. R., Zenn, M., & Georgiade, G. (2004). A randomized controlled comparison of electro-acupoint stimulation or ondansetron versus placebo for the prevention of postoperative nausea and vomiting. *Anesth Analg, 99,* 1070–1075.

Gan, T. J., Meyer, T., Apfel, C. C., Chung, F., Davis, P. J., Eubanks, S., Kovac, A., Philip, B. K., Sessler, D. I., Temo, J., Tramèr, M. R., & Watcha, M. (2003). Consensus guidelines for managing postoperative nausea and vomiting. *Anesth Analg, 97,* 62–71.

Garcia, J., Ervin, F. R., & Koelling, R. A. (1966). Learning with prolonged delay of reinforcement. *Psychonom Sci, 5,* 121–122.

Garcia, J., & Hankins, W. G. (1977). On the origin of food aversion paradigms. In L. M. Barker, M. R. Best, & M. Domjan (Eds.), *Learning mechanisms in food selection* (pp. 3–22). Waco, TX: Baylor University Press.

Garcia, J., Hankins, W. G., & Coil, J. D. (1976). Koalas, men, and other conditioned gastronomes. In N. W. Milgram, L. Krames, & T. Alloway (Eds.), *Food aversion learning* (pp. 195–218). New York: Plenum Press.

Garcia, J., Hankins, W. G., & Rusiniak, K. W. (1974). Behavioral regulation of the milieu interne in man and rat. *Science, 185,* 824–831.

Garcia, J., Kimeldorf, D. J., & Koelling, R. A. (1955). Conditioned aversion to saccharin resulting from exposure to gamma radiation. *Science, 122,* 157–158.

Garcia, J., & Koelling, R. A. (1966). Relation of cue to consequence in avoidance learning. *Psychonom Sci, 4,* 123–124.

Garcia, J., & Koelling, R. A. (1967). A comparison of aversions induced by x-rays, toxins, and drugs in the rat. *Radiat Res Suppl, 7,* 439–450.

Garcia, J., Lasiter, P. S., Bermudez-Rattoni, F., & Deems, D. A. (1985). A general theory of aversion learning. *Ann N Y Acad Sci, 443,* 8–21.

Garcia, J., Quick, D. F., & White, B. (1984). Conditioning disgust and fear from mollusk to monkey. In D. Alkon & J. Farley (Eds.), *Primary neural substrates of learning and behavioral change* (pp. 47–61). Cambridge, UK: Cambridge University Press.

Gardner, C. J., Armour, D. R., Beattie, D. T., Gale, J. D., Hawcock, A. B., Kilpatrick, G. J.,Twissell, D. J., & Ward, P. (1996). GR205171: A novel antagonist with high affinity for the tachykinin NK_1 receptor, and potent broad-spectrum anti-emetic activity. *Regul Pept, 65,* 45–53.

Garthright, W. E., Archer, D. L., & Kvenberg, J. E. (1988). Estimates of incidence and costs of intestinal infectious diseases in the United States. *Public Health Rep, 103,* 107–115.

Geldof, H., Van Der Schee, E. J., Van Blankenstein, M., & Grashuis, J. L. (1986). Electrogastrographic study of gastric myoelectrical activity in patients with unexplained nausea and vomiting. *Gut, 27,* 799–808.

Gentilcore, D., Chaikomin, R., Jones, K. L., Russo, A., Feinle-Bisset, C., Wishart, J. M., Rayner, C. K., & Horowitz M. (2006). Effects of fat on gastric emptying of and the glycemic, insulin, and incretin responses to a carbohydrate meal in type 2 diabetes. *J Clin Endocrinol Metab, 91,* 2062–2067.

Gerhart, D. J. (1991). Emesis, learned aversion, and chemical defense in octocorals: A central role for prostaglandins? *Am J Physiol Regul Integr Comp Physiol, 260,* R839–843.

German, V. F., Corrales, R., Ueki, L. F., & Nadel, J. A. (1982). Reflex stimulation of tracheal mucus gland secretion by gastric irritation in cats. *J Appl Physiol, 52,* 1153–1155.

Gianaros, P. J., Quigley, K. S., Muth, E. R., Levine, M. E., Vasko, R. C., Jr., & Stern, R. M. (2003). Relationship between temporal changes in cardiac parasympathetic activity and motion sickness severity. *Psychophysiology, 40,* 39–44.

Gianaros, P. J., Stern, R. M., Morrow, G. R., & Hickok, J. T. (2001). Relationship of gastric myoelectrical and cardiac parasympathetic activity to chemotherapy-induced nausea. *J Psychosom Res, 50,* 263–266.

Gibbs, R. A., Weinstock, G. M., Metzker, M. L., Muzny, D. M., Sodergren, E. J., Scherer, S., Scott, G., Steffen, D., Worley, K. C., Burch, P. E., et al. (2004). Genome sequence of the Brown Norway rat yields insights into mammalian evolution. *Nature, 428,* 493–521.

Gil, A., Nachum, Z., Dachir, S., Chapman, S., Levy, A., Shupak, A., Adir, Y., & Tal, D. (2005). Scopolamine patch to prevent seasickness: Clinical response vs. plasma concentration in sailors. *Aviat Space Environ Med, 76,* 766–770.

Gilardi, J. D., Duffey, S. S., Munn, C. A., & Tell, L. A. (1999). Biochemical functions of geophagy in parrots: Detoxification of dietary toxins and cytoprotective effects. *J Chem Ecol, 25,* 897–919.

Gillies, G. E., Linton, E. A., & Lowry, P. J. (1982). Corticotropin releasing activity of the new CRF is potentiated several times by vasopressin. *Nature, 299,* 355–357.

Girod, V., Bouvier, M., & Grelot, L. (2000). Characterization of lipopolysaccharide-induced emesis in conscious piglets: Effects of cervical vagotomy, cyclooxygenase inhibitors and a 5-HT(3) receptor antagonist. *Neuropharmacology, 39,* 2329–2335.

Glander, K. E. (1994). Non-human primate self medication with wild plant foods. In N. Etkin (Ed.), *Eating on the wild side* (pp. 227–239). Tucson: University of Arizona Press.

Glendinning, J. I. (2007). How do predators cope with chemically defended foods? *Biol Bull, 213,* 252–266.

Glendinning, J. I., Yiin, Y. M., Ackroff, K., & Sclafani, A. (2008). Intragastric infusion of denatonium conditions flavor aversions and delays gastric emptying in rodents. *Physiol Behav, 93,* 757–765.

Glinoer, D. (1998). Thyroid hyperfunction during pregnancy. *Thyroid, 8,* 859–864.

Gnecchi Ruscone, T., Guzzetti, S., Lombardi, F., & Lombardi, R. (1986). Lack of association between prodromes nausea and vomiting, and specific electrocardiographic patterns of acute myocardial infarction. *Int J Cardiol, 11,* 17–23.

Goadsby, P.J. (1999) Autoregulation and autonomic control of the cerebral circulation: implications and pathophysiology. In C. J. Mathias and R. Bannister (Eds.), *Autonomic failure: A textbook of clinical disorders of the autonomic nervous system* (4th ed., pp. 85–91). New York: Oxford University Press.

Goiny, M., & Uvnäs-Moberg, K. (1987). Effects of dopamine receptor antagonists on gastrin and vomiting responses to apomorphine. *Naunyn Schmiedebergs Arch Pharmacol, 336,* 16–19.

Golding, J. F. (2006). Motion sickness susceptibility. *Auton Neurosci, 129,* 67–76.

Golding, J. F., & Stott, J. R. R. (1997). Comparison of the effects of a muscarinic receptor antagonist and hyoscine (scopolamine) on motion sickness, skin conductance and heart rate. *Br J Clin Pharmacol, 43,* 633–637.

Gonlachanvit, S., Chen, Y. H., Hasler, W. L., Sun, W. M., & Owyang, C. (2003a). Ginger reduces hyperglycemia-evoked gastric dysrhythmias in healthy humans: Possible role of endogenous prostaglandins. *J Pharmacol Exp Ther, 307,* 1098–1103.

Gonlachanvit, S., Hsu, C. W., Boden, G. H., Knight, L. C., Maurer, A. H., Fisher, R. S., & Parkman, H. P. (2003b). Effect of altering gastric emptying on postprandial plasma glucose concentrations following a physiologic meal in type-II diabetic patients. *Dig Dis Sci, 48,* 488–497.

Gonsalves, S. F., Landgraf, B. E., Ciardelli, T. L., & Borison, H. L. (1991). Early toxicity of recombinant interleukin-2 in cats. *Arch Int Pharmacodyn Ther, 310,* 175–185.

Goodwin, T. M. (2000). Human chorionic gonadotropin and hyperemesis gravidarum. In G. Koren and R. Bishai (Eds.), *Nausea and vomiting of pregnancy: State of the art 2000* (pp. 15–22). Montreal: Transcontinental Inc.

Gordon, C. R., Ben-Aryeh, H., Szargel, R., Attias, J., Rolnick, A., & Laufer, D. (1989). Salivary changes associated with seasickness. *J Auton Nerv Syst, 26*, 37–42.

Gorgiladze, G. I., & Bryanov, I. I. (1989). Space motion sickness. *Kosm Biol Aviakosm Med, 23*, 4–14.

Gralla, R., Lichinitser, M., Van Der Vegt, S., Sleeboom, H., Mezger, J., Peschel, C., Tonini, G., Labianca, R., Macciocchi, A., & Aapro, M. (2003). Palonosetron improves prevention of chemotherapy-induced nausea and vomiting following moderately emetogenic chemotherapy: Results of a double-blind randomized phase III trial comparing single doses of palonosetron with ondansetron. *Ann Oncol, 4*, 1570–1577.

Grant, P. J., Hughes, J. R., Dean, H. G., Davies, J. A., & Prentice, C. R. (1986). Vasopressin and catecholamine secretion during apomorphine-induced nausea mediate acute changes in haemostatic function in man. *Clin Sci (Lond), 71*, 621–624.

Grant, V. L. (1987). Do conditioned taste aversions result from activation of emetic mechanisms? *Psychopharmacology (Berl), 93*, 405–415.

Graves, T. (1992). Emesis as a complication of cancer chemotherapy: Pathophysiology, importance, and treatment. *Pharmacotherapy, 11*, 337–345.

Graybiel, A. (1980). Space motion sickness: Skylab revisited. *Aviat Space Environ Med, 51*, 814–822.

Green, H. H. (1925). Perverted appetites. *Physiol Rev, 5*, 336–346.

Greenwood, M. H., Lader, M. H., Kantameneni, B. D., & Curzon, G. (1975). The acute effects of oral (—)-tryptophan in human subjects. *Br J Clin Pharmacol, 2*, 165–172.

Grelot, L., Dapzol, J., Esteve, E., Frugiere, A., Bianchi, A. L., Sheldrick, R. L., Gardner, C. J., & Ward, P. (1998). Potent inhibition of both the acute and delayed emetic responses to cisplatin in piglets treated with GR205171, a novel highly selective tachykinin NK1 receptor antagonist. *Br J Pharmacol, 124*, 1643–1650.

Grelot, L., Girod, V., Dapzol, J., Maffrand, J. P., & Serradeil-Le Gal, C. (2001). A non-peptide vasopressin V(1a) receptor antagonist, SR 49059, does not prevent cisplatin-induced emesis in piglets. *Fundam Clin Pharmacol, 15*, 189–200.

Grelot, L., Le Stunff, H., Milano, S., Blower, P. R., & Romain, D. (1996). Repeated administration of the 5-HT3 receptor antagonist granisetron reduces the incidence of delayed cisplatin-induced emesis in the piglet. *J Pharmacol Exp Ther, 279*, 255–261.

Grelot, L., & Miller, A. D. (1997). Neural control of respiratory muscle activation during vomiting. In A. B. Miller, A. L. Bianchi, & B. P. Bishop (Eds.), *Neural control of the respiratory muscles* (pp. 239–248). Boca Raton, FL: CRC Press.

Grill, H. J. (1985). Introduction: Physiological mechanisms in conditioned taste aversions. *Ann NY Acad Sci, 443*, 67–88.

Grill, H. J., & Norgren, R. (1978a). The taste reactivity test: 1. Mimetic responses to gustatory stimuli in neurologically normal rats. *Brain Res, 143*, 263–279.

Grill, H. J., & Norgren, R. (1978b). The taste reactivity test: 2. Mimetic responses to gustatory stimuli in chronic thalamic and chronic decerebrate rats. *Brain Res, 143*, 281–297.

Groop, L. C., Luzi, L., DeFronzo, R. A., & Melander, A. (1989). Hyperglycaemia and absorption of sulphonylurea drugs. *Lancet, 2*(8655), 129–130.

Gross, P. M., Wall, K. M., Pang, J. J., Shaver, S. W., & Wainman, D. S. (1990). Microvascular specializations promoting rapid interstitial solute dispersion in nucleus tractus solitarius. *Am J Physiol Regul Integr Comp Physiol, 259*, R1131–1138.

Gross, S., Librach, C., & Cecutti, A. (1989). Maternal weight loss associated with hyperemesis gravidarum: A predictor of fetal outcome. *Am J Obstet Gynecol, 160,* 906–909.

Grossman, M. I., Woolmy, J. R., Dutton, D. F., & Ivy, A. C. (1945). The effect of nausea on gastric secretion and a study of the mechanism concerned. *Gastroenterology, 4,* 347–351.

Grunberg, S. M., Deuson, R. R., Mavros, P., Geling, O., Hansen, M., Cruciani, G., Daniele, B., De Pouvourville, G., Rubenstein, E. B., & Daugaard, G. (2004). Incidence of chemotherapy-induced nausea and emesis after modern antiemetics. *Cancer, 100,* 2261–2268.

Gustavson, C. R. (1977). Comparative and field aspects of learned food aversions. In L. M. Barker, M. R. Best, & M. Domjan (Eds.), *Learning mechanisms in food selection* (pp. 23–43). Waco, TX: Baylor University Press.

Gustavson, C. R., Garcia, J., Hankins, W. G., & Rusiniak, K. W. (1974). Coyote predation control by aversive conditioning. *Science, 184,* 581–583.

Gylys, J. A., Doran, K. M., & Buyniski, J. P. (1979). Antagonism of cisplatin induced emesis in the dog. *Res Commun Chem Pathol Pharmacol, 23,* 61–68.

Habermann, J., Eversmann, T., Erhardt, F., Gottsmann, M., Ulbrecht, G., & Scriba, P. C. (1978). Increased urinary excretion of triiodothyronine (T3) and thyroxine (T4) and decreased serum thyreotropic hormone (TSH) induced by motion sickness. *Aviat Space Environ Med, 49,* 58–61.

Habib, A. S., Chen, Y. T., Taguchi, A., Hu, X. H., & Gan, T. J. (2006a). Postoperative nausea and vomiting following inpatient surgeries in a teaching hospital: A retrospective database analysis. *Curr Med Res Opin, 22,* 1093–1099.

Habib, A. S., Itchon-Ramos, N., Phillips-Bute, B. G., Gan, T. J., & Duke Women's Anesthesia Research Group. (2006b). Transcutaneous acupoint electrical stimulation with the Reliefband for the prevention of nausea and vomiting during and after cesarean delivery under spinal anesthesia. *Anesth Analg, 102,* 581–584.

Haig, D. (1993). Genetic conflicts in human pregnancy. *Q Rev Biol, 68,* 495–532.

Hainsworth, J. D., & Hesketh, P. J. (1992). Single-dose ondansetron for the prevention of cisplatin-induced emesis: Efficacy results. *Semin Oncol, 19,* 14–19.

Halford, J. C., Wanninayake, S. C., & Blundell, J. E. (1998). Behavioral satiety sequence (BSS) for the diagnosis of drug action on food intake. *Pharmacol Biochem Behav, 61,* 159–168.

Hall, G., & Symonds, M. (2006). Overshadowing and latent inhibition of context aversion conditioning in the rat. *Auton Neurosci, 129,* 42–49.

Hamilton, J. W., Bellahsene, B. E., Reicherlderfer, M., Webster, J. H., & Bass, P. (1986). Human electrogastrograms: Comparison of surface and mucosal recordings. *Dig Dis Sci, 31,* 33–39.

Hammer, J., Howell, S., Bytzer, P., Horowitz, M., & Talley, N. J. (2003). Symptom clustering in subjects with and without diabetes mellitus: A population-based study of 15,000 Australian adults. *Am J Gastroenterol, 98,* 391–398.

Hanson, J. S., & McCallum, R. W. (1985). The diagnosis and management of nausea and vomiting: A review. *Am J Gastroenterol, 80,* 210–218.

Hao, S., Sternini, C., & Raybould, H. E. (2008). Role of CCK1 and Y2 receptors in activation of hindbrain neurons induced by intragastric administration of bitter taste receptor ligands. *Am J Physiol Regul Integr Comp Physiol, 294,* R33–38.

Harding, R. K. (1995). 5-HT3 receptor antagonists and radiation-induced emesis: Preclinical data. In D. J. Reynolds, P. L. R. Andrews, & C. J. Davis (Eds.), *Serotonin and the scientific basis of anti-emetic therapy* (pp. 127–133). Oxford: Oxford Clinical Communications.

Harding, R. K., & McDonald, T. J. (1989). Identification and characterization of the emetic effects of peptide YY. *Peptides, 10,* 21–24.

Harm, D. H. (1990). Physiology of motion sickness symptoms. In G. H. Crampton (Ed.), *Motion and space sickness* (pp. 153–177). Boca Raton, FL: CRC Press.

Harm, D. H. (2002). Motion sickness neurophysiology, physiological correlates, and treatment. In K. M. Stanney (Ed.), *Handbook of virtual environments: Design, implementation, and applications* (pp. 637–661). Mahwah, NJ: Lawrence Erlbaum Associates.

Harmon, D., O'Connor, P., Gleasa, O., & Gardiner, J. (2000). Menstrual cycle irregularity and the incidence of nausea and vomiting after laparoscopy. *Anaesthesia, 55,* 1164–1167.

Harris, M. C., & Loewy, A. D. (1990). Neural regulation of vasopressin-containing hypothalamic neurons and the role of vasopressin in cardiovascular function. In A. D. Loewy & K. M. Spyer (Eds.), *Central regulation of autonomic functions* (pp. 224–246). New York: Oxford University Press.

Harrison, W. A., Lipe, W. A., & Decker, W. J. (1972). Apomorphine-induced emesis in the dog: Comparison of routes of administration. *J Am Vet Med Assoc, 160,* 85–86.

Hasegawa, S., Takeda, N., Morita, M., Horii, A., Koizuka, I., Kubo, T., & Matsunaga, T. (1992). Vestibular, central, and gastral triggering of emesis: A study on individual susceptibility in rats. *Acta Otolaryngol, 112,* 927–931.

Hasler, W. L. (2007). Type 1 diabetes and gastroparesis: Diagnosis and treatment. *Curr Gastroenterol Rep, 9,* 261–269.

Hasler, W. L. (2009). Methods of gastric electrical stimulation and pacing: A review of their benefits and mechanisms of action in gastroparesis and obesity. *Neurogastroenterol Motil, 21,* 229–243.

Hasler, W. L., Kim, M. S., Chey, W. D., Stevenson, V., Stein, B., & Owyang, C. (1995a). Central cholinergic and alpha-adrenergic mediation of gastric slow wave dysrhythmias evoked during motion sickness. *Am J Physiol Gastrointest Liver Physiol, 268,* G539–547.

Hasler, W. L., Soudah, H. C., Dulai, G., & Owyang, C. (1995b). Mediation of hyperglycemia-evoked gastric slow wave dysrhythmias by endogenous prostaglandin. *Gastroenterology, 108,* 727–736.

Hatcher, R. A. (1924). The mechanism of vomiting. *Physiological Reviews, 4,* 479–504.

Hatcher, R. A., & Weiss, S. (1923). Studies on vomiting. *J Pharm Exper Ther, 22,* 139–193.

Haug, T. T., Mykletun, A., & Dahl, A. A. (2002). The prevalence of nausea in the community: Psychological, social, and somatic factors. *Gen Hosp Psychiatry, 24,* 81–86.

Haut, M. W., Beckwith, B., Laurie, J. A., & Klatt, N. (1991). Post chemotherapy nausea and vomiting in cancer patients receiving outpatient chemotherapy. *J Psychosocial Oncol, 9,* 117–130.

Hawthorn, J. (1995). *Understanding and management of nausea and vomiting.* Oxford: Blackwell.

Hawthorn, J., Andrews, P. L. R., Ang, V. T. Y., & Jenkins, J. S. (1988). Differential release of vasopressin and oxytocin in response to abdominal vagal afferent stimulation of apomorphine in the ferret. *Brain Res, 438,* 193–198.

Hawthorn, J., & Cunningham, D. (1990). Dexamethasone can potentiate the antiemetic action of a 5HT$_3$ receptor antagonist on cyclophosphamide induced vomiting in the ferret. *Br J Cancer, 61,* 56–60.

Hawthorn, J., Ostler, K. J., & Andrews, P. L. R. (1988). The role of the abdominal visceral innervation and 5-hydroxytryptamine M-receptors in vomiting induced by the cytotoxic drugs cyclophosphamide and cis-platin in the ferret. *Q J Exp Physiol, 73,* 7–21.

Haxby, J. V., Hoffman, E. A., & Gobbini, M. I. (2000). The distributed human neural system for face perception. *Trends Cogn Sci, 4,* 223–233.

Heim, M. E., & Queisser, W. (1982). Antiemetic effects of the cannabinoid levonantradol hydrochloride in patients receiving cancer chemotherapy. In E. A. Mirand, W. B. Hutchinson, & E. Mihich (Eds.), *Proceedings of the 13th International Cancer Congress, September 8–15, 1982, Seattle, Washington.* New York: A.R. Liss, 1983.

Henry, T. R., Bakay, R. A., Votaw, J. R., Pennell, P. B., Epstein, C. M., Faber, T. L., Grafton, S. T., & Hoffman, J. M. (1998). Brain blood flow alterations induced by therapeutic vagus nerve stimulation in partial epilepsy: 1. Acute effects at high and low levels of stimulation. *Epilepsia, 39,* 983–990.

Hesketh, P. J. (2000). Comparative review of 5-HT$_3$ receptor antagonists in the treatment of acute chemotherapy-induced nausea and vomiting. *Cancer Invest, 18,* 163–173.

Hesketh, P. J. (2008). Chemotherapy-induced nausea and vomiting. *N Engl J Med, 358,* 2482–2494.

Hesketh, P. J., Grunberg, S. M., Gralla, R. J., Warr, D. G., Roila, F., de Wit, R., Chawla, S. P., Carides, A. D., Ianus, J., Elmer, M. E., Evans, J. K., Beck, K., Reines, S., & Horgan, K. J. (2003a). The oral neurokinin-1 antagonist aprepitant for the prevention of chemotherapy-induced nausea and vomiting: A multinational, randomized, double-blind, placebo-controlled trial in patients receiving high-dose cisplatin—Aprepitant Protocol 052 Study Group. *J Clin Oncol, 21,* 4112–4119.

Hesketh, P. J., Kris, M. G., Grunberg, S. M., Beck, T., Hainsworth, J. D., Harker, G., Aapro, M. S., Gandara, D., & Lindley, C. M. (1997). Proposal for classifying the acute emetogenicity of cancer chemotherapy. *J Clin Oncol, 15,* 103–109.

Hesketh, P., Navari, R., Grote, T., Gralla, R., Hainsworth, J., Kris, M., Anthony, L., Khojasteh, A., Tapazoglou, E., Benedict, C., & Hahne, W. (1996). Double-blind, randomized comparison of the antiemetic efficacy of intravenous Dolasetron mesylate and intravenous ondansetron in the prevention of acute cisplatin-induced emesis in patients with cancer: Dolasetron Comparative Chemotherapy-induced Emesis Prevention Group. *J Clin Oncol, 14,* 2242–2249.

Hesketh, P. J., Van Belle, S., Aapro, M., Tattersall, F. D., Naylor, R. J., Hargreaves, R., Carides, A. D., Evans, J. K., & Horgan, K. J. (2003b). Differential involvement of neurotransmitters through the time course of cisplatin-induced emesis as revealed by therapy with specific receptor antagonists. *Eur J Cancer, 39,* 1074–1080.

Hickok, J. T., Roscoe, J. A., & Morrow, G. R. (2001). The role of patients' expectations in the development of anticipatory nausea related to chemotherapy. *J Pain Symptom Manage, 22,* 843–850.

Hickok, J. T., Roscoe, J. A., Morrow, G. R., King, D. K., Atkins, J. N., & Fitch, T. R. (2003). Nausea and emesis remain a significant problem of chemotherapy despite prophylaxis with 5-hydroxytryptamine-3 antiemetics: A University of Rochester James P. Wilmot Cancer Center Community Clinical Oncology Program Study of 360 cancer patients treated in the community. *Cancer, 97,* 2880–2886.

Higa, G. M., Auber, M. L., Altaha, R., Piktel, D., Kurian, S., Hobbs, G., & Landreth, K. (2006). 5-Hydroxyindoleacetic acid and substance P profiles in patients receiving emetogenic chemotherapy. *J Oncol Pharm Pract, 12,* 201–209.

Hikami, K., Hasegawa, Y., & Matsuzawa, T. (1990). Social transmission of food preferences in Japanese monkeys (Macaca fuscata) after mere exposure or aversion
training. *J Comp Psychol, 104,* 233–237.

Hill, D. R., Shaw, T. M., Graham, W., & Woodruff, G. N. (1990). Autoradiographical
detection of cholecystokinin-A receptors in primate brain using 125I-Bolton Hunter
CCK-8 and 3H-MK-329. *J Neurosci, 10,* 1070–1081.

Hillsley, K., & Grundy, D. (1999). Plasticity in the mesenteric afferent response to cisplatin following vagotomy in the rat. *J Auton Nerv Syst, 76,* 93–98.

Himi, N., Koga, T., Nakamura, E., Kobashi, M., Yamane, M., & Tsujioka, K. (2004).
Differences in autonomic responses between subjects with and without nausea while
watching an irregularly oscillating video. *Auton Neurosci, 116,* 46–53.

Hinder, R. A., & Kelly, K. A. (1977). Human gastric pacesetter potential: Site of origin,
spread, and response to gastric transection and proximal gastric vagotomy. *Am J
Surg, 133,* 29–33.

Hirsch, J. (1994). Impact of postoperative nausea and vomiting in the surgical setting.
Anaesthesia, 49, 30–33.

Hladik, C. M., & Chivers, D. J. (1994). Foods and the digestive system. In D. J. Chivers
& P. Langer (Eds.), *The digestive system in mammals* (pp. 65–73). Cambridge, UK:
Cambridge University Press.

Hobbs, S. H., Clingerman, H., & Elkins, R. L. (1976). Illness-induced taste aversions in
normal and bulbectomized hamsters. *Physiol Behav, 17,* 235–238.

Holbrook, J. D., Gill, C. H., Zebda, N., Spencer, J. P., Leyland, R., Rance, K. H., Trinh, H.,
Balmer, G., Kelly, F. M., Yusaf, S. P., Courtney, N., Luck, J., Rhodes, A., Modha, S.,
Moore, S. E., Sanger, G. J., & Gunthorpe, M. J. (2009). Characterisation of 5-HT$_3$C,
5-HT$_3$D and 5-HT$_3$E receptor subunits: Evolution, distribution, and function. *J
Neurochem, 108,* 384–396.

Holmes, A. M., Rudd, J. A., Tattersall, F. D., Aziz, Q., & Andrews, P. L. R. (2009).
Opportunities for the replacement of animals in the study of nausea and vomiting:
Replacement in a multi-system reflex. *Br J Pharmacol, 167,* 865–880.

Holzäpfel, A., Festa, A., Stacher-Janotta, G., Bergmann, H., Shnawa, N., Brannath, W.,
Schernthaner, G., & Stacher G. (1999). Gastric emptying in Type II (non-insulin-
dependent) diabetes mellitus before and after therapy readjustment: No influence of
actual blood glucose concentration. *Diabetologia, 42,* 1410–1412.

Hook, E. B. (1978). Dietary cravings and aversions during pregnancy. *Am J Clin Nutr,
31,* 1355–1362.

Horn, C. C. (2008). Why is the neurobiology of nausea and vomiting so important?
Appetite, 50, 430–434.

Horn, C. C. (2009) Brain Fos expression induced by the chemotherapy agent cisplatin
in the rat is partially dependent on an intact abdominal vagus. *Autonom Neurosci,
148,* 76–82.

Horn, C. C., Ciucci, M., & Chaudhury, A. (2007). Brain Fos expression during 48 h after
cisplatin treatment: Neural pathways for acute and delayed visceral sickness. *Auton
Neurosci, 132,* 44–51.

Horn, C. C., Richardson, E. J., Andrews, P. L. R., & Friedman, M. I. (2004). Differential
effects on gastrointestinal and hepatic vagal afferent fibers in the rat by the anticancer agent cisplatin. *Auton Neurosci, 115,* 74–81.

Hornby, P. J. (2001). Central neurocircuitry associated with emesis. *Am J Med,
111*(Suppl. 8A), 106S–112S.

Horowitz, M., Harding, P. E., Maddox, A. F., Wishart, J. M., Akkermans, L. M., Chatterton, B. E., & Shearman, D. J. (1989). Gastric and esophageal emptying in patients with type 2 (non-insulin-dependent) diabetes mellitus. *Diabetologia, 32,* 151–159.

Horowitz, M., Jones, K. L., Harding, P. E., and Wishart, J. M. (2002a). Relationship between the effects of cisapride on gastric emptying and plasma glucose concentrations in diabetic gastroparesis. *Digestion, 65,* 41–46.

Horowitz, M., O'Donovan, D., Jones, K. L., Feinle, C., Rayner, C. K., & Samsom, M. (2002b). Gastric emptying in diabetes: Clinical significance and treatment. *Diabet Med, 19,* 177–194.

Horowitz, M., & Samsom, M. (Eds.). (2004). *Gastrointestinal function in diabetes mellitus.* Chichester, UK: Wiley.

Houpt, T. A., Pittman, D. W., Barranco, J. M., Brooks, E. H., & Smith, J. C. (2003). Behavioral effects of high-strength static magnetic fields on rats. *J Neurosci, 23,* 1498–1505.

Hsu, J. J., Clark-Glena, R., Nelson, D. K., & Kim, C. H. (1996). Nasogastric enteral feeding in the management of hyperemesis gravidarum. *Obstet Gynecol, 88,* 343–346.

Hu, S., Grant, W. F., Stern, R. M., & Koch, K. L. (1991). Motion sickness severity and physiological correlates during repeated exposures to a rotating optokinetic drum. *Aviat Space Environ Med, 62,* 308–314.

Hu, S., & Hui, L. (1997). Adaptation to optokinetic rotation-induced motion sickness without experiencing nausea. *Perceptual and Motor Skills, 84,* 1235–1240.

Hu, S., & Stern, R. M. (1999). The retention of adaptation to motion sickness eliciting stimulation. *Aviat Space Environ Med, 70,* 766–768.

Hu, S., Stern, R. M., & Koch, K. L. (1991). Effects of pre-exposures to a rotating optokinetic drum on adaptation to motion sickness. *Aviat Space Environ Med, 62,* 53–56.

Hu, S., Stern, R. M., & Koch, K. L. (1992). Electrical acustimulation relieves vection-induced motion sickness. *Gastroenterology, 102,* 1854–1858.

Hu, S., Stern, R. M., Vasey, M. W., & Koch, K. L. (1989). Motion sickness and gastric myoelectrical activity as a function of speed of rotation of a circular vection drum. *Aviat Space Environ Med, 60,* 411–414.

Hu, S., Stritzel, R., Chandler, A., & Stern, R. M. (1995). P6 acupressure reduces symptoms of vection-induced motion sickness. *Aviat Space Environ Med, 66,* 631–634.

Huang, Y. J., Maruyama, Y., Lu, K. S., Pereira, E., & Roper, S. D. (2005). Mouse taste buds release serotonin in response to taste stimuli. *Chem Senses, 30*(Suppl. 1), i39–40.

Hultin, L., Lindsrom, G., & Lehmann, A. (2005). In vivo imaging of tachykinin NK1 receptor agonist induced reflux in rats. *Neurogastroenterol Motil, 17*(Suppl. 2), 60.

Hummel, T., von Mering, R., Huch, R., & Kölble, N. (2002). Olfactory modulation of nausea during early pregnancy. *Brit J Obstet Gynecol, 109,* 1394–1397.

Hursti, T. J., Borjeson, S., Hellstrom, P. M., Avall-Lundqvist, E., Stock, S., Steineck, G., & Peterson, C. (2005). Effect of chemotherapy on circulating gastrointestinal hormone levels in ovarian cancer patients: Relationship to nausea and vomiting. *Scand J Gastroenterol, 40,* 654–661.

Hursti, T. J., Fredrikson, M., Steineck, G., Borjeson, S., Furst, C. J., & Peterson, C. (1993). Endogenous cortisol exerts antiemetic effect similar to that of exogenous corticosteroids. *Br J Cancer, 68,* 112–114.

Hutchison, S. L., Jr. (1973). Taste aversion in albino rats using centrifugal spin as an unconditioned stimulus. *Psychol Rep, 33,* 467–470.

Iber, F. L., Parveen, S., Vandrunen, M., Sood, K. B., Reza, F., Serlovsky, R., & Reddy, S. (1993). Relation of symptoms to impaired stomach, small bowel, and colon motility in long-standing diabetes. *Dig Dis Sci, 38,* 45–50.

Ikegaya, Y., & Matsuki, N. (2002). Vasopressin induces emesis in Suncus murinus. *Jpn J Pharmacol, 89,* 324–326.

Intagliata, N., & Koch, K. L. (2007). Gastroparesis in type 2 diabetes mellitus: Prevalence, etiology, diagnosis, and treatment. *Curr Gastroenterol Rep, 9,* 270–279.

Ito, S.-I., & Craig, A. D. (2003). Vagal input to lateral area 3a in cat cortex. *J Neurophysiol, 90,* 143–154.

Ivy, A. C., & Vloedman, D. A. (1925). The small intestine in hunger. *Am J Physiol, 72,* 99–106.

Jackson, T. R., & Smith, J. W. (1978). A comparison of two aversion treatment methods for alcoholism. *J Stud Alcohol, 39,* 187–191.

Jacob, T. J., Franser, C., Wang, L., Walker, V., & O'Connor, S. (2003). Psychophysical evaluation of responses to pleasant and mal-odour stimulation in human subjects: Adaptation, dose-response, and gender differences. *Int J Psychophysiol, 48,* 67–80.

Jacobs, H. L., & Sharma, K. N. (1969). Taste versus calories: Sensory and metabolic signals in the control of food intake. *Annals of the New York Academy of Science, 157,* 1084–1125.

Jacobsen, P. B., Andrykowski, M. A., Redd, W. H., Die-Trill, M., Hakes, T. B., Kaufman, R. J., Currie, V. E., & Holland, J. C. (1988). Nonpharmacologic factors in the development of posttreatment nausea with adjuvant chemotherapy for breast cancer. *Cancer, 61,* 379–385.

Janatuinen, E., Pikkarainen, P., Laakso, M., & Pyorala, K. (1993). Gastrointestinal symptoms in middle-aged diabetic patients. *Scand J Gastroenterol, 28,* 427–432.

Janes, R. J., Muhonen, T., Karjalainen, U. P., & Wiklund, T. (1998). Urinary 5-hydroxy-indoleacetic acid (5-HIAA) excretion during multiple-day high-dose chemotherapy. *Eur J Cancer, 34,* 196–198.

Janig, W. (1990). Functions of the sympathetic innervation of the skin. In A. D. Loewy & K. M. Spyer (Eds.), *Central regulation of autonomic functions* (pp. 334–348). Oxford and New York: Oxford University Press.

Järnfelt-Samsioe, A., Samsioe, G., & Velinder, G. (1983). Nausea and vomiting in pregnancy: A contribution to its epidemiology. *Gynecol Obstet Invest, 16,* 221–229.

Jebbink, R. J., Samsom, M., Bruijs, P. P., Bravenboer, B., Akkermans, L. M., Vanberge-Henegouwen, G. P., & Smout, A. J. (1994). Hyperglycemia induces abnormalities of gastric myoelectrical activity in patients with type I diabetes mellitus. *Gastroenterology, 107,* 1390–1397.

Jednak, M. A., Shadigian, E. M., Kim, M. S., Woods, M. L., Hooper, F. G., Owyang, C., & Hasler, W. L. (1999). Protein meals reduce nausea and gastric slow wave dysrhythmic activity on first trimester pregnancy. *Am J Physiol Gastrointest Liver Physiol, 277,* G855–G861.

Jeng-Weei Lin, J., Parker, D. E., Lahav, M., & Furness, T. A. (2005). Unobtrusive vehicle motion prediction cues reduced simulator sickness during passive travel in a driving simulator. *Ergonomics, 48,* 608–624.

Jett, M., Brinkley, W., Neill, R., Gemski, P., & Hunt, R. (1990). Staphylococcus aureus enterotoxin B challenge of monkeys: Correlation of plasma levels of arachidonic acid cascade products with occurrence of illness. *Infect Immun, 58,* 3494–3499.

Jewell, D., & Young, G. (2003). Interventions for nausea and vomiting in early pregnancy. *Cochrane Database of Systematic Reviews, 4* (Online): CD000145.

Jodal, M., & Lundgren, O. (1989). Neurohumoral control of gastrointestinal blood flow. In S. G. Schultz, J. D. Wood, & B. B. Rauner (Eds.), *Handbook of physiology, the gastrointestinal system: Vol. 1. Motility and circulation* (Part 2, pp. 1667–1712). Bethesda, MD: American Physiological Society.

Johanson, J. F., Drossman, D. A., Panas, R., Wahle, A., & Ueno R. (2008). Clinical trial: phase 2 study of lubiprostone for irritable bowel syndrome with constipation. *Aliment Pharmacol Ther 27*, 685–696.

Jokela, R. M., Cakmakkaya, O. S., Danzeisen, O., Korttila, K. T., Kranke, P., Malhotra, A., Paura, A., Radke, O. C., Sessler, D. I., Soikkeli, A., Roewer, N., & Apfel, C.C. (2009). Ondansetron has similar clinical efficacy against both nausea and vomiting. *Anaesthesia 64*, 147–151.

Johannsen, U. J., Summers, R., & Mark, A. L. (1981). Gastric dilation during stimulation of cardiac sensory receptors. *Circulation, 63*, 960–964.

Jokerst, M. D., Gatto, M., Fazio, R., Gianaros, P. J., Stern, R. M., & Koch, K. L. (1999a). Effects of gender of subjects and experimenter on susceptibility to motion. *Aviat Space Environ Med, 70*, 962–965.

Jokerst, M. D., Gatto, M., Fazio, R., Stern, R. M., & Koch, K. L. (1999b). Slow deep breathing prevents the development of tachygastria and symptoms of motion sickness. *Aviat Space Environ Med, 70*, 1189–1192.

Jones, K. L., Horowitz, M., Carney, B. I., Wishart, J. M., Guha, S., & Green L. (1996). Gastric emptying in early noninsulin-dependent diabetes mellitus. *J Nucl Med, 37*, 1643–1648.

Jones, K. R., & Jones, G. E. (1985). Pre- and postprandial EGG variation. In R. M. Stern & K. L. Koch (Eds.), *Electrogastrography* (pp. 165–181). New York: Praeger.

Jones, M. (2007). Are we so different? How apes eat. In M. Jones, *Feast: Why humans share food* (pp. 23–43). Oxford: Oxford University Press.

Jones, W. H. S. (Trans.). (1923). *Hippocrates* (Loeb ed., Vol. 1). Cambridge: Harvard University Press.

Jones, W. H. S. (Trans.). (1967). *Hippocrates* (Loeb ed., Vol. 4). Cambridge: Harvard University Press.

Jordan, V., Mac Donald, J., Crichton, S., Stone, P., & Ford, H. (1995). The incidence of hyperemesis gravidarum is increased among Pacific Islanders living in Wellington. *N Z Med J, 108*, 342–344.

Kabalak, A. A., Akcay, M., Akcay, F., & Gogus, N. (2005). Transcutaneous electrical acupoint stimulation versus ondansetron in the prevention of postoperative vomiting following pediatric tonsillectomy. *J Altern Complement Med, 11*, 407–413.

Kaivola, S., Parantainen, J., Osterman, T., & Timonen, H. (1983). Hangover headache and prostaglandins: Prophylactic treatment with tolfenamic acid. *Cephalalgia, 3*, 31–36.

Kallen, B. (2000). Hyperemesis gravidarum during pregnancy and delivery outcome: A registry study. In G. Koren and R. Bishai (Eds.), *Nausea and vomiting of pregnancy: State of the art 2000* (pp. 36–40). Toronto: Motherisk.

Kan, K. K., Jones, R. L., Ngan, M. P., & Rudd, J. A. (2004). Excitatory action of prostanoids on the ferret isolated vagus nerve preparation. *Eur J Pharmacol, 491*, 37–41.

Kan, K. K., Rudd, J. A., & Wai, M. K. (2006). Differential action of anti-emetic drugs on defecation and emesis induced by prostaglandin E2 in the ferret. *Eur J Pharmacol, 544*, 153–159.

Kaplan, I. (1964). Motion sickness on railroads. *Ind Med Surg, 33*, 648–651.

Kapur, P. A. (1991). The big "little problem." *Anesth Analg, 73*, 243–245.

Kassander, P. (1958). Asymptomatic gastric retention in diabetics (gastroparesis diabeticorum). *Ann Intern Med, 48,* 797–812.

Kavaliers, M., Choleris, E., Agamo, A., Braun, W. J., Colwell, D. D., Muglia, L. J., Ogawa, S., & Pfaff, D. W. (2006). Inadvertent social information and the avoidance of parasitized male mice: A role for oxytocin. *Proc Nat Acad Sci USA, 103,* 4293–4298.

Kaya, N., Shen, T., Lu, S. G., Zhao, F. L., & Herness, S. (2004). A paracrine signaling role for serotonin in rat taste buds: Expression and localization of serotonin receptor subtypes. *Am J Physiol Regul Integr Comp Physiol, 286,* R649–658.

Kayashima, N., & Hayama, T. (1975). Reproducibility of copper sulfate emesis by oral administration in dogs. *Nippon Yakurigaku Zasshi, 71,* 169–173.

Kayashima, N., & Hayama, T. (1976). Reproducibility of emesis by orally administrated copper sulfate in cats. *Nippon Yakurigaku Zasshi, 72,* 287–291.

Keeton, R. W. (1925). Nausea and related sensations elicited by duodenal stimulation. *Arch Int Med, 35,* 687–697.

Kelly, K. A. (1977). Neural control of gastric electric and motor activity. In F. P Brooks & P. W. Evers (Eds.), *Nerves and the gut* (pp. 223–232). Thorofare, NJ: Slack.

Kenny, G. N. (1994). Risk factors for postoperative nausea and vomiting. *Anaesthesia, 49,* S6–10.

Kern, M. K., & Shaker, R. (2002). Cerebral cortical registration of subliminal visceral stimulation. *Gastroenterology, 122,* 290–298.

Keshavarzian, A., Iber, F. L., & Vaeth, J. (1987). Gastric emptying in patients with insulin-requiring diabetes mellitus. *Am J Gastroenterol, 82,* 29–35.

Kiefer, S. W., & Orr, M. R. (1992). Taste avoidance, but not aversion, learning in rats lacking gustatory cortex. *Behav Neurosci, 106,* 140–146.

Kiernan, B. D., Soykan, I., Lin, Z., Dale, A., & McCallum, R. W. (1997). A new nausea model in humans produces mild nausea without electrogastrogram and vasopressin changes. *Neurogastroenterol Motil, 9,* 257–263.

Kim, C. H., Azpiroz, F., & Malagelada, J.-R. (1986). Characteristics of spontaneous and drug-induced gastric dysrhythmias in a chronic canine model. *Gastroenterology, 90,* 421–427.

Kim, C. H., Hanson, R. B., Abell, T. L., & Malagelada, J.-R. (1989). Effect of inhibition of prostaglandin synthesis on epinephrine-induced gastroduodenal electro-mechanical changes in humans. *Mayo Clin Proceed, 64,* 149–157.

Kim, C. H., Kennedy, F. P., Camilleri, M., Zinsmeister, A. R., & Ballard, D. J. (1991). The relationship between clinical factors and gastrointestinal dysmotility in diabetes mellitus. *Gastrointestinal Motil, 3,* 268–272.

Kim, M. S., Chey, W. D., Owyang, C., & Hasler, W. L. (1997). Role of plasma vasopressin as a mediator of nausea and gastric slow wave dysrhythmias in motion sickness. *Am J Physiol Gastrointest Liver Physiol, 272,* G853–862.

Kim, T. W., Beckett, E. A. H., Hanna, R., Koh, S. D., Ördög, T., Ward, S. M., Sanders, K. M. (2002). Regulation of pacemaker frequency in the murine gastric antrum. *J Physiol (Lond), 538,* 145–157.

Kim, Y. Y., Kim, H. J., Kim, E. N., Ko, H. D., & Kim, H. T. (2005). Characteristic changes in the physiological components of cybersickness. *Psychophysiology, 42,* 616–625.

Kimeldorf, D. J., Garcia, J., & Rubadeau, D. O. (1960). Radiation-induced conditioned avoidance behavior in rats, mice, and cats. *Radiat Res, 12,* 710–718.

Kimura, M., Amino, N., Tamaki, H., Ito, E., Mitsuda, N., Miyai, K., & Tanizawa, O (1993). Gestational thyrotoxicosis and hyperemesis gravidarum: Possible role of hCG with higher stimulating activity. *Clin Endocrinol (Oxf), 38,* 345–350.

King, G. L. (1988). Characterization of radiation-induced emesis in the ferret. *Radiat Res, 114,* 599–612.

King, G. L., & Landauer, M. R. (1990). Effects of zacopride and BMY25801 (batano-pride) on radiation-induced emesis and locomotor behavior in the ferret. *J Pharmacol Exp Ther, 253,* 1026–1033.

Kinney, N. E., Wright, J. W., & Harding, J. W. (1993). Motion-induced aversions during and after recovery from olfactory nerve section in mice. *Physiol Behav, 53,* 631–633.

Kinzig, K. P., D'Alessio, D. A., & Seeley, R. J. (2002). The diverse roles of specific GLP-1 receptors in the control of food intake and the response to visceral illness. *J Neurosci, 22,* 10470–10476.

Kirsch, I. (1999). Response expectancy: An introduction. In I. Kirsch (Ed.), *How expectancies shape experience* (pp. 3–13). Washington, DC: American Psychological Association.

Klebanoff, M. A., Koslowe, P. A., Kaslow, R., & Rhoads, G. G. (1985). Epidemiology of vomiting in early pregnancy. *Obstet Gynecol, 66,* 612–616.

Klosterhalfen, S., Kellermann, S., Pan, F., Stockhorst, U., Hall, G., & Enck, P. (2005a). Effects of ethnicity and gender on motion sickness susceptibility. *Aviat Space Environ Med, 76,* 1051–1057.

Klosterhalfen, S., Kellermann, S., Stockhorst, U., Wolf, J., Kirschbaum, C., Hall, G., & Enck, P. (2005b). Latent inhibition of rotation chair-induced nausea in healthy male and female volunteers. *Psychosom Med, 67,* 335–340.

Klosterhalfen, S., Pan, F., Kellermann, S., & Enck, P. (2006). Gender and race as determinants of nausea induced by circular vection. *Gend Med, 3,* 236–242.

Knight, B., Mudge, C., Openshaw, S., White, A., & Hart, A. (2001). Effect of acupuncture on nausea of pregnancy: A randomized, control trial. *Obstet Gynecol, 97,* 184–188.

Knox, A. P., Strominger, N. L., Battles, A. H., & Carpenter, D. O. (1993). Behavioral studies of emetic sensitivity in the ferret. *Brain Res Bull, 31,* 477–484.

Ko, G. T., Chan, W. B., Chan, J. C., Tsang, L. W., & Cockram, C. S. (1999). Gastrointestinal symptoms in Chinese patients with Type 2 diabetes mellitus. *Diabet Med, 16,* 670–674.

Kobrinsky, N. L. (1988). Regulation of nausea and vomiting in cancer chemotherapy: A review with emphasis on opiate mediators. *The Am J Ped Hematol/Oncol, 103,* 209–213.

Kobrinsky, N. L., Pruden, P. B., Cheang, M. S., Levitt, M., Bishop, A. J., & Tenenbein, M. (1988). Increased nausea and vomiting induced by naloxone in patients receiving cancer chemotherapy. *The Am J Ped Hematol/Oncol, 103,* 206–208.

Koch, K. L. (1993). Motion sickness. In M. H. Sleisenger (Ed.), *The handbook of nausea and vomiting* (pp. 43–60). Pawling, NY: Caduceus Medical Publishers.

Koch, K. L. (1998). Clinical approaches to unexplained nausea and vomiting. *Adv Gastroenterol Hepatol Clin Nutr, 3,* 163–178.

Koch, K. L. (2000a). Therapy of nausea and vomiting. In M. M. Wolfe (Ed.), *Therapy of digestive disorders* (pp. 731–746). Phildaelphia: W. B. Saunders, Co.

Koch, K. L. (2000b). Unexplained nausea and vomiting. *Curr Treat Options Gastroenterol, 4,* 303–314.

Koch, K. L. (2001a). Electrogastrography: Physiological basis and clinical application in diabetic gastropathy. *Diabetes Technol Ther, 3,* 51–62.

Koch, K. L. (2001b). Nausea: An approach to a symptom. *Clin Persp Gastroenterol,* 285–297.

Koch, K. L. (2003). Diagnosis and treatment of neuromuscular disorders of the stomach. *Curr Gastroenterol Rep, 5,* 323–330.

Koch, K. L. (2006). Nausea and vomiting. In M. M. Wolfe (Ed.), *Therapy of digestive disorders* (2nd ed., pp. 1003–1117). Philadelphia: Elsevier.

Koch, K. L., & Bingaman, S. (1998). Gastric electrical activity, gastric emptying, and the water load test in evaluating patients with functional dyspepsia symptoms [Abstract]. *Am J Gastroenterol, 93,* 1642.

Koch, K. L., Bingaman, S., Xu, L., Summy-Long, J., Haberer, L. J., & Pritchard, J. F. (1996a). Effect of ondansetron on morphine-induced nausea, gastric myoelectrical activity, and plasma vasopressin levels in healthy humans. *Gastroenterology, 110,* A696.

Koch, K. L., Bingaman, S., Xu, L., Summy-Long, J., Haberer, L. J., & Pritchard, J. F. (1996b). Titrated morphine sulphate infusions: A model for inducing nausea in humans [Abstract]. *Clin Pharmacol Ther, 59,* 194.

Koch, K. L., & Frissora, C. L. (2003). Nausea and vomiting during pregnancy. *Gastroenterol Clin North Am, 32,* 201–234.

Koch, K. L., Hong, S.-P., & Xu, L. (2000). Reproducibility of gastric myoelectrical activity and the water load test in patients with dysmotility-like dyspepsia symptoms and in control subjects. *J Clin Gastroenterol, 31,* 125–129.

Koch, K. L., & Stern, R. M. (1993). Electrogastrography. In D. Kumar and D. Wingate (Eds.), *An illustrated guide to gastrointestinal motility* (pp. 290–307). London: Churchill Livingstone.

Koch, K. L., & Stern, R. M. (1994). Electrogastrographic data acquisition and analysis: The Penn State experience. In J. Z. Chen & R. W. McCallum (Eds.), *Electrogastrography: Principles and applications* (pp. 31–44). New York: Raven Press.

Koch, K. L., & Stern, R. M. (2004). *Handbook of electrogastrography.* New York: Oxford University Press.

Koch, K. L., Stern, R. M., Dwyer, A., & Vasey, M. (1987). Temporal relationships between tachygastria and symptoms of motion sickness [Abstract]. *Gastroenterology, 92,* 1473.

Koch, K. L., Stern, R. M., Stewart, W. R., & Vasey, M. W. (1989). Gastric emptying and gastric myoelectrical activity in patients with diabetic gastroparesis: Effect of long-term domperidone treatment. *Am J Gastroenterol, 84,* 1069–1075.

Koch, K. L., Stern, R. M., Vasey, M., Botti, J. J., Creasy, G. W., & Dwyer, A. (1990a). Gastric dysrhythmias and nausea of pregnancy. *Dig Dis Sci, 35,* 961–968.

Koch, K. L., Stern, R. M., Vasey, M. W., Seaton, J. F., Demers, L. M., & Harrison, T. S. (1990b). Neuroendocrine and gastric myoelectrical responses to illusory self-motion in humans. *Am J Physiol, 258,* E304–310.

Koch, K. L., Stewart, W. R., & Stern, R. M. (1987). Effects of barium meals on gastric electromechanical activity in man: A fluoroscopic-electrogastrographic study. *Dig Dis Sci, 32,* 1217–1222.

Koch, K. L., Summy-Long, J., Bingaman, S., Sperry, N., & Stern, R. M. (1990c). Vasopressin and oxytocin responses to illusory self-motion and nausea in man. *J Clin Endocrinol Metab, 71,* 1269–1275.

Koch, K. L., Xu, L., Bingaman, S., Summy-Long, J., Seton, J., Stern, R. M., Joslyn, A., & Williams, M. (1993). Effects of ondansetron on morphine-induced nausea, vasopressin, and gastric myoelectrical activity in healthy humans [Abstract]. *Gastroenterology, 104,* 535.

Koch, K. L., Xu, L., & Hong, S.-P. (2000). Spectrum of gastric dysrhythmias and gastric emptying in 54 patients with chronic unexplained nausea and vomiting [Abstract]. *Gastroenterology, 118,* 849.

Koch, K. L., Xu, L., & Noar, M. (2001). Gastric myoelectrical and emptying activity in patients with gastroesophageal reflux disease (GERD) and dysmotility-like functional dyspepsia (GERD+): Effect of water load test. *Am J Gastroenterol, 96,* 526.

Kohl, R. L. (1985). Endocrine correlates of susceptibility to motion sickness. *Aviat Space Environ Med, 56,* 1158–1165.

Kohl, R. L. (1987). Hormonal responses of metoclopramide-treated subjects experiencing nausea or emesis during parabolic flight. *Aviat Space Environ Med, 58,* A266–269.

Kohl, R. L. (1990). Endocrinology of space/motion sickness. In G. H. Crampton (Ed.), *Motion and space sickness.* Boca Raton, FL: CRC Press.

Koivuranta, M., Laara, E., Snare, L., & Alahuhta, S. (1997). A survey of postoperative nausea and vomiting. *Anaesthesia, 52,* 443–449.

Kong, M. F., & Horowitz, M. (1999). Gastric emptying in diabetes mellitus: Relationship to blood-glucose control. *Clin Geriatr Med, 15,* 321–338.

Konsman, J. P., Parnet, P., & Dantzer, R. (2002). Cytokine-induced sickness behaviour: Mechanisms and implications. *Trends Neurosci, 25,* 154–159.

Koren, G., & Bishai, R. (2000). *Nausea and vomiting of pregnancy: State of the art 2000.* Toronto: Motherisk.

Koren, G., Pastuszak, A., & Ito, S. (1998). Drugs in pregnancy. *New Engl J Med, 338,* 1128–1137.

Krane, R. V., Sinnamon, H. M., & Thomas, G. J. (1976). Conditioned taste aversions and neophobia in rats with hippocampal lesions. *Comp Physiol Psychol, 90,* 680–693.

Kraus, T., Hösl, K., Kiess, O., Schanze, A., Kornhuber, J., & Forster, C. (2007). BOLD fMRI deactivation of limbic and temporal brain structures and mood enhancing effect by transcutaneous vagus nerve stimulation. *J Neural Transm, 114,* 1485–1493.

Kreis, M. E. (2006). Postoperative nausea and vomiting. *Auton Neurosci, 129,* 86–91.

Kris, M. G. (2003). Why do we need another antiemetic? Just ask. *J Clin Oncol, 21,* 4077–4080.

Kris, M. G., Hesketh, P. J., Somerfield, M. R., Feyer, P., Clark-Snow, R., Koeller, J. M., Morrow, G. R., Chinnery, L. W., Chesney, M. J., Gralla, R. J., & Grunberg, S. M. (2006). American Society of Clinical Oncology guideline for antiemetics in oncology: Update 2006. *J Clin Oncol, 24,* 2932–2947.

Krishnamani, R., & Mahaney, W. C. (2000). Geophagy among primates: Adaptive significance and ecological consequences. *Anim Behav, 59,* 899–915.

Kucharczyk, J. (1991). Humoral factors in nausea and emesis. In J. Kucharczyk, J. D. Stewart, & A. D. Miller (Eds.), *Nausea and vomiting: Recent research and clinical advances* (pp. 59–75). Boca Raton, FL: CRC Press.

Kühn, C. G. (Ed.). (1827–1833). *Cl. Galeni, Opera Omnia* (Repografischer Nachdruck der Ausg. Leipzig, 1821–1833). (Reprinted, 1965, Hildesheim: Georg Olms).

Kuo, B., Koch, K., Chey, W. D., Wo, J. M., Sitrin, M., Hasler, W., Lackner, J., Katz, L., Landrigan, B., Selover, K., Hutson, A., Barthel, D., Semler, J., & Parkman, H. P. (2006). SmartPill, a novel ambulatory diagnostic test for measuring gastric emptying in health and disease [Abstract]. *Gastroenterology, 130,* A434.

Kuo, B., McCallum, R. W., Koch, K. L., Sitrin, M. D., Wo, J. M., Chey, W. D., Hasler, W. L., Lackner, J. M., Katz, L. A., Semler, J. R., Wilding, G. E., & Parkman, H. P. (2008). Comparison of gastric emptying of a non-digestible capsule to a radio-labeled meal in healthy and gastroparetic subjects. *Aliment Pharmacol Ther, 27,* 86–96.

Kushner, R. F., Gleason, B., & Shanta-Retelny, V. (2004). Reemergence of pica following gastric bypass surgery for obesity: A new presentation of an old problem. *J Am Diet Assoc, 104,* 1393–1397.

Kyoung, M.C., Kashyap, P. C., Dutta, N., Stoltz, G., Ördög, T., Shea-Donohue, T., Bauer, A. J., Linden, D. R., Szurszewski, J. H., Gibbons, S. J., & Farrugia, G. (2010). CD206-positive M2 macrophages that express heme oxigenase-1 protect against diabetic gastroparesis in mice. *Gastroenterology, 138,* 2399–2409.

LaBaw, W., Holton, C., Tewell, K., & Eccles, D. (1975). The use of self-hypnosis by children with cancer. *Am J Clin Hypnosis, 17,* 233–238.

Lacroix, R., Eason, E., & Melzack, R. (2000). Nausea and vomiting during pregnancy: A prospective study of its frequency, intensity, and pattern of change. *Am J Obstet Gynecol, 182,* 931–937.

Lacy, B. E., Crowell, M. D., & Koch, K. L. (2002). The Stomach: Normal function and clinical disorders. In M. M. Schuster, M. D. Crowell, & K. L. Koch (Eds.), *Atlas of gastrointestinal motility in health and disease* (pp. 135–150). Hamilton: B. C. Decker.

Lacy, B. E., & Levy, L. C. (2007). Lubiprostone: A chloride channel activator. *J Clin Gastroenterol, 41,* 345–351.

Ladabaum, U., Koshy, S. S., Woods, M. L., Hooper, F. G., Owyang, C., & Hasler, W. L. (1998). Differential symptomatic and electrogastrographic effects of distal and prox-imal human gastric distension. *Am J Physiol Gastrointest Liver Physiol, 275,* G418–424.

Ladabaum, U., Minoshima, S., Hasler, W. L., Cross, D., Chey, W. D., & Owyang, C. (2001). Gastric distension correlates with activation of multiple cortical and subcor-tical regions. *Gastroenterology, 120,* 369–376.

Ladabaum, U., Minoshima, S., & Owyang, C. (2000). Pathobiology of visceral pain: Molecular mechanisms and therapeutic implications: 5. Central nervous system processing of somatic and visceral sensory signals. *Am J Physiol Gastrointest Liver Physiol, 279,* G1–G6.

Ladabaum, U., Roberts, T. P., & McGonigle, D. J. (2007). Gastric fundic distension activates fronto-limbic structures but not primary somatosensory cortex: A func-tional magnetic resonance imaging study. *Neuroimage, 34,* 724–732.

Lamm, S. H. (2000). The epidemiological assessment of the safety and efficacy of Bendectin. In G. Koren and R. Bishai (Eds.), *Nausea and vomiting of pregnancy: State of the art 2000* (pp. 100–103). Montreal: Transcontinental Inc.

Landas, S., Fischer, J., Wilkin, L. D., Mitchell, L. D., Johnson, A.K., Turner, J. W., Theriac, M., & Moore, K. C. (1985). Demonstration of regional blood-brain barrier permeability in human brain. *Neurosci Lett, 57,* 251–256.

Landauer, M. R., Balster, R. L., & Harris, L. S. (1985). Attenuation of cyclophosph-amide-induced taste aversions in mice by prochlorperazine, delta 9-tetrahydrocan-nabinol, nabilone, and levonantradol. *Pharmacol Biochem Behav, 23,* 259–266.

Lang, I. M. (1988). Cisplatin and myoelectric activity. *Dig Dis Sci, 33,* 1342–1343.

Lang, I. M. (1990). Digestive tract motor correlates of vomiting and nausea. *Can J Physiol Pharmacol, 68,* 242–253.

Lang, I. M., Dana, N., Medda, B. K., & Shaker, R. (2002). Mechanisms of airway protection during retching, vomiting, and swallowing. *Am J Physiol Gastrointest Liver Physiol, 283,* G529–G536.

Lang, I. M., & Marvig, J. (1989). Functional localization of specific receptors mediating gastrointestinal motor correlates of vomiting. *Am J Physiol Gastrointest Liver Physiol, 256,* G92–99.

Lang, I. M., Marvig, J., & Sarna, S. K. (1988). Comparison of gastrointestinal responses to CCK-8 and associated with vomiting. *Am J Physiol Gastrointest Liver Physiol, 254,* G254–263.

Lang, I. M., Marvig, J., Sarna, S. K., & Condon, R. E. (1986). Gastrointestinal myoelectric correlates of vomiting in the dog. *Am J Physiol Gastrointest Liver Physiol, 251,* G830–838.

Lang, I. M., Sarna, S. K., and Condon, R. E. (1986). Gastrointestinal motor correlates of vomiting in the dog: Quantification and characterization as an independent phenomenon. *Gastroenterology, 90,* 4–47.

Lang, I. M., Sarna, S. K., & Dodds, W. J. (1993). Pharyngeal, esophageal, and proximal gastric responses associated with vomiting. *Am J Physiol Gastrointest Liver Physiol, 265,* G963–972.

Lang, I. M., Sarna, S. K., & Shaker, R. (1999). Gastrointestinal motor and myoelectric correlates of motion sickness. *Am J Physiol Gastrointest Liver Physiol, 277,* G642–652.

Lang, R. E., Heil, J. W., Ganten, D., Hermann, K., Unger, T., & Rascher, W. (1983). Oxytocin unlike vasopressin is a stress hormone in the rat. *Neuroendocrinology, 37,* 314–316.

Langley, J. N. (1921). *The autonomic nervous system.* Cambridge, UK: W. Heffer & Sons.

Laszlo, L. (Ed.). (1983). *Antiemetics and cancer chemotherapy.* Baltimore: Williams & Wilkins.

Lau, A. H., Kan, K. K., Lai, H. W., Ngan, M. P., Rudd, J. A., Wai, M. K., & Yew, D. T. (2005a). Action of ondansetron and CP-99,994 to modify behavior and antagonize cisplatin-induced emesis in the ferret. *Eur J Pharmacol, 506,* 241–247.

Lau, A. H., Ngan, M. P., Rudd, J. A., & Yew, D. T. (2005b). Differential action of domperidone to modify emesis and behaviour induced by apomorphine in the ferret. *Eur J Pharmacol, 516,* 247–252.

Lau, A. H., Rudd, J. A., & Yew, D. T. (2005). Action of ondansetron and CP-99, 994 on cisplatin-induced emesis and locomotor activity in Suncus murinus (house musk shrew). *Behav Pharmacol, 16,* 605–612.

Laufer, B. (1930). *Geophagy* (pp. 99–198; Field Museum Natural History Publ. 80, Anthropological Series 18). Chicago: Field Museum Natural History.

Lawal, A., Kern, M., Sanjeevi, A., Hofmann, C., & Shaker, R. (2005). Cingulate cortex: A closer look at its gut-related functional topography. *Am J Physiol Gastrointest Liver Physiol, 289,* G722–730.

Lawes, I. N. C. (1991). The central connections of the area postrema define the paraventricular system involved in antinoxious behaviours. In J. Kucharczyk, D. J. Stewart, & A. D. Miller (Eds.), *Nausea and vomiting: Recent research and clinical advances* (pp. 77–101). Boca Raton, FL: CRC Press.

Lawler, I. R., Foley, W. J., Pass, G. J., & Eschler, B. M. (1998). Administration of a 5HT3 receptor antagonist increases the intake of diets containing Eucalyptus secondary metabolites by marsupials. *J Comp Physiol B, 168,* 611–618.

Leake, C. D. (1952). *The old Egyptian medical papyri* (Logan Clendening Lectures on the History and Philosophy of Medicine, Second Series). Lawrence: University of Kansas Press. (Reprinted, 1994, Chicago: Ares Publishers).

Leatherdale, B. A., Green, D. J., Harding, L. K., Griffin, D., & Bailey, C. J. (1982). Guar and gastric emptying in non-insulin dependent diabetes. *Acta Diabetol Lat, 19,* 339–343.

Lee, A. (2006). *Adverse drug reaction* (2nd ed.). London: Pharmaceutical Press.

Lee, M., & Feldman, M. (1993). Nausea and vomiting. In M. H. Sleisenger & J. S. Fordtran (Eds.), *Gastrointestinal disease: Pathophysiology/Diagnosis/Management* (Vol. 1, pp. 509–523). Philadelphia: W. B. Sanders Company.

Lefebvre, R. A., Willems, J. L., & Bogaert, M. G. (1981). Gastric relaxation and vomiting by apomorphine, morphine, and fentanyl in the conscious dog. *Eur J Pharmacol, 69,* 139–145.

Lehmann, R., Honegger, R. A., Feinle, C., Fried, M., Spinas, G. A., & Schwizer, W. (2003). Glucose control is not improved by accelerating gastric emptying in patients with type 1 diabetes mellitus and gastroparesis; A pilot study with cisapride as a model drug. *Exp Clin Endocrinol Diabetes, 111,* 255–261.

Lentz, J. M., & Collins, W. E. (1977). Motion sickness susceptibility and related behavioral characteristics in men and women. *Aviat Space Environ Med, 48,* 316.

Lerman, Y., Sadovsky, G., Goldberg, E., Kedem, R., Peritz, E., & Pines, A. (1992). Motion sickness-like symptoms among tank simulator drivers. *Israel J Med Sci, 28,* 610–615.

Leslie, R. A. (1986). Comparative aspects of the area postrema: Fine-structural considerations help to determine its function. *Cell Mol Neurobiol, 6,* 95–120.

Leslie, R. A., McDonald, T. J., & Robertson, H. A. (1988). Autoradiographic localization of peptide YY and neuropeptide Y binding sites in the medulla oblongata. *Peptides, 9,* 1071–1076.

Leslie, R. A., Reynolds, D. J. M., & Lawes, I. N. C. (1992). Central connections of the nuclei of the vagus nerve. In S. Ritter, R. C. Ritter, & C. D. Barnes (Eds.), *Neuroanatomy and physiology of abdominal vagal afferents* (pp. 81–98). Boca Raton, FL: CRC Press.

Leventhal, H., Easterling, D. V., Nerenz, D. R., & Love, R. R. (1988). The role of motion sickness in predicting anticipatory nausea. *J Behav Med, 11,* 117–130.

Levick, J. R. (1991). *An introduction to cardiovascular physiology.* London: Butterworth & Co.

Levine, A. S., Sievert, C. E., Morley, J. E., Gosnell, B. A., & Silvis, S. E. (1984). Peptidergic regulation of feeding in the dog (Canis familiaris). *Peptides, 5,* 675–679.

Levine, M. E., Chillas, J. C., Stern, R. M., & Knox, G. W. (2000). The effects of 5-HT$_3$ receptor antagonists on gastric tachyarrhythmia and the symptoms of motion sickness. *Aviat Space Environ Med, 71,* 1111–1114.

Levine, M. E., Gillis, M., Koch, S. Y., Voss, A. C., Stern, R. M., & Koch, K. L. (2008). Protein and ginger for the treatment of chemotherapy-induced delayed nausea and gastric dysrhythmia. *J Altern Complement Med, 14,* 545–551.

Levine, M. E., Muth, E. R., Williamson, M. J., & Stern, R. M. (2004). Protein-predominant meals inhibit the development of gastric tachyarrhythmias, nausea, and the symptoms of motion sickness. *Aliment Pharmacol Ther, 19,* 583–590.

Levine M. E., Stern, R. M., & Koch, K. L. (2006). The effects of manipulating expectations through placebo and nocebo administration on gastric tachyarrhythmia and motion-induced nausea. *Psychosom Med, 68,* 478–486.

Levine, M. G., & Esser, D. (1988). Total parenteral nutrition for the treatment of severe hyperemesis gravidarum: Maternal nutritional effects and fetal outcome. *Obstet Gynecol, 72,* 102–107.

Levitt, M., Warr, D., Yelle, L., Rayner, H. L., Lofters, W. S., Perrault, D. J.,Wilson, K. S., Latreille, J., Potvin, M., Warner, E., Pritchard, K. I., Palmer, M., Zee, B., & Pater, J. L. (1993). Ondansetron compared with dexamethasone and metoclopramide as antiemetics in the chemotherapy of breast cancer with cyclophosphamide, methotrexate, and fluorouracil. *N Engl J Med, 328,* 1081–1084.

Levy, R. A., Jones, D. R., & Carlson, E. H. (1981). Biofeedback rehabilitation of airsick aircrew. *Aviat Space Environ Med, 52,* 118.

Lewis, J. J., & Crossland, J. (1970). *Lewis's Pharmacology* (4th ed.). Baltimore: Williams and Wilkins.

Lewis, T. (1942). *Pain.* London: Macmillan.

Li, X., Jiang, Z. L., Wang, G. H., & Fan, J. W. (2005). Plasma vasopressin, an etiologic factor of motion sickness in rat and human? *Neuroendocrinology, 81,* 351–359.

Liau, C. T., Chu, N. M., Liu, H. E., Deuson, R., Lien, J., & Chen, J. S. (2005). Incidence of chemotherapy-induced nausea and vomiting in Taiwan: Physicians' and nurses' estimation vs. patients' reported outcomes. *Support Care Cancer, 13,* 277–286.

Liberski, S. M., Koch, K. L., Atnip, R. G., & Stern, R. M. (1990) Ischemic gastroparesis: Resolution after revascularization. *Gastroenterology, 99,* 252–257.

Lidell, H. G., Scott, R., & Jones, H. S. (1968). *A Greek-English lexicon.* Oxford: Clarendon Press.

Lien, H. C., Sun, W. M., Chen, Y. H., Kim, H., Hasler, W., & Owyang, C. (2003). Effects of ginger on motion sickness and gastric slow-wave dysrhythmias induced by circular vection. *Am J Physiol Gastrointest Liver Physiol, 284,* G481–489.

Limebeer, C. L., Litt, D. E., & Parker, L. A. (2009). Effect of 5-HT(3) antagonist and a 5-HT(1A) agonist on fluoxetine-induced conditioned gaping reactions in rats. *Psychopharmacology (Berl), 203,* 763–770.

Limebeer, C. L., & Parker, L. A. (1999). Delta-9-tetrahydrocannabinol interferes with the establishment and the expression of conditioned rejection reactions produced by cyclophosphamide: A rat model of nausea. *Neuroreport, 10,* 3769–3772.

Limebeer, C. L., & Parker, L. A. (2000). The antiemetic drug ondansetron interferes with lithium-induced conditioned rejection reactions, but not lithium-induced taste avoidance in rats. *J Exp Psychol Anim Behav Process, 26,* 371–384.

Limebeer, C. L., & Parker, L. A. (2003). The 5-HT1A agonist 8-OH-DPAT dose-dependently interferes with the establishment and the expression of lithium-induced conditioned rejection reactions in rats. *Psychopharmacology (Berl), 166,* 120–126.

Lin, C., Chen, J. D. Z., Schirmer, B. D., & McCallum, R. W. (2000). Postprandial response of gastric slow waves: Correlation of serosal recordings with the electrogastrogram. *Dig Dis Sci, 45,* 645–651.

Lin, Z., Sarosiek, I., Forster, J., & McCallum, R. W. (2006). Symptom responses, long-term outcomes, and adverse events beyond 3 years of high-frequency gastric electrical stimulation for gastroparesis. *Neurogastroenterol Motil, 18,* 18–27.

Lin, Z. Y., McCallum, R. W., Schirmer, B. D., & Chen, J. D. Z. (1998). Effects of pacing parameters in the entrainment of gastric slow waves in patients with gastroparesis. *Am J Physiol Gastrointest Liver Physiol, 274,* G186–G191.

Lindberg, G., Nordesjö, G., & Hellström-Lindberg, E. (1996). Nausea during intensive chemotherapy is not associated with tachygastria [Abstract]. *Neurogastroenterol Motil, 20,* 180.

Lindquist, N., & Hay, M. E. (1995). Can small rare prey be chemically defended? The case for marine larvae. *Ecology, 76,* 1347–1358.

Liu, J., Kashimura, S., Hara, K., & Zhang, G. (2001). Death following cupric sulphate emesis. *J Toxicol Clin Toxicol, 39,* 161–163.

Liu, Q., Yang, Q., Sun, W., Vogel, P., Heydorn, W., Yu, X-Q., Hu, Z., Yu, W., Jonas, B., Pineda, R., Calderon-Gay, V., Germann, M., O'Neill, E., Brommage, R., Cullinan, E., Platt, K., Wilson, A., Powell, D., Sands, A., Zambrowicz, B., & Shi, Z. (2008). Discovery and characterisation of novel tryptophan hydroxylase inhibitors that selectively inhibit serotonin synthesis in the gastrointestinal tract. *J Pharmacol Exp Ther, 325,* 47–55.

Liu, Y. L., Malik, N. M., Sanger, G. J., & Andrews, P. L. (2006). Ghrelin alleviates cancer chemotherapy-associated dyspepsia in rodents. *Cancer Chemother Pharmacol, 58,* 326–333.

Liu, Y. L., Malik, N., Sanger, G. J., Friedman, M. I., & Andrews, P. L. R. (2005). Pica: A model of nausea? Species differences in response to cisplatin. *Physiol Behav, 85,* 271–277.

Lockette, W., & Farrow, S. (1993). Characteristics of a genetic polymorphism associated with development of motion sickness. *Aviat Space Environ Med, 64,* 454.

Lockwood, D. R., Kwon, B., Smith, J. C., & Houpt, T. A. (2003). Behavioral effects of static high magnetic fields on unrestrained and restrained mice. *Physiol Behav, 78,* 635–640.

Loewy, A. D. (1990a). Anatomy of the autonomic nervous system: An overview. In A. D. Loewy & K. M. Spyer (Eds.), *Central regulation of autonomic functions* (pp. 3–16). New York: Oxford University Press.

Loewy, A. D. (1990b). Central autonomic pathways. In A. D. Loewy & K. M. Spyer (Eds.), *Central regulation of autonomic functions* (pp. 88–103). New York: Oxford University Press.

Logue, A. W. (1991). *The psychology of eating and drinking.* New York: W. H. Freeman.

Lopez, L. B., Ortega Soler, C. R., & de Portela, M. L. (2004). Pica during pregnancy: A frequently underestimated problem. *Arch Latinoam Nutr, 54,* 17–24.

Lu, C. L., Wu, Y. T., Yeh, T. C., Chen, L. F., Chang, F. Y., Lee, S. D., Ho, L. T., & Hsideh, J. C. (2004). Neuronal correlates of gastric pain induced by fundus distension: A 3T-fMRI study. *Neurogastroenterol Motil, 16,* 575–587.

Lucertini, M., & Lugli, V. (2004). The Italian Air Force rehabilitation programme for air-sickness. *Acta Otorhinolaryngol Ital, 24,* 181–187.

Lucot, J. B. (1998). Pharmacology of motion sickness. *J Vestib Res, 18,* 61–66.

Lucot, J. B., Obach, R. S., McLean, S., & Watson, J. W. (1997). The effect of CP-99,994 on the responses to provocative motion in the cat. *Br J Pharmacol, 120,* 116–120.

Lumsden, K., & Holden, W. S. (1969). The act of vomiting in man. *Gut, 10,* 173–179.

Lurken, M. S., Kashyap, P., Parkman, H. P., Abell, T. L., Hasler, W. L., Koch, K. L., Pasricha, P. J., Tonascia, J., Smyrk, T. C., Hamilton, F. A., & Farrugia, G. (2008). The pathological basis of gastroparesis. *Gastroenterology 134,* P254.

MacGregor, I. L., Gueller, R., Watts, H. D., & Meyer, J. H. (1976). The effect of acute hyperglycemia on gastric emptying in man. *Gastroenterology, 70,* 190–196.

Magee, L. A., Mazzotta, P., & Koren, G. (2002). Evidence-based view of safety and effectiveness of pharmacologic therapy for nausea and vomiting of pregnancy (NVP). *Am. J Obstet Gynecol, 186,* S256–261.

Mahadevan, U., & Kane, S. (2006). American gastroenterological association institute medical position statement on the use of gastrointestinal medications in pregnancy. *Gastroenterology, 131,* 278–282.

Maleki, D., Locke, G. R., Camilleri, M., Zinsmeister, A. R., Yawn, B. P., Leibson, C., & Melton, I. J. (2000). Gastrointestinal tract symptoms among persons with diabetes mellitus in the community. *Arch Intern Med, 160,* 2808–2816.

Malik, N. M., Liu, Y. L., Cole, N., Sanger, G. J., & Andrews, P. L. R. (2007). Differential effects of dexamethasone, ondansetron, and a tachykinin NK1 receptor antagonist (GR205171) on cisplatin-induced changes in behaviour, food intake, pica, and gastric function in rats. *Eur J Pharmacol, 555,* 164–173.

Malik, N. M., Moore, G. B., Kaur, R., Liu, Y. L., Wood, S. L., Morrow, R. W., Sanger, G. J., & Andrews, P. L. R. (2008). Adaptive upregulation of gastric and hypothalamic ghrelin receptors and increased plasma ghrelin in a model of cancer chemotherapy-induced dyspepsia. *Regul Pept, 148,* 33–38.

Malik, N. M., Moore, G. B., Smith, G., Liu, Y. L., Sanger, G. J., & Andrews, P. L. R. (2006). Behavioural and hypothalamic molecular effects of the anti-cancer agent cisplatin in the rat: A model of chemotherapy-related malaise? *Pharmacol Biochem Behav, 83,* 9–20.

Manning, A., & Stamp Dawkins, M. (1998). *An introduction to animal behaviour.* Cambridge, UK: Cambridge University Press.

Marchioro, G., Azzarello, G., Viviani, F., Barbato, F., Pavanetto, M., Rosetti, F., Pappagallo, G. L., & Vinante, O. (2000). Hypnosis in the treatment of anticipatory nausea and vomiting in patients receiving cancer chemotherapy. *Oncology, 59,* 100–104.

Marino, L. (2007). Cetacean brains: How aquatic are they? *Anat Rec (Hoboken), 290,* 694–700.

Markham, C., Diamond, S. G., & Treciokas, L. J. (1974). Carbidopa in Parkinson disease and in nausea and vomiting of levodopa. *Arch Neurol, 31,* 128–133.

Marks, P. J., Vipond, I. B., Carlisle, D., Deakin, D., Fey, R. E., & Caul, E. O. (2000). Evidence for airborne transmission of Norwalk-like virus (NLV) in a hotel restaurant. *Epidemiol Infect, 124,* 481–487.

Marsh, K. J., Wallis, I. R., & Foley, W. J. (2007). Behavioral contributions to the regulated intake of plant secondary metabolites in koalas. *Oecologia, 154,* 283–290.

Marsland, A. L., Gianaros, P. J., Prather, A. A., Jennings, J. R., Neumann, S. A., & Manuck, S. B. (2007). Stimulated production of proinflammatory cytokines covaries inversely with heart rate variability. *Psychosom Med, 69,* 709–716.

Marten, P. A., Brown, T. A., Barlow, D. H., Borkovec, T. D., Shear, K. M., & Lydiard, R. B. (1993). Evaluation of the ratings comprising the associated symptom criterion of DSM-III-R Generalized Anxiety Disorder. *J Nerv Ment Dis, 181,* 676–682.

Martin, R. D. (2007). The evolution of human reproduction: A primatological perspective. *Am J Phys Anthropol* (Suppl. 45), 59–84.

Martin, R. P., Wisenbaker, J., & Huttunen, M. O. (1999). Nausea during pregnancy: Relation to early childhood temperament behavioral problems at 12 years. *J Abnor Child Psychol, 27,* 323–329.

MASCC (2004). Multinational Association of Supportive Care in Cancer, Antiemesis Tool: Instructions. Metairie, LA: Author.

Masson, G. M., Anthony, F., & Chau, E. (1985). Serum chorionic gonadotropin (hCG) schwangerschaftsprotein one (sp1), progesterone, and oestradiol levels in patients with nausea and vomiting in early pregnancy. *Br J Obstet Gynaecol, 92,* 211–215.

Mathews, A. (1990). The cognitive function of anxiety. *Behav Res Ther, 28,* 455–468.

Mathias, J. R., & Clench, M. H. (1998). Relationship of reproductive hormones and neuromuscular disease of the gastrointestinal tract. *Dig Dis, 16,* 3–13.

Matsuki, N., Ueno, S., Kaji, T., Ishihara, A., Wang, C. H., & Saito, H. (1988). Emesis induced by cancer chemotherapeutic agents in the Suncus murinus: A new experimental model. *Jpn J Pharmacol, 48,* 303–306.

Matsumoto, S., Kawasaki, Y., Mikami, M., Nakamoto, M., Tokuyasu, H., Kometani, Y., Chikumi, H., Hitsuda, Y., Matsumoto, Y., & Sasaki, T. (1999). [Relationship between cancer chemotherapeutic drug-induced delayed emesis and plasma levels of substance P in two patients with small cell lung cancer]. *Gan To Kagaku Ryoho, 26,* 535–538.

Matthews, L. H. (1949). The origin of stomach oil in the petrels, with comparative observations on the avian proventriculus. *The Ibis, 91,* 373–392.

Mattsson, J. L., & Yochmowitz, M. G. (1980). Radiation-induced emesis in monkeys. *Radiat Res, 82,* 191–199.

Max, B. (1992). This and that: The essential pharmacology of herbs and spices. *Trends in Pharmacol Sci, 13,* 15–20.

Mazda, T., Yamamoto, H., Fujimura, M., & Fujimiya, M. (2004). Gastric distension-induced release of 5-HT stimulates c-fos expression in specific brain nuclei via 5-HT3 receptors in conscious rats. *Am J Physiol Gastrointest Liver Physiol, 287,* G228–235.

Mazzotta, P., & Magee, L. A. (2000). A risk-benefit assessment of pharmacological and non-pharmacological treatments for nausea and vomiting of pregnancy. *Drugs, 59,* 781–800.

Mazzotta, P., Stewart, D., Atanackovic, G., Koren, G., & Magee, L. A. (2000). Psychosocial morbidity among women with NVP: Prevalence and association with anti-emetic therapy. *J Psychosom Obstet Gynecol, 21,* 129–136.

McAllister, K. H., & Pratt, J. A. (1998). GR205171 blocks apomorphine and amphetamine-induced conditioned taste aversions. *Eur J Pharmacol, 353,* 141–148.

McCaffrey, R. J. (1985). Appropriateness of kaolin consumption as an index of motion sickness in the rat. *Physiol Behav, 35,* 151–156.

McCaffrey, R. J., & Graham, G. (1980). Age-related differences for motion sickness in the rat. *Exp Aging Res, 6,* 555–561.

McCallum, R., Lin, Z., Wetzel, P., Sarosiek, I., & Forster, J. (2005). Clinical response to gastric electrical stimulation in patients with post surgical gastroparesis. *Clin Gastroenterol Hepatol, 3,* 49–54.

McCallum, R. W., Chen, J. D. Z., Lin, Z., Schirmer, B., Williams, R., & Ross, R. (1998). Gastric pacing improves emptying and symptoms in patients with gastroparesis. *Gastroenterology, 114,* 456–461.

McCann, M. J., Verbalis, J. G., & Stricker, E. M. (1989). LiCl and CCK inhibit gastric emptying and feeding and stimulate OT secretion in rats. *Am J Physiol Regul Integr Comp Physiol, 256,* R463–468.

McCarthy, L. E., & Borison, H. L. (1984). Cisplatin-induced vomiting eliminated by ablation of the area postrema in cats. *Cancer Treat Rep, 68,* 401–404.

McClure, J. A., & Fregly, A. R. (1972). Effect of environmental temperature on sweat onset during motion sickness. *Aerosp Med, 43,* 959–967.

McCutcheon, B., Ballard, M., & McCaffrey, R. J. (1992). Intraperitoneally injected cholecystokinin-octapeptide activates pica in rats. *Physiol Behav, 51,* 543–547.

McKeigue, P. M., Lamm, S. H., Linn, S., & Kutcher, J. S. (1994). Bendectin and birth defects: 1. A meta-analysis of the epidemiologic studies. *Teratology, 50,* 27–37.

McLellan, D. L., & Park, D. M. (1973). Failure to vomit in hereditary ataxia: Report of a family. *Neurology, 23,* 725–728.

McMahon, L. R., & Wellman, P. J. (1997). Decreased intake of a liquid diet in nonfood-deprived rats following intra-PVN injections of GLP-1 (7–36) amide. *Pharmacol Biochem Behav, 58,* 673–677.

McMillan, S. C. (1989). The relationship between age and intensity of cancer-related symptoms. *Oncol Nurs Forum, 16,* 237–241.

McMurray, G. A. (1950). Experimental study of a case of insensitivity to pain. *AMA Arch Neurol Psychiatry, 64,* 650–667.

Megens, A. A., Ashton, D., Vermeire, J. C., Vermote, P. C., Hens, K. A., Hillen, L. C., Fransen, J. F., Mahieu, M., Heylen, L., Leysen, J. E., Jurzak, M. R., & Janssens, F. (2002). Pharmacological profile of (2r-trans)-4-[1-[3,5-bis(trifluromethyl)benzoyl]-2-(phenylmethyl)-4-piperidinyl]-n-(2,6-dimethylphenyl)-1-acetamide (s)-hydroxyb-utanedioate (R116301), an orally and centrally active neurokinin-a receptor antagonist. *J Pharmacol Exp Ther, 302,* 696–709.

Mehendale, S., Aung, H., Wang, C. Z., Tong, R., Foo, A., Xie, J. T., & Yuan, C. S. (2007). Scutellaria baicalensis and a constituent falvinoid baicalein, attenuate ritanovir-induced gastrointestinal side-effects. *J Pharm Pharmacol, 59,* 1567–1572.

Mehendale, S., Aung, H., Wang, A., Yin, J. J., Wang, C. Z., Xie, J. T., & Yuan, C. S. (2005). American ginseng berry extract and ginsenoside attenuate cisplatin-induced kaolin intake in rats. *Cancer Chemother Pharmacol, 56,* 63–69.

Mehendale, S. R., Aung, H. H., Yin, J. J., Lin, E., Fishbein, A., Wang, C. Z., Xie, J. T., & Yuan, C. S. (2004). Effects of antioxidant herbs on chemotherapy-induced nausea and vomiting in a rat-pica model. *Am J Chin Med, 32,* 897–905.

Mele, P. C., McDonough, J. R., McLean, D. B., & O'Halloran, K. P. (1992). Cisplatin-induced conditioned taste aversion: Attenuation by dexamethasone but not zaco-pride or GR38032F. *Eur J Pharmacol, 218,* 229–236.

Melzack R., Rosberger, Z., Hollingsworth, M. L., & Thirwell, M. (1985). New approaches to measuring nausea. *CMAJ, 133,* 755–758, 761.

Merck. (2003). *Emend* [Technical report 9565000]. Whitehouse Station, NJ: Merck & Co.

Merck. (2010). Retrieved January 16, 2010, from http://www.merck.com/product/usa/pi_circulars/e/emend/emend_pi.pdf

Miaskiewicz, S. L., Stricker, E. M., & Verbalis, J. G. (1989). Neurohypophyseal secretion in response to cholecystokinin but not meal-induced gastric distention in humans. *J Clin Endocrinol Metab, 68,* 837–843.

Michl, T., Jocic, M., Schuligoi, R., & Holzer, P. (2001). Role of tachykinin receptors in the central processing of afferent input from the acid-threatened rat stomach. *Regul Pept, 102,* 119–126.

Migdalis, L., Thomaides, T., Chairopoulos, C., Kalogeropoulou, C., Charalabides, J., & Mantzara, F. (2001). Changes of gastric emptying rate and gastrin levels are early indicators of autonomic neuropathy in type II diabetic patients. *Clin Auton Res, 11,* 259–263.

Milano, S., Blower, P., Romain, D., & Grelot, L. (1995). The piglet as a suitable animal model for studying the delayed phase of cisplatin-induced emesis. *J Pharmacol Exp Ther, 274,* 951–961.

Miller, A. D. (1991). Motion-induced nausea and vomiting. In J. Kucharczyk, D. J. Stewart, & A. D. Miller (Eds.), *Nausea and vomiting: Recent research and clinical advances* (pp. 13–41). Boca Raton, FL: CRC Press.

Miller, A. D. (1993). Neuroanatomy and physiology. In M. H. Sleisenger (Ed.), *Handbook of nausea and vomiting* (pp. 1–9). New York: Parthenon.

Miller, A. D., & Leslie, R. A. (1994). The area postrema and vomiting. *Front Neuroendocrinol, 15,* 301–320.

Miller, A. D., Nonaka, S., Siniaia, M. S., & Jakus, J. (1995). Multifunctional ventral respiratory group: Bulbospinal expiratory neurons play a role in pudendal discharge during vomiting. *J Auton Nerv Syst, 54,* 253–260.

Miller, A. D., Rowley, H. A., Roberts, T. P., & Kucharczyk, J. (1996). Human cortical activity during vestibular- and drug-induced nausea detected using MSI. *Ann N Y Acad Sci, 781,* 670–672.

Miller, K. E., & Muth, E. R. (2004). Efficacy of acupressure and acustimulation bands for the prevention of motion sickness. *Aviat Space Environ Med, 75,* 227–234.

Mintchev, M. P., & Bowes, K. L. (1994). Capabilities and limitations of electrogastrograms. In J. Z. Chen & R. W. McCallum (Eds.), *Electrogastrography: Principles and applications* (pp. 155–169). New York: Raven Press.

Mintchev, M. P., Kingma, Y. J., & Bowes, K. L. (1993). Accuracy of cutaneous recordings of gastric electrical activity. *Gastroenterology, 104,* 1273–1280.

Mintchev, M. P., Sanmiguel, C.P., Otto, S.J., & Bowles, K. L. (1998). Microprocessor controlled movement of liquid gastric content using sequential neural electrical stimulation. *Gut, 43,* 607–611.

Minton, N., Swift, R., Lawlor, C., Mant, T., & Henry, J. (1993). Ipecacuanha-induced emesis: A human model for testing antiemetic drug activity. *Clin Pharmacol Ther, 54,* 53–57.

Mircic, G., Jankovic, S., & Beleslin, D. (1998). Differences in the effects of vasopressin and oxytocin on feline gastric corpus motility: Selective action of vasopressin on longitudinal muscle. *Pharmacol Res, 37,* 383–394.

Mitchell, D. (1976). Experiments on neophobia in wild and laboratory rats: A reevaluation. *J Comp Physiol Psychol, 90,* 190–197.

Mitchell, D., Beatty, E. T., & Cox, P. K. (1977). Behavioral differences between two populations of wild rats: Implications for domestication research. *Behav Biol, 19,* 206–216.

Mitchell, D., Krusemark, M. L., & Hafner, D. (1977). Pica: A species relevant behavioral assay of motion sickness in the rat. *Physiol Behav, 18,* 125–130.

Mitchell, D., Laycock, J. D., & Stephens, W. F. (1977). Motion sickness-induced pica in the rat. *Am J Clin Nutr, 30,* 147–150.

Mitchell, D., Wells, C., Hoch, N., Lind, K., Woods, S. C., & Mitchell, L. K. (1976). Poison induced pica in rats. *Physiol Behav, 17,* 691–697.

Mitchell, D., Winter, W., & Morisaki, C. M. (1977). Conditioned taste aversions accompanied by geophagia: Evidence for the occurrence of "psychological" factors in the etiology of pica. *Psychosom Med, 39,* 401–412.

Mjörnheim, A. C., Finizia, C., Blohmé, G., Attvall, S., Lundell, L., & Ruth, M. (2003). Gastrointestinal symptoms in type 1 diabetic patients, as compared in a general population: A questionnaire-based study. *Digestion, 68,* 102–108.

Mogil, J. S. (2009). Animal models of pain: Progress and challenges. *Nat Rev Neurosci, 10,* 283–294.

Mokri, B. (2004). Spontaneous low cerebrospinal pressure/volume headaches. *Curr Neurol Neurosci Rep, 4,* 117–124.

Moldovan, C., Dumitrascu, D. L., Demian, L., Brisc, C., Vatca, L., & Magheru, S. (2005). Gastroparesis in diabetes mellitus: An ultrasonographic study. *Rom J Gastroenterol, 14,* 19–22.

Money, K. E. (1990). Motion sickness and evolution. In G. H. Crampton (Ed.), *Motion and space sickness* (pp. 1–7). Boca Raton, FL: CRC Press.

Money, K. E., & Cheung, B. S. (1983). Another function of the inner ear: Facilitation of the emetic response to poisons. *Aviat Space Environ Med, 54,* 208–211.

Monnier, L., Lapinski, H., & Colette, C. (2003). Contributions of fasting and postprandial plasma glucose increments to the overall diurnal hyperglycemia of type 2 diabetic patients: Variations with increasing levels of HbA(1c). *Diabetes Care, 26,* 881–885.

Monstein, H. J., Truedsson, M., Ryberg, A., & Ohlsson, B. (2008). Vasopressin receptor mRNA expression in the human gastrointestinal tract. *Eur Surg Res, 40,* 34–40.

Montana, J. G., Buckley, G. M., Cooper, N., Dyke, H. J., Gowers, L., Gregory, J. P., Hellewell, P. G., Kendall, H. J., Lowe, C., Maxey, R., Miotla, J., Naylor, R. J., Runcie, K. A., Tuladhar, B., & Warneck, J. B. (1998). Aryl sulfonamides as selective PDE4 inhibitors. *Bioorg Med Chem Lett, 8,* 2635–2640.

Morest, D. K. (1960). A study of the structure of the area postrema with Golgi methods. *Am J Anat, 107,* 291–303.

Morgan, C. L. (1894). *An introduction to comparative psychology.* London: W. Scott.

Mori, M., Amino, N., Tamaki, H., Miyai, K., & Tanizawa, O. (1988). Morning sickness and thyroid function in normal pregnancy. *Obstet Gynecol, 72,* 355–359.

Morita, M., Takeda, N., Kubo, T., & Matsunaga, T. (1988a). Pica as an index of motion sickness in rats. *ORL J Otorhinolaryngol Relat Spec, 50,* 188–192.

Morita, M., Takeda, N., Kubo, T., Yamatodani, A., Wada, H., & Matsunaga, T. (1988b). Effects of anti-motion sickness drugs on motion sickness in rats. *ORL J Otorhinolaryngol Relat Spec, 50,* 330–333.

Morrow, G. R. (1984a). Methodology in behavioral and psychosocial cancer research: The assessment of nausea and vomiting; Past problems, current issues, and suggestions for future research. *Cancer, 53,* 2267–2280.

Morrow, G. R. (1984b). Susceptibility to motion sickness and the development of anticipatory nausea and vomiting in cancer patients undergoing chemotherapy. *Cancer Treat Rep, 68,* 1177–1178.

Morrow, G. R. (1985). The effect of a susceptibility to motion sickness on the side effects of cancer chemotherapy. *Cancer, 55,* 2766–2770.

Morrow, G. R. (1989). Chemotherapy-related nausea and vomiting: Etiology and management. *Cancer, 39,* 89–104.

Morrow, G. R. (1992) A patient report measure for the quantification of chemotherapy induced nausea and emesis: Psychometric properties of the Morrow assessment of nausea and emesis (MANE). *Br J Cancer Suppl, 66,* S72–S74.

Morrow, G. R. (1993). Psychological aspects of nausea and vomiting: Anticipation of chemotherapy. In M. H. Sleisenger (Ed.), *Handbook of nausea and vomiting* (pp. 11–25). New York: Parthenon.

Morrow, G. R., Andrews, P. L. R., Hickok, J. T., & Stern, R. (2000). Vagal changes following cancer chemotherapy: Implications for the development of nausea. *Psychophysiology, 37,* 378–384.

Morrow, G. R., Angel, C., & DuBeshter, B. (1992). Autonomic changes during cancer chemotherapy induced nausea and emesis. *Br J Cancer* (Suppl. 19), S42–45.

Morrow, G. R., & Dobkin, P. L. (1988). Anticipatory nausea and vomiting in cancer patients undergoing chemotherapy treatment: Prevalence, etiology, and behavioral interventions. *Clin Psychol Rev, 8,* 517–556.

Morrow, G. R., Hickok, J. T., Andrews, P. L. R., & Stern, R. M. (2002a) Reduction in serum cortisol after platinum based chemotherapy for cancer: A role for the HPA axis in treatment-related nausea? *Psychophysiology, 39,* 491–495.

Morrow, G. R., Hickok, J. T., DuBeshter, B., & Lipshultz, S. E. (1999). Changes in clinical measures of autonomic nervous system function related to cancer chemotherapy-induced nausea. *J Auton Nerv Syst, 78,* 57–63.

Morrow, G. R., & Morrell, C. (1982). Behavioral treatment for the anticipatory nausea and vomiting induced by cancer chemotherapy. *N Engl J Med, 307,* 1476–1480.

Morrow, G. R., Roscoe, J. A., Hickok, J. T., Andrews, P. L. R., & Matteson, S. (2002b). Nausea and emesis: Evidence for a biobehavioral perspective. *Support Care Cancer, 10,* 96–105.

Morrow, G. R., & Rosenthal, S. N. (1996). Models, mechanisms, and management of anticipatory nausea and emesis. *Oncology, 53*(Suppl. 1), 4–7.

Morrow, G. R., Waight, J., & Black, P. M. (1991). Anticipatory nausea development in cancer patients: Replication and extension of a learning model. *Br J Psychol, 82,* 61–72.

Morton, D. B., & Griffiths, P. H. (1985). Guidelines on the recognition of pain, distress, and discomfort in experimental animals and a hypothesis for assessment. *Vet Rec, 116,* 431–436.

Moulton, E. A., Burstein, R., Tully, S., Hargreaves, R., Becerra, L., & Borsook, D. (2008). Interictal dysfunction of a brainstem descending modulatory center in migraine patients. *PLosOne, 3,* e3799.

Mowrey, D. B., & Clayson, D. E. (1982). Motion sickness, ginger, and psychophysics. *Lancet, 1*(8273), 655–657.

Muth, E. R. (2006) Motion and space sickness: Intestinal and autonomic correlates. *Auton Neurosci, 129,* 58–66.

Muth, E. R., Stern, R. M., & Koch, K. L. (1996). Effects of vection-induced motion sickness on gastric myoelectric activity and oral-cecal transit time. *Dig Dis Sci, 41,* 330–334.

Muth, E. R., Stern, R. M., Thayer, J. F., & Koch, K. L. (1996) Assessment of the multiple dimensions of nausea: The Nausea Profile. *J Psychosom Res, 40,* 511–520.

Muth, E. R., Stern, R. M., Uijtdehaage, S. H. J., & Koch, K. L. (1994). Effects of Asian ancestry on susceptibility to vection-induced motion sickness. In J. Z. Chen & R. W. McCallum (Eds.), *Electrogastrography: Principles and applications* (pp. 227–234). New York: Raven Press.

Nachman, M., & Ashe, J. H. (1974). Effects of basolateral amygdala lesions on neophobia, learned taste aversions, and sodium appetite in rats. *J Comp Physiol Psychol, 87,* 622–643.

Naitoh, T., & Wassersug, R. J. (1992). The emetic response of urodel amphibians. *Zoolog Sci, 9,* 713–718.

Naitoh, T., Wassersug, R. J., & Leslie, R. A. (1989). The physiology, morphology, and ontogeny of emetic behavior in anuran amphibians. *Physiolog Zool, 62,* 819–843.

Narayanan, J. T., Watts, R., Haddad, N., Labar, D. R., Li, P. M., & Filippi, C. G. (2002). Cerebral activation during vagus nerve stimulation: A functional MR study. *Epilepsia, 43,* 1509–1514.

Navari, R. M. (2003). Pathogenesis-based treatment of chemotherapy-induced nausea and vomiting: Two new agents. *J Support Oncol, 1,* 89–103.

Navari, R., Gandara, D., Hesketh, P., Hall, S., Mailliard, J., Ritter, H., Friedman, C., & Fitts, D. (1995a). Comparative clinical trial of granisetron and ondansetron in the prophylaxis of cisplatin-induced emesis: The Granisetron Study Group. *J Clin Oncol, 13,* 1242–1248.

Navari, R. M., Madajewicz, S., Anderson, N., Tchekmedyian, N. S., Whaley, W., Garewal, H., Beck, T. M., Chang, A. Y., Greenberg, B., Caldwell, K. C. et al. (1995b). Oral ondansetron for the control of ciplatin-induced delayed emesis: A large, multicenter, double-blind, randomized comparative trial of ondansetron versus placebo. *J Clin Oncol, 13*, 2408–2416.

NCI (2009). Acute/Delayed emesis etiology [updated October 2, 2009]. Retrieved January 16, 2010, from http://www.cancer.gov/cancertopics/pdq/supportivecare/nausea/HealthProfessional/page6

Neidhart, J. A., Gagen, M., Wilson, H. E., & Young, D. C. (1981). Comparative trial of the antiemetic effects of THC and haloperidol. *J Clin Pharmacol, 21*, 38s–42s.

Nesse R. M., & Williams G. C. (1998). Evolution and the origins of disease. *Scientific American, 279*, 86–93.

Newson, B., Ahlman, H., Dahlstrom, A., & Nyhus, L. M. (1982). Ultrastructural observations in the rat ileal mucosa of possible epithelial "taste cells" and submucosal sensory neurons. *Acta Physiol Scand, 114*, 161–164.

Newson, B., Ahlman, H., Dahlstrom, A., Das Gupta, T. K., & Nyhus, L. M. (1979). Are there sensory neurons in the mucosa of the mammalian gut? *Acta Physiol Scand, 105*, 521–523.

Neymark, N., & Crott, R. (2005). Impact of emesis on clinical and economic outcomes of cancer therapy with highly emetogenic chemotherapy regimens: A retrospective analysis of three clinical trials. *Support Care Cancer, 10*, 812–818.

Niedringhaus, M., Jackson, P. G., Evans, S. R., Verbalis, J. G., Gillis, R. A., & Sahibzada, N. (2008a). Dorsal motor nucleus of the vagus: A site for evoking simultaneous changes in crural diaphragm activity, lower esophageal sphincter pressure, and fundus tone. *Am J Physiol Regul Integr Comp Physiol, 294*, R121–131.

Niedringhaus, M., Jackson, P. G., Pearson, R., Shi, M., Dretchen, K., Gillis, R. A., & Sahibzada, N. (2008b). Brainstem sites controlling the lower esophageal sphincter and crural diaphragm in the ferret: A neuroanatomical study. *Auton Neurosci, 144*, 50–60.

Niijima, A., & Yamamoto, T. (1994). The effects of lithium chloride on the activity of the afferent nerve fibres from the abdominal visceral organs in the rat. *Brain Res Bull, 35*, 141–145.

Noar, M. K., & Koch, K. L. (2003). Effect of radiofrequency ablation on gastric dysrhythmias and gastric emptying in patients with gastroesophageal reflux disease (GERD) and functional dyspepsia [Abstract]. *Gastroenterology, 124*, A98.

Noar, M. D., Koch, K. L., & Levine, M. (2004). Functional gastric outlet obstruction detected by electrogastrogram and gastric emptying: Results in patients with gastroparesis and gastroesophageal reflux disease (GERD); Resolution of abnormalities by balloon dilation of pylorus. Retrieved June 12, 2009, from http://www.3cpmcompany.com/pdf/ddw%202004%20egg%20obstruction%20tx2.pdf

Noar, M. D., & Noar, E. (2008). Gastroparesis associated with GERD and corresponding reflux symptoms may be corrected by radiofrequency ablation (RF) of the cardia and esophagogastric junction. *Surg Endosc, 22*, 2440–2444.

Norheim, A. J., Pedersen, E. J., Fønnebø, V., & Berge, L. (2001). Acupressure treatment of morning sickness in pregnancy: A randomized, double-blind, placebo-controlled study. *Scand J Prim Health Care, 19*, 43–47.

North, R. A., Whitehead, R., & Larkins, R. G. (1991). Stimulation by human chorionic gonadotropin of prostaglandin synthesis by early human placental tissue. *J Clin Endocrinol Metab, 73*, 60–70.

Nowlis, G. H., Frank, M. E., & Pfaffmann, C. (1980). Specificity of acquired aversions to taste qualities in hamsters and rats. *J Comp Physiol Psychol, 94,* 932–942.

Nunn, J. F. (1996). *Ancient Egyptian medicine.* Norman: University of Oklahoma Press.

Nussey, S. S., Hawthorn, J., Page, S. R., Ang, V. T., & Jenkins, J. S. (1988). Responses of plasma oxytocin and arginine vasopressin to nausea induced by apomorphine and ipecacuanha. *Clin Endocrinol (Oxf), 28,* 297–304.

Nussey, S. S., & Whitehead, S. A. (2001). *Endocrinology: An integrated approach.* Exeter, UK: BIOS Scientific Publishers.

O'Brien, B., Relyea, M. J., & Taerum, T. (1996). Efficacy of P6 acupressure in the treatment of nausea and vomiting during pregnancy. *Am J Obstet Gynecol, 174,* 708–715.

O'Donnell, S., Webb, J. K., & Shine, R. (2010). Conditioned taste aversion enhances the survival of an endangered predator imperilled by a toxic invader. *J Appl Ecol, 47,* 558–565.

Oertel, B. G., Schneider, A., Rohr, M., Schmidt, H., Tegeder, I., Geisslinger, G., & Lötsch, J. (2007). The partial 5-hydroxytryptamine 1A receptor agonist buspirone does not antagonise morphine-induced respiratory depression in humans. *Clin Pharmacol Ther, 81,* 59–68.

Olivares, M., Araya, M., Pizarro, F., & Uauy, R. (2001). Nausea threshold in apparently healthy individuals who drink fluids containing graded concentrations of copper. *Reg Toxicol Pharmacol, 33,* 271–275.

Olson, B. R., Freilino, M., Hoffman, G. E., Stricker, E. M., Sved, A. F., & Verbalis, J. G. (1993). c-Fos expression in rat brain and brainstem nuclei in response to treatments that alter food intake and gastric motility. *Mol Cell Neurosci, 4,* 93–106.

Olszewski, P. K., Shi, Q., Billington, C. J., & Levine, A. S. (2000). Opioids affect acquisition of LiCl-induced conditioned taste aversion: Involvement of OT and VP systems. *Am J Physiol Regul Integr Comp Physiol, 279,* R1504–1511.

Oman, C. M., Lichtenberg, B. K., & Money, K. E. (1990). Symptoms and signs of space motion sickness on SPACELAB-1. In G. H. Crampton (Ed.), *Motion and space sickness* (pp. 217–246). Boca Raton, FL: CRC Press.

Onions, C. T. (Ed.). (1973). *The shorter Oxford English dictionary on historical principles.* London: Oxford University Press.

Onishi, T., Mori, T., Yanagihara, M., Furukawa, N., & Fukuda, H. (2007). Similarities of the neuronal circuit for the induction of fictive vomiting between ferrets and dogs. *Auton Neurosci, 136,* 20–30.

Ördög, T. (2008). Interstitial cells of Cajal in diabetic gastroenteropathy. *Neurogastroenterol Motil, 20,* 8–18.

Ördög, T., Takayama, I., Cheung, W. K., Ward, S. M., & Sanders, K. M. (2000). Remodeling of networks of interstitial cells of Cajal in a murine model of diabetic gastroparesis. *Diabetes, 49,* 1731–1739.

Orr, L. E., & McKernan, J. F. (1981). Antiemetic effects of delta-9-tetrahydrocannabinol in chemotherapy-associated nausea and emesis as compared to placebo and compazine. *J Clin Pharmacol, 21,* 76s–80s.

Osinski, M. A., Seifert, T. R., Shaughnessy, T. K., Gintant, G. A., & Cox, B. F. (2003). Emetic liability testing in ferrets. In S. J. Enna, M. Williams, J. W. Ferkany, T. Kenakin, R. D. Porsolt & J. P. Sullivan (Eds.), *Current protocols in pharmacology* (pp. 5.31.1–5.31.8). New York: John Wiley and Sons.

Osinski, M. A., Uchic, M. E., Seifert, T., Shaughnessy, T. K., Miller, L. N., Nakane, M., Cox, B. F., Brioni, J. D., & Moreland, R. B. (2005). Dopamine D2, but not D4, receptor agonists are emetogenic in ferrets. *Pharmacol Biochem Behav, 81,* 211–219.

Ostler, G. (1962). *The little Oxford dictionary of current English* (3rd ed.; rev. by J. S. Coulson). Oxford: Clarendon Press; New York: Oxford University Press.

Otto, B., Riepl, R. L., Klosterhalfen, S., & Enck, P. (2006). Endocrine correlates of acute nausea and vomiting. *Auton Neurosci, 129,* 17–21.

Owyang, C., & Hasler, W. L. (2002). Physiology and pathophysiology of the interstitial cells of Cajal: From bench to bedside: 6. Pathogenesis and therapeutic approaches to human gastric dysrhythmias. *Am J Physiol Gastrointest Liver Physiol, 283,* G6–15.

Ozaki, A., & Sukamoto, T. (1999). Improvement of cisplatin-induced emesis and delayed gastric emptying by KB-R6933, a novel 5-HT3 receptor antagonist. *Gen Pharmacol, 33,* 283–288.

Ozaki, N., Sengupta, J. N., & Gebhart, G. F. (1999). Mechanosensitive properties of gastric vagal afferent fibers in the rat. *J Neurophysiol, 82,* 2210–2220.

Pacak, K., & Palkovits, M. (2001). Stressor specificity of central neuroendocrine responses: Implications for stress-related disorders. *Endocr Rev, 22,* 502–548.

Page, A. J., & Blackshaw, L. A. (1998). An in vitro study of the properties of vagal afferent fibres innervating the ferret oesophagus and stomach. *J Physiol, 512,* 907–916.

Page, A. J., Slattery, J. A., Milte, C., Laker, R., O'Donnell, T., Dorian, C., Brierley, S. M., & Blackshaw, L. A. (2007). Ghrelin selectively reduces mechanosensitivity of upper gastrointestinal vagal afferents. *Am J Physiol Gastrointest Liver Physiol, 292,* G1376–1384.

Page, S. R., Peterson, D. B., Crosby, S. R., Ang, V. T., White, A., Jenkins, J. S., & Nussey, S. S. (1990). The responses of arginine vasopressin and adrenocorticotrophin to nausea induced by ipecacuanha. *Clin Endocrinol (Oxf), 33,* 761–770.

Parker, D. E., & Parker, K. L. (1990). Adaptation to the simulated stimulus rearrangement of weightlessness. In G. G. Crampton (Ed.), *Motion and space sickness* (pp. 247–262). Boca Raton, FL: CRC Press.

Parker, L. A. (1998). Emetic drugs produce conditioned rejection reactions in the taste reactivity test. *J Psychophysiol, 12,* 3–13.

Parker, L. A. (2003). Taste avoidance and taste aversion: Evidence for two different processes. *Learn Behav, 31,* 165–172.

Parker, L. A. (2006). The role of nausea in taste avoidance learning in rats and shrews. *Auton Neurosci, 125,* 34–41.

Parker, L. A., & Joshi, A. (1998). Naloxone-precipitated morphine withdrawal induced place aversions: Effect of naloxone at 24 hours postmorphine. *Pharmacol Biochem Behav, 61,* 331–333.

Parker, L. A., & Kemp, S. W. (2001). Tetrahydrocannabinol (THC) interferes with conditioned retching in Suncus murinus: An animal model of anticipatory nausea and vomiting (ANV). *Neuroreport, 12,* 749–751.

Parker, L. A., Kwiatkowska, M., Burton, P., & Mechoulam, R. (2004). Effect of cannabinoids on lithium-induced vomiting in the Suncus murinus (house musk shrew). *Psychopharmacology (Berl), 171,* 156–161.

Parker, L. A., & Limebeer, C. L. (2006). Conditioned gaping in rats: A selective measure of nausea. *Auton Neurosci, 129,* 36–41.

Parker, L. A., Limebeer, C. L., & Kwiatkowska, M. (2005). Cannabinoids: Effects on vomiting and nausea in animal models. In R. Mechoulam (Ed.), *Cannabinoids as therapeutics* (pp. 183–200). Boston: Birkhäuser Verlag.

Parker, L. A., & Mechoulam, R. (2003). Cannabinoid agonists and antagonists modulate lithium-induced conditioned gaping in rats. *Integr Physiol Behav Sci, 38,* 133–145.

Parker, L. A., Mechoulam, R., & Schlievert, C. (2002). Cannabidiol, a non-psychoactive component of cannabis and its synthetic dimethylheptyl homolog suppress nausea in an experimental model with rats. *Neuroreport, 13,* 567–570.

Parker, L. A., Mechoulam, R., Schlievert, C., Abbott, L., Fudge, M. L., & Burton, P. (2003). Effects of cannabinoids on lithium-induced conditioned rejection reactions in a rat model of nausea. *Psychopharmacology (Berl), 166,* 156–162.

Parker, L. A., Rana, S. A., & Limebeer, C. L. (2008). Conditioned nausea in rats: Assessment by conditioned disgust reactions, rather than conditioned taste avoidance. *Can J Exp Psychol, 62,* 198–209.

Parkes, J. D. (1986). A neurologist's view of nausea and vomiting. In C. B. Davis, G. V. Lake-Bakaar, & D. G. Grahame-Smith (Eds.), *Nausea and vomiting: Mechanisms and treatment* (pp. 160–166). Berlin: Springer-Verlag.

Parkman, H. P., Hasler, W. L., & Fisher, R. S. (2004). American Gastroenterological Association technical review on the diagnosis and treatment of gastroparesis. *Gastroenterology, 127,* 1592–1622.

Parkman, H. P., Miller, M., Trate, D., Knight, L. C., Urbain, J. L., Maurer, A. H., & Fisher, R. S. (1997). Electrogastrography and gastric emptying scintigraphy are complementary for assessment of dyspepsia. *J Clin Gastroenterol, 24,* 214–219.

Parrott, R. F., & Forsling, M. L. (1992). CCK-A receptors mediate the effect of cholecystokinin on vasopressin but not on cortisol in pigs. *Am J Physiol Regul Integr Comp Physiol, 262,* R1154–1157.

Parrott, R. F., & Forsling, M. L. (1994). The CCKA receptor antagonist devazepide inhibits the effect of apomorphine on vasopressin release in pigs. *Gen Pharmacol, 25,* 1337–1340.

Passik, S. D., Kirsh, K. L., Rosenfeld, B., McDonald, M. V., & Theobald, D. E. (2001). The changeable nature of patients' fears regarding chemotherapy: Implications for palliative care. *J Pain Symptom Manage, 21,* 113–120.

Paul, M. A., MacLellan, M., & Gray, G. (2005). Motion-sickness medications for aircrews: Impact on psychomotor performance. *Aviat Space Environ Med, 76,* 560–565.

Paule, M. G., Chelonis, J. J., Blake, D. J., & Dornhoffer, J. L. (2004). Effects of drug countermeasures for space motion sickness on working memory in humans. *Neurotoxicol Teratol, 26,* 825–837.

Pavlov, I. P. (1927). *Conditioned reflexes: An investigtion of the physiological activity of the cerebral cortex.* London: Oxford University Press/Humphrey Milford.

Payne, W. W., & Poulton, E. P. (1927). Experiments on visceral sensation: Part 1. The relation of pain to activity in the oesophagus. *J Physiol, 63,* 217–241.

Payne, W. W., & Poulton, E. P. (1928). Experiments on visceral sensation: Part 2. The sensation of "nausea" and "sinking"; oesophageal reflexes and counter irritation. *J Physiol, 65,* 157–172.

Pecoraro, N., Ginsberg, A. B., Warne, J. P., Gomez, F., La Fleur, S. E., & Dallman, M. F. (2006). Diverse basal and stress-related phenotypes of Sprague Dawley rats from three vendors. *Physiol Behav, 89,* 598–610.

Peeters, A., Van de Wyngaert, F., Van Lierde, M., Sindic, C. J., & Laterre, E. C. (1993). Wernicke's encephalopathy and central pontine myelinolysis induced by hyperemesis gravidarum. *Acta Neurol Belg, 93,* 276–282.

Pelchat, M. L., & Rozin, P. (1982). The special role of nausea in the acquisition of food dislikes by humans. *Appetite, 3,* 341–351.

Penfield, W., & Rasmussen, T. (1950). *The cerebral cortex of man.* Macmillan: New York.

Peng, M. T. (1963). Locus of emetic action of epinephrine and DOPA in dogs. *J Pharm Exp Ther, 139,* 345.

Peng, S. Y., Wa, K. C., Wang, J. J., Chuang, J. H., Peng, S. K., & Lai, Y. H. (2007). Predicting postoperative nausea and vomiting with the application of an artificial neural network. *Br J Anaesthesiol, 98,* 60–65.

Pepper, G. V., & Craig-Roberts, S. (2006). Rates of nausea and vomiting in pregnancy and dietary characteristics across populations. *Proc Biol Sci, 273,* 2675–2679.

Percie Du Sert, N., Chu, K. M., Wai, M. K., Rudd, J. A., & Andrews, P. L. (2009). Reduced normogastric electrical activity associated with emesis: A telemetric study in ferrets. *World J Gastroenterol, 15,* 6034–6043.

Percie Du Sert, N., Chu, K. M., Wai, M. K., Rudd, J. A., & Andrews, P. L. R (2010a). Telemetry in a motion-sickness model implicates the abdominal vagus in a motion–induced gastric dysrhythmia. *Exp Physiol, 95,* 768–773.

Percie Du Sert, N., Rudd, J. A., & Andrews, P. L. R. (2008). The effects of vasopressin (AVP) and oxytocin (OXY) on the isolated gastrointestinal tract in emetic (ferret, Suncus murinus) and non emetic (rat) species. *J Pharmacol Sci, 106*(Suppl. 1), 258P.

Percie Du Sert, N., Rudd, J. A., Apfel, C. C., & Andrews, P. L. R. (2010b) Cisplatin-induced emesis: systematic review and meta-analysis of the ferret model and the effects of 5-HT3 receptor antagonists. *Cancer Chemother Pharmacol,* in press.

Perera, A. D., Verbalis, J. G., Mikuma, N., Majumdar, S. S., & Plant, T. M. (1993). Cholecystokinin stimulates gonadotropin-releasing hormone release in the monkey (Macaca mulatta). *Endocrinology, 132,* 1723–1728.

Peroutka, S. J., & Snyder, S. H. (1982). Antiemetics: neurotransmitter receptor binding predicts therapeutic actions. *Lancet, 20,* 658–659.

Perry, M. R., Rhee, J., & Smith, W. L. (1994). Plasma levels of peptide YY correlate with cisplatin-induced emesis in dogs. *J Pharm Pharmacol, 46,* 553–557.

Petrakis, I. E., Vrachassotakis, N., Sciacca, V., Vassilakis, S. I., & Chalkiadakis, G. (1999). Hyperglycaemia attenuates erythromycin-induced acceleration of solid-phase gastric emptying in idiopathic and diabetic gastroparesis. *Scand J Gastroenterol, 34,* 396–403.

Phillips, R. J., & Powley, T. L. (2000). Tension and stretch receptors in gastrointestinal smooth muscle: Re-evaluating vagal mechanoreceptor electrophysiology. *Brain Res Rev, 34,* 1–26.

Phillips, W. T., Schwartz, J. G., & McMahan, C. A. (1992). Rapid gastric emptying of an oral glucose solution in type 2 diabetic patients. *J Nucl Med, 33,* 1496–1500.

Phillips, W. T., Schwartz, J. G., & McMahan, C. A. (1993). Reduced postprandial blood glucose levels in recently diagnosed non-insulin-dependent diabetics secondary to pharmacologically induced delayed gastric emptying. *Dig Dis Sci, 38,* 51–58.

Pi-Sunyer, F. X., Aronne, L. J., Heshmati, H. M., Devin, J., & Rosenstock, J. (2006). Effect of rimonabant, a cannabinoid-1 receptor blocker, on weight and cardiometabolic risk factors in overweight or obese patients: RIO-North America; A randomized controlled trial. *JAMA, 295,* 761–775.

Pittman, Q. J., & Spencer, S. J. (2005). Neurohypophysial peptides: Gatekeepers in the amygdala. *Trends Endocrinol Metab, 16,* 343–344.

Pole, M., Einarson, A., Pairaudeau, N., Einarson, T., & Koren, G. (2000). Drug labeling and risk perceptions of terato teratogenicity: A survey of pregnant Canadian women and their health professionals. *J Clin Pharmacol, 40,* 573–577.

Poli-Bigelli, S., Rodrigues-Pereira, J., Carides, A. D., Julie Ma, G., Eldridge, K., Hipple, A., Evans, J. K., Horgan, K. J., & Lawson, F. (2003). Addition of the neurokinin

1 receptor antagonist aprepitant to standard antiemetic therapy improves control of chemotherapy-induced nausea and vomiting: Results from a randomized, double-blind, placebo-controlled trial in Latin America. *Cancer, 97,* 3090–3098.

Polland, W. S., & Bloomfield, A. L. (1931). Experimental referred pain from the gastro-intestinal tract: Part 1. The esophagus. *J Clin Invest, 10,* 435–452.

Pollick, A. S., & de Waal, F. B. M. (2007). Ape gestures and language evolution. *Proc Nat Acad Sci USA, 104,* 8184–8189.

Pongrojpaw, D., Somprasit, C., & Chanthasenanont, A. (2007). A randomized comparison of ginger and dimenhydrinate in the treatment of nausea and vomiting in pregnancy. *J Med Assoc Thai, 90,* 1703–1709.

Popov, A. P. (1943). Special vestibular training. In W. E. Voyachek et al. (Eds.), *Fundamentals of aviation medicine* (pp. 191–206). Toronto: University of Toronto Press.

Potter, P. (Trans.). (1995). *Hippocrates* (Loeb ed., Vol. 8). Cambridge, MA: Harvard University Press.

Prakash, C., Lustman, P. J., Freedland, K. E., & Clouse, R. E. (1998). Tricyclic antidepressants for functional nausea and vomiting: Clinical outcome in 37 patients. *Dig Dis Sci, 43,* 1951–1956.

Pratt, J. A., & Stolerman, I. P. (1984). Pharmacologically specific pretreatment effects on apomorphine-mediated conditioned taste aversions in rats. *Pharmacol Biochem Behav, 20,* 507–511.

Prescott, M. (2006). *Primate sensory capabilities and communication signals: Implications for care and use in the laboratory.* London: National Centre for the Replacement, Refinement and Reduction of Animals in Research. Retrieved April 8, 2009, from http://www.nc3rs.org.uk/news.asp?id=187

Preziosi, P., D'Amato, M., Del Carmine, R., Martire, M., Pozzoli, G., & Navarra, P. (1992). The effects of 5-HT3 receptor antagonists on cisplatin-induced emesis in the pigeon. *Eur J Pharmacol, 221,* 343–350.

Proctor, G. B., & Carpenter, G. H. (2007). Regulation of salivary gland function by autonomic nerves. *Auton Neurosci, 133,* 3–18.

Profet M. (1988). The evolution of pregnancy sickness as protection to the embryo against Pleistocene teratogens. *Evolutionary Theory, 8,* 177–190.

Profet, M. (1992). Pregnancy sickness as adaptation: A deterrent to maternal ingestion of teratogens. In J. Barkow, L. Cosmides, & J. Tooby (Eds.), *The adapted mind* (pp. 327–365). New York: Oxford University Press.

Purkis, I. F. (1964). Factors that influence postoperative vomiting. *Can Anaesth Soc J, 11,* 335–353.

Pusch, F., Berger, A., Wildling, E., Zimpfer, M., Moser, M., Sam, C., & Krafft, P. (2002). Preoperative orthostatic dysfunction is associated with an increased incidence of postoperative nausea and vomiting. *Anesthesiology, 96,* 1381–1385.

Qu, R., Furukawa, N., & Fukuda, H. (1995) Changes in extrahepatic biliary motilities with emesis in dogs. *J Auton Nerv Syst, 56,* 87–96.

Quigley, E. M. M., Hasler, W. L., & Parkman, H. P. (2001). AGA technical review on nausea and vomiting. *Gastroenterology, 120,* 263–286.

Rabin, B. M., & Hunt, W. A. (1992). Relationship between vomiting and taste aversion learning in the ferret: Studies with ionizing radiation, lithium chloride, and amphetamine. *Behav Neural Biol, 58,* 83–93.

Rabin, B. M., Hunt, W. A., Bakarich, A. C., Chedester, A. L., & Lee, J. (1986a). Angiotensin II-induced taste aversion learning in cats and rats and the role of the area postrema. *Physiol Behav, 36,* 1173–1178.

Rabin, B. M., Hunt, W. A., Chedester, A. L., & Lee, J. (1986b). Role of the area postrema in radiation-induced taste aversion learning and emesis in cats. *Physiol Behav, 37,* 815–818.

Ramhamadany, E. M., Fowler, J., & Baird, I. M. (1989). Effect of the gastric balloon versus sham procedure on weight loss in obese subjects. *Gut, 30,* 1054–1057.

Ramsbottom, N., & Hunt, J. N. (1970). Studies of the effect of metoclopramide and apomorphine on gastric emptying and secretion in man. *Gut, 11,* 989–993.

Rana, S. A., & Parker, L. A. (2008). Differential effects of neurotoxin-induced lesions of the basolateral amygdala and central nucleus of the amygdala on lithium-induced conditioned disgust reactions and conditioned taste avoidance. *Behav Brain Res, 189,* 284–297.

Rao, R. H., & Spathis, G. S. (1987). Intramuscular glucagon as a provocative stimulus for the assessment of pituitary function: Growth hormone and cortisol responses. *Metabolism, 36,* 658–663.

Rathmann, W., Enck, P., Frieling, T., & Gries, F. A. (1991). Visceral afferent neuropathy in diabetic gastroparesis. *Diabetes Care, 14,* 1086–1089.

Reason, J. T. (1967). *An investigation of some factors contributing to individual variation in motion sickness susceptibility* (Flying Personnel Research Communication, Report No. 1277). London: Ministry of Defence.

Reason, J. T., & Brand, J. J. (1975). *Motion sickness.* London: Academic Press.

Reavley, C. M., Golding, J. F., Cherkas, L. F., Spector, T. D., & MacGregor, A. J. (2006). Genetic influences on motion sickness susceptibility in adult women: A classical twin study. *Aviat Space Environ Med, 77,* 1148–1152.

Regan, E. C., & Price, K. R. (1994). The frequency of occurrence and severity of side-effects of immersion virtual reality. *Aviat Space Environ Med, 65,* 527–530.

Reichardt, B., Üngörgil, S., Riepl, R. L., Schedlowski, M., Lehnert, P., & Enck, P. (1997). ACTH- and ADH- profiles during motion sickness screened by continuous blood sampling. *Gastroenterology, 112,* A811.

Reichardt, B., Ayan, T., Otto, C., Klosterhalfen, S., Riepl, R. L., Probst, T., Lehnert, P., & Enck, P. (1998). Short-term changes of ACTH and ADH levels during nausea development. *Neurogastroeneterology, 10,* 93.

Reid, K., Palmer, J. L., Wright, R. J., Clemes, S. A., Troakes, C., Somal, H. S., House, F., & Stott, J. R. R. (2000). Comparison of the neurokinin-1 antagonist GR205171, alone and in combination with the 5-HT$_3$ antagonist ondansetron, hyoscine, and placebo in the prevention of motion-induced nausea in man. *Br J Clin Pharmacol, 50,* 61–64.

Reid, R. M. (1992). Cultural and medical perspectives on geophagia. *Med Athropol, 13,* 337–351.

Renaud, L. P., Tang, M., McCann, M. J., Stricker, E. M., & Verbalis, J. G. (1987). Cholecystokinin and gastric distension activate oxytocinergic cells in rat hypothalamus. *Am J Physiol Regul Integr Comp Physiol, 253,* R661–665.

Reschke, M. F., Harm, D. L., Parker, D. E., Sandoz, G. R., Homick, J. L., & Vanderploeg, J. M. (1994). Neurophysiologic aspects: Space motion sickness. In A. E. Nicogossian, C. L. Huntoon, & S. L. Pool (Eds.), *Space physiology and medicine* (pp. 228–260). Philadelphia: Lea & Febiger.

Reschke, M. F., Somers, J. T., & Ford, G. (2006). Stroboscopic vision as a treatment for motion sickness: Strobe lighting vs. shutter glasses. *Aviat Space Environ Med, 77,* 2–7.

Revusky, S., & Martin, G. M. (1988). Glucocorticoids attenuate taste aversions produced by toxins in rats. *Psychopharmacology (Berl), 96,* 400–407.

Rhodes, V. A., Watson, P. M., & Johnson, M. H. (1984). Development of reliable and valid measures of nausea and vomiting. *Cancer Nursing, 7,* 33–41.

Ricci, J. A., Siddique, R., Stewart, W. F., Sandler, R. S., Sloan, S., & Farup, C. E. (2000). Upper gastrointestinal symptoms in a U.S. national sample of adults with diabetes. *Scand J Gastroenterol, 35,* 152–159.

Rice, T. (2000). *Voyages of discovery.* London: Scriptum Eds.

Richards, W., Hillsley, K., Eastwood, C., & Grundy, D. (1996). Sensitivity of vagal mucosal afferents to cholecystokinin and its role in afferent signal transduction in the rat. *J Physiol, 497*(Pt. 2), 473–481.

Richardson, C. T., Walsh, J. H., Hicks, M. I., & Fordtran, J. S. (1976). Studies on the mechanisms of food stimulated gastric acid secretion in normal human subjects. *J Clin Invest, 58,* 623–631.

Richardson, J., Smith, J. E., McCall, G., Richardson, A., Pilkington, K., & Kirsch, I. (2007). Hypnosis for nausea and vomiting in cancer chemotherapy: A systematic review of the research evidence [Review]. *Eur J Cancer Care, 16,* 402–412.

Riddle, O., & Burns, F. H. (1931). A conditioned emetic reflex in the pigeon. *Proc Soc Exp Biol Med, 28,* 979–981.

Riezzo, G., Clemente, C., Leo, S., & Russo, F. (2005). The role of electrogastrography and gastrointestinal hormones in chemotherapy-related dyspeptic symptoms. *J Gastroenterol, 40,* 1107–1115.

Riezzo, G., Pezzolla, F., Darconza, G., & Giorgio, I. (1992). Gastric myoelectrical activity in the first trimester of pregnancy: A cutaneous electrogastrographic study. *Am J Gastroenterol, 87,* 702–707.

Riley, A. L., & Freeman, K. B. (2004). Conditioned taste aversion: A database. *Pharmacol Biochem Behav, 77,* 655–656.

Riley, T. R., Chinchilli, V. M., Shoemaker, M., & Koch, K. L. (2001). Is nausea associated with chronic hepatitis C infection? *Am J Gastroenterol, 96,* 3356–3360.

Risinger, F. O., & Cunningham, C. L. (2000). DBA/2J mice develop stronger lithium chloride-induced conditioned taste and place aversions than C57BL/6J mice. *Pharmacol Biochem Behav, 67,* 17–24.

Robertson, G. L. (1977). The regulation of vasopressin function in health and disease. *Recent Prog Horm Res, 33,* 333–385.

Robichaud, A., Savoie, C., Stamatiou, P. B., Tattersall, F. D., & Chan, C. C. (2001). PDE4 inhibitors induce emesis in ferrets via a noradrenergic pathway. *Neuropharmacology, 40,* 262–269.

Robinson, B. W., & Mishkin, M. (1968). Alimentary responses to forebrain stimulation in monkeys. *Exp Brain Res, 4,* 330–366.

Rock, E. M., Benzaquen, J., Limebeer, C., & Parker, L. A. (2009). Potential of the rat model of conditioned gaping to detect nausea produced by roipram, a phosphodiesterase-4 (PDE4) inhibitor. *Pharmacol Biochem Behav, 91,* 537–541.

Rodriguez, M., Lopez, M., Symonds, M., & Hall, G. (2000). Lithium-induced context aversion in rats as a model of anticipatory nausea in humans. *Physiol Behav, 71,* 571–579.

Roila, F., Hesketh, P. J., & Herrstedt, J. (2006). Prevention of chemotherapy- and radiotherapy-induced emesis: Results of the 2004 Perugia International Antiemetic Consensus Conference. *Ann Oncol, 17,* 20–28.

Roldan, G., & Bures, J. (1994) Tetrodotoxin blockade of amygdala overlapping with poisoning impairs acquisition of conditioned taste aversion in rats. *Behav Brain Res, 65,* 213–219.

Rolls, E. T. (2004). The functions of the orbitofrontal cortex. *Brain Cogn, 55,* 11–29.

Roos, I. A., Fairlie, D. P., & Whitehouse, M. W. (1981). A peculiar toxicity manifested by platinum(II) amines in rats: Gastric distension after intraperitoneal administration. *Chem Biol Interact, 35,* 111–117.

Root-Bernstein, R., & Root-Bernstein, M. (1997). *Honey, mud, maggots, and other medical marvels: The science behind folk's remedies and old wives' tales.* Boston: Houghton Mifflin.

Roscoe, J. A., Bushunow, P., Jean-Pierre, P., Heckler, C. E., Purnell, J. Q., Peppone, L. J., Chen, Y., Ling, M. N. and Morrow, G. R. (2009). Acupressure bands are effective in reducing radiation therapy-related nausea. *J Pain Symptom Manage, 38,* 381–389.

Roscoe, J. A., Bushunow, P., Morrow, G. R., Hickok, J. T., Kuebler, P. J., Jacobs, A., & Bannerjee, T. K. (2004). Patient expectation is a strong predictor of severe nausea after chemotherapy: A University of Rochester Community Clinical Oncology Program study of patients with breast carcinoma. *Cancer, 101,* 2701–2708.

Roscoe, J. A., Hickok, J. T., & Morrow, G. R. (2000). Patient expectations as predictor of chemotherapy-induced nausea. *Ann Behav Med, 22,* 121–126.

Roscoe J. A., Morrow, G. R., Hickok, J. T., & Stern, R. M. (2000). Nausea and vomiting remain a significant clinical problem: Trends over time in controlling chemotherapy-induced nausea and vomiting in 1413 patients treated in community clinical practices. *J Pain Symptom Manage, 20,* 113–121.

Rosztoczy, A., Roka, R., Varkonvi, T. T., Lengvel, C., Izbeki, F., Lonovies, J., & Wittmann, T. (2004). Regional differences in the manifestation of gastrointestinal motor disorders in type 1 diabetic patients with autonomic neuropathy. *Z Gastroenterol, 42,* 1295–1300.

Rouzade, M. L., Fioramonti, J., & Bueno, L. (1998). A model for evaluation of gastric sensitivity in awake rats. *Neurogastroenterol Motil, 10,* 157–163.

Rowe, J. W., Shelton, R. L., Helderman, J. H., Vestal, R. E., & Robertson, G. L. (1979). Influence of the emetic reflex on vasopressin release in man. *Kidney Int, 16,* 729–735.

Rozengurt, E. (2006). Taste receptors in the gastrointestinal tract: 1. Bitter taste receptors and alpha-gustducin in the mammalian gut. *Am J Physiol Gastrointest Liver Physiol, 291,* G171–177.

Rub, R., Andrews, P. L. R., & Whitehead, S. A. (1992). Vomiting: Incidence, causes, ageing, and sex. In A. L. Bianchi, L. Grelot, A. D. Miller, & G. L. King (Eds.), *Mechanisms and control of emesis* (pp. 363–364). Montrouge, France: Colloque INSERM/John Libbey Eurotext.

Rubio-Pérez, M. J., Aranda Aguilar, E., Barneto Aranda, I., Lomas Garrido, M., & Gonzalez Mancha, R. (1992). Efficacia antiemetica de la metroclopramida en la dilatacion gastrica inducida por cisplatino en ratas Wistar. *Neoplasia, 10,* 40–43.

Rudd, J. A., & Andrews, P. L. R. (2005). Mechanisms of acute, delayed, and anticipatory emesis induced by anticancer therapies. In P. Hesketh (Ed.), *Management of nausea and vomiting in cancer and cancer treatment* (pp. 15–66). Sudbury, MA: Jones and Bartlett.

Rudd, J. A., Cheng, C. H., Naylor, R. J., Ngan, M. P., & Wai, M. K. (1999). Modulation of emesis by fentanyl and opioid receptor antagonists in Suncus murinus (house musk shrew). *Eur J Pharmacol, 374,* 77–84.

Rudd, J. A., Jordan, C. C., & Naylor, R. J. (1994). Profiles of emetic action of cisplatin in the ferret: A potential model of acute and delayed emesis. *Eur J Pharmacol, 262,* R1–2.

Rudd, J. A., & Naylor, R. J. (1995). Opioid receptor involvement in emesis and anti-emesis. In D. J. Reynolds, P. L. R. Andrews, & C. J. Davis (Eds.), *Serotonin and the scientific basis of anti-emetic therapy* (pp. 208–221). Oxford: Oxford Clinical Communications.

Rudd, J. A., Ngan, M. P., & Wai, M. K. (1998). 5-HT$_3$ receptors are not involved in conditioned taste aversions induced by 5-hydroxytryptamine, ipecacuanha, or cis-platin. *Eur J Pharmacol, 352,* 143–149.

Rudd, J. A., Ngan, M. P., Wai, M. K., King, A. G., Witherington, J., Andrews, P. L. R., & Sanger, G. J. (2006). Anti-emetic activity of ghrelin in ferrets exposed to the cyto-toxic anti-cancer agent cisplatin. *Neurosci Lett, 392,* 79–83.

Rudd, J. A., Yamamoto, K., Yamatodani, A., & Takeda, N. (2002). Differential action of ondansetron and dexamethasone to modify cisplatin-induced acute and delayed kaolin consumption ("pica") in rats. *Eur J Pharmacol, 454,* 47–52.

Rundles, R. (1945). Diabetic neuropathy: General review with report of 125 cases. *Medicine, 24,* 111–160.

Rupniak, N. M., & Williams, A. R. (1994). Differential inhibition of foot tapping and chromodacryorrhoea in gerbils by CNS penetrant and non-penetrant tachykinin NK1 receptor antagonists. *Eur J Pharmacol, 265,* 179–183.

Rupniak, N. M., Tye, S. J., & Iversen, S. D. (1990). Drug-induced purposeless chewing: Animal model of dyskinesia or nausea? *Psychopharmacology (Berl), 102,* 325–328.

Ryan, J. L., Heckler, C., Dakhil, S. R., Kirschner, J., Flynn, P. J., Hickok, J. T.,& Morrow, G. R. (2009). *Ginger for chemotherapy-related nausea in cancer patients: A URCC CCOP randomized, double-blind, placebo-controlled clinical trial of 644 cancer patients* [Abstract]. American Society of Clinical Oncology Meeting.

Sacks, O. (1981). *Migraine.* London: Pan Books.

Saeki, M., Sakai, M., Saito, R., Kubota, H., Ariumi, H., Takano, Y., Yamatodani, A., & Kamiya, H. (2001). Effects of HSP-117, a novel tachykinin NK1-receptor antagonist, on cisplatin-induced pica as a new evaluation of delayed emesis in rats. *Jpn J Pharmacol, 86,* 359–362.

Safari, H. R., Fassett, M. J., Souter, I. C., Alsulyman, O. M., & Goodwin, T. M. (1998). The efficacy of methylprednisolone in the treatment of hyperemesis gravidarum: A randomized, double-blind, controlled trial. *Am J Obstet Gynecol, 179,* 921–924.

Sahakian, V., Rouse, D., Sipes, S., Rose, N., & Niebyl, J. (1991). Vitamin B6 is effective therapy for nausea and vomiting of pregnancy: A randomized, double-blind, place-bo-controlled study. *Obstet Gynecol, 78,* 33–36.

Sanders, K. M. (1984). Role of prostaglandins in regulating gastric motility. *Am J Physiol Gastrointest Liver Physiol, 247,* G117–126.

Sanders, K. M., Bauer, A. J., & Publicover, N. G. (1983). Regulation of gastric antral slow wave frequency by prostagladins. In C. Roman (Ed.), *Gastrointestinal motility* (pp. 77–85). Lancaster, UK: MTP Press.

Sanger, G. J., & Andrews, P. L. R. (2006). Treatment of nausea and vomiting: Gaps in our knowledge. *Auton Neurosci, 129,* 3–16.

Santucci, D., Corazzi, G., Francia, N., Antonelli, A., Aloe, L., & Alleva, E. (2000). Neurobehavioural effects of hypergravity conditions in the adult mouse. *Neuroreport, 11,* 3353–3356.

Santucci, D., Francia, N., Aloe, L., & Alleva, E. (2002). Neurobehavioural responses to hypergravity environment in the CD-1 mouse. *J Gravit Physiol, 9,* P39–40.

Saper, C. B. (2002). The central autonomic nervous system: Conscious visceral percep-tion and autonomic pattern generation. *Ann Rev Neurosci, 25,* 433–469.

Sarna, S. K. (1989). Motor correlates of functional gastrointestinal symptoms. *Gastroenterol Int, 2,* 122–126.

Sasaki, H., Nagulesparan, M., Dubois, A., Straus, E., Samloff, I. M., Lawrence, W. H., Johnson, G. C., Sievers, M. L., & Unger, R. H. (1983). Hypergastrinemia in obese noninsulin-dependent diabetes: A possible reflection of high prevalence of vagal dysfunction. *J Clin Endocrinol Metab, 56,* 744–750.

Sato, T., Igarashi, N., Minami, S., Okabe, T., Hashimoto, H., Hasui, M., & Kato, E. (1988). Recurrent attacks of vomiting, hypertension, and psychotic depression: A syndrome of periodic catecholamine and prostaglandin discharge. *Acta Endocrinol (Copenh), 117,* 189–197.

Sawhney, M. S., Prakash, C., Lustman, P. J., & Clouse, R. E. (2007). Tricyclic antidepressants for chronic vomiting in diabetic patients. *Dig Dis Sci, 52,* 418–424.

Sawai, S., Sakakibara, R., Kanai, K., Kawaguchi, N., Uchiyama, T., Yamamoto, T., Ito, T., Liu, Z., & Hattori, T. (2006). Isolated vomiting due to a unilateral dorsal vagal complex lesion. *Eur Neurol, 56,* 246–248.

Schafe, G. E., & Bernstein, I. L. (1998). Forebrain contribution to the induction of a brainstem correlate of conditioned taste aversion: 2. Insular (gustatory) cortex. *Brain Res, 800,* 40–47.

Schofferman, J. A. (1976). A clinical comparison of syrup of ipecac and apomorphine use in adults. *JACEP, 5,* 22–25.

Schrager, V. L., & Ivy, A. C. (1928). Symptoms produced by distention of the gallbladder and biliary ducts. *Surg Gynecol Obstet, 47,* 1–13.

Schulze, K., & Christensen, J. (1977). Lower sphincter of the opossum esophagus in pseudopregnancy. *Gastroenterology, 73,* 1082–1085.

Schvarcz, E., Palmér, M., Aman, J., Horowitz, M., Stridsberg, M., & Berne, C. (1997). Physiological hyperglycemia slows gastric emptying in normal subjects and patients with insulin-dependent diabetes mellitus. *Gastroenterology, 113,* 60–66.

Schvarcz, E., Palmer, M., Ingberg, C. M., Aman, J., & Berne, C. (1996). Increased prevalence of upper gastrointestinal symptoms in long-term type 1 diabetic mellitus. *Diabet Med, 13,* 478–481.

Schwartz, J. G., Green, G. M., Guan, D., McMahan, C. A., & Phillips, W. T. (1996). Rapid gastric emptying of a solid pancake meal in type II diabetic patients. *Diabetes Care, 19,* 468–471.

Schwartz, J. G., Guan, D., Green, G. M., & Phillips, W. T. (1994). Treatment with an oral proteinase inhibitor slows gastric emptying and acutely reduces glucose and insulin levels after a liquid meal in type II diabetic patients. *Diabetes Care, 17,* 255–262.

Schwartz, M. D., Jacobsen, P. B., & Bovbjerg, D. H. (1996). Role of nausea in the development of aversions to a beverage paired with chemotherapy treatment in cancer patients. *Physiol Behav, 59,* 659–663.

Schwartzberg, L. S. (2007). Chemotherapy-induced nausea and vomiting: Which antiemetic for which therapy? *Oncology (Williston Park), 21,* 946–953.

Scuderi, P. E. (2003). Pharmacology of antiemetics. *International anesthesiology clinics, 41*(4): 41–66.

Scurlock, J., & Anderson, J. B. (2005). *Diagnoses in Assyrian and Babylonian medicine.* Urbana: University of Illinois Press.

Seeley, R. J., Blake, K., Rushing, P. A., Benoit, S., Eng, J., Woods, S. C., & D'Alessio, D. (2000). The role of CNS glucagon-like peptide-1 (7–36) amide receptors in mediating the visceral illness effects of lithium chloride. *J Neurosci, 20,* 1616–1621.

Sem-Jacobsen, C. W. (1968). *Depth-electrographic stimulation of the human brain and behaviour*. Springfield, IL: Charles C. Thomas.

Semmens, J. P. (1971). Female sexuality and life situations: An etiologic psycho-socio-sexual profile of weight gain and nausea and vomiting of pregnancy. *Obstet Gynecol, 38,* 555–563.

Serradeil-Le Gal, C., Wagnon, J., Valette, G., Garcia, G., Pascal, M., Maffrand, J. P., & Le Fur, G. (2002). Nonpeptide vasopressin receptor antagonists: Development of selective and orally active V1a, V2, and V1b receptor ligands. *Prog Brain Res, 139,* 197–210.

Serrador, J. M., Schlegel, T. T., Black, F. O., & Wood, S. J. (2005). Cerebral hypoperfusion precedes nausea during centrifugation. *Aviat Space Environ Med, 76,* 91–96.

Sewards, T. V. (2004). Dual separate pathways for the sensory and hedonic aspects of taste. *Brain Res Bull, 62,* 271–283.

Shapiro, R. E., & Miselis, R. R. (1985). The central neural connections of the area postrema of the rat. *J Comp Neurol, 234,* 344–364.

Sharma, M., Rai, K., Sharma, S. S., & Gupta, Y. K. (2000). Effect of antioxidants on pyrogallol-induced delay in gastric emptying in rats. *Pharmacology, 60,* 90–96.

Sharma, S. S., & Gupta, Y. K. (1998). Reversal of cisplatin-induced delay in gastric emptying in rats by ginger (Zingiber officinale). *J Ethnopharmacol, 62,* 49–55.

Shelton, R. L., Kinney, R. M., & Robertson, G. L. (1977). Emesis: A species specific stimulus for vasopressin (VP) release. *Clin Res, 25,* 301A.

Shrim, A., Boskovic, R., Maltepe, C., Navios, Y., Garcia-Bournissen, F., & Koren, G. (2006). Pregnancy outcome following large doses of vitamin B6 in the first trimester. *J Obstet Gynaecol, 26,* 749–751.

Shupak, A., & Gordon, C. R. (2006). Motion sickness advances in pathogenesis, prediction, prevention, and treatment. *Aviat Space Environ Med, 77,* 1213–1223.

Sims, D. W., Andrews, P. L., & Young, J. Z. (2000). Stomach rinsing in rays. *Nature, 404,* 566.

Simpson, S. W., Goodwin, T. M., Robins, S. B., Rizzo, A. A., Howes, R. A., Buckwalter, D. K., & Buckwalter, J. G. (2001). Psychological factors and hyperemesis gravidarum. *J Women's Health, Gender Based Medicine, 10,* 471–477.

Singer, L. K., York, D. A., Berthoud, H. R., & Bray, G. A. (1999). Conditioned taste aversion produced by inhibitors of fatty acid oxidation in rats. *Physiol Behav, 68,* 175–179.

Singh, L., Field, M. J., Hughes, J., Kuo, B. S., Suman-Chauhan, N., Tuladhar, B. R., Wright, D. S., & Naylor, R. J. (1997). The tachykinin NK_1 receptor antagonist PD154075 blocks cisplatin-induced delayed emesis in the ferret. *Eur J Pharmacol, 321,* 209–216.

Sinha, R. (1968). Effect of vestibular Coriolis reaction on respiration and blood-flow changes in man. *Aerosp Med, 39,* 837–844.

Sipols, A. J., Brief, D. J., Ginter, K. L., Saghafi, S., & Woods, S. C. (1992). Neuropeptide Y paradoxically increases food intake yet causes conditioned flavor aversions. *Physiol Behav, 51,* 1257–1260.

Skidgel, R. A., & Erdös, E. G. (2006) Histamine, bradykinin, and their antagonists. In L. L. Brunton, J. S. Lazo, & K. L. Parker (Eds.), *Goodman & Gilman's pharmacological basis of therapeutics* (11th ed., pp. 629–651). New York: McGraw-Hill.

Slotnick, R. N. (2001). Safe, successful nausea suppression in early pregnancy with P6 acustimulation. *J Reprod Med, 36,* 811–814.

Smith, C. C., & Brizzee, K. R. (1961). Cineradiographic analysis of vomiting in the cat. *Gastroenterology, 40,* 654–664.

Smith, C., Crowther, C., Beilby, J., & Dandeaux, J. (2000). The impact of nausea and vomiting on women: A burden of early pregnancy. *Aust N Z J Obstet Gynaecol, 4,* 397–401.

Smith, J. E., Friedman, M. I., & Andrews, P. L. R. (2001). Conditioned food aversion in Suncus murinus (house musk shrew): A new model for the study of nausea in a species with an emetic reflex. *Physiol Behav, 73,* 593–598.

Smith, J. E., Paton, J. F., & Andrews, P. L. R. (2002). An arterially perfused decerebrate preparation of Suncus murinus (house musk shrew) for the study of emesis and swallowing. *Exp Physiol, 87,* 563–574.

Smith, P. M., Lowes, V. L., & Ferguson, A. V. (1994). Circulating vasopressin influences area postrema neurons. *Neuroscience, 59,* 185–194.

Smith, U. (1996). Gastric emptying in type 2 diabetes: Quick or slow? *Diabet Med, 13*(Suppl. 5), S31–33.

Smith, W. D. (Trans.). (1994). *Hippocrates* (Loeb ed., Vol. 7). Cambridge, MA: Harvard University Press.

Smith, W. L., Alphin, R. S., Jackson, C. B., & Sancilio, L. F. (1989). The antiemetic profile of zacopride. *J Pharm Pharmacol, 41,* 101–105.

Smyth, J. F., Coleman, R. E., Nicolson, M., Gallmeier, W. M., Leonard, R. C., Cornbleet, M. A., Allan, S. G., Upadhyaya, P. K., & Bruntsch, U. (1991). Does dexamethasone enhance control of acute cisplatin induced emesis by ondansetron? *BMJ, 303,* 1423–1426.

Soanes, C., & Stevenson, A. (Eds.). (2006). *Oxford dictionary of English* (2nd ed.). Oxford: Oxford University Press.

Sogabe, M., Okahisa, T., Tsujigami, K., Okita, Y., Hayashi, H., Taniki, T., Hukuno, H., Nakasono, M., Muguruma, N., Okamura, S., & Ito, S. (2005). Ultrasonographic assessment of gastric motility in diabetic gastroparesis before and after attaining glycemic control. *J Gastroenterol, 40,* 583–590.

Sorensen, P. S., & Hammer, M. (1985). Vasopressin in plasma and ventricular cerebrospinal fluid during dehydration, postural changes, and nausea. *Am J Physiol Regul Integr Comp Physiol, 248,* R78–83.

Sorensen, P. S., Hammer, M., & Gjerris, F. (1982). Cerebrospinal fluid vasopressin in benign intracranial hypertension. *Neurology NY, 32,* 1255–1259.

Spangeus, A., El-Salhy, M., Suhr, O., Eriksson, J., & Lithner, F. (1999). Prevalence of gastrointestinal symptoms in young and middle-aged diabetic patients. *Scand J Gastroenterol, 34,* 1196–1202.

Spealman, R. D. (1983). Maintenance of behavior by postponement of scheduled injections of nicotine in squirrel monkeys. *J Pharmacol Exp Ther, 227,* 154–159.

Spiegl, F. (1996). *Fritz Spiegl's sick notes: An alphabetical browsing-book of derivatives, abbreviations, mnemonics, and slang for amusement and edification of medics, nurses, patients, and hypochondriacs.* New York: Parthenon.

Spinks, A. B., Wasiak, J., Villanueva, E. V., & Bernath, V. (2004). Scopolamine for preventing and treating motion sickness. *Cochrane Database of Systematic Reviews, 3* (Online): CD002851.

Spizer, T. R. (1995). Clinical evidence for 5-HT3 receptor antagonist efficacy in radiation-induced emesis. In D. J. Reynolds, P. L. R. Andrews, & C. J. Davis (Eds.), *Serotonin and the scientific basis of anti-emetic therapy* (pp. 134–141). Oxford: Oxford Clinical Communications.

St Andre, J., Albanos, K., & Reilly, S. (2007). C-fos expression in the rat following lithium chloride induced-illness. *Brain Res, 1135,* 122–128.

Stadler, M., Bardiau, F., Seidel, L., Albert, A., & Boogaerts, J. G. (2003). Difference in risk factors for postoperative nausea and vomiting. *Anesthesiology, 98,* 46–52.

Stamp Dawkins, M. (2003). Behaviour as a tool in the assessment of animal welfare. *Zoology (Jena), 106,* 383–387.

Stanghellini, V., Tosetti, C., & Paternico, A. (1996). Risk indicators of delayed gastric emptying of solids in patients with functional dyspepsia. *Gastroenterology, 110,* 1036–1045.

Stanney, K. M., Hale, K. S., Nahmens, I., & Kennedy, R. S. (2003). What to expect from immersive virtual environment exposure: Influence of gender, body mass index, and past experience. *Human Factors, 45,* 504–520.

Starling, E. H. (1905). Croonian Lecture: On the chemical correlation of the functions of the body. *Lancet, 2,* 339–341, 423–425, 501–503, 579–583.

Steinbrook, R. A. (2001). An opioid antagonist for postoperative ileus. *N Engl J Med, 345,* 988–989.

Steiner, J. E. (1973). The gustofacial response: Observation on normal and anencephalic newborn infants. In J. F. Bosma (Ed.), *Fourth Symposium on Oral Sensation and Perception: Development in the fetus and infant* (pp. 254–278). Bethesda, MD: U.S. Department of Health, Education, and Welfare.

Stephan, F. K., Smith, J. C., & Fisher, E. (1999). Profound conditioned taste aversion induced by oral consumption of 2-deoxy-D-glucose. *Physiol Behav, 68,* 221–226.

Stephan, T., Deutschlander, A., Nolte, A., Schneider, E., Wiesmann, M., Brandt, T., & Dieterich, M. (2005). Functional MRI of galvanic vestibular stimulation with alternating currents at different frequencies. *Neuroimage, 26,* 721–732.

Stern, R. M. (2002). The psychophysiology of nausea. *Acta Biologica Hungarica, 53,* 389–399.

Stern, R. M., Hu, S., Anderson, R. B., Leibowitz, H. W., & Koch, K. L. (1990). The effects of fixation and restricted visual field on vection-induced motion sickness. *Aviat Space Environ Med, 61,* 712–715.

Stern, R. M., Hu, S., LeBlanc, R., & Koch, K. L. (1993). Chinese hyper-susceptibility to vection-induced motion sickness. *Aviat Space Environ Med, 64,* 827–830.

Stern, R. M., Hu, S., Uijtdehaage, S. H. J., Muth, E. R., Xu, L. H., & Koch, K. L. (1996). Asian hypersusceptibility to motion sickness. *Human Heredity, 46,* 7–14.

Stern, R. M. Hu, S., Vasey, M. W., & Koch, K. L. (1989). Adaptation to vection-induced symptoms of motion sickness. *Aviat Space Environ Med, 60,* 566–571.

Stern, R. M., Jokerst, M. D., Levine, M. E., & Koch, K. L. (2001a). The stomach's response to unappetizing food: Cephalic-vagal effects on gastric myoelectric activity. *Neurogastroenterol Motil, 13,* 151–154.

Stern, R. M., Jokerst, M. D., Muth, E. R., & Hollis, C. (2001b). Acupressure relieves the symptoms of motion sickness and reduces abnormal gastric activity. *Altern Ther Health Med, 7,* 91–94.

Stern, R. M., & Koch, K. L. (1994). Using the electrogastrogram to study motion sickness. In J. Z. Chen & R. W. McCallum (Eds.), *Electrogastrography: Principles and applications* (pp. 199–218). New York: Raven Press Ltd.

Stern, R. M., & Koch, K. L. (2006) Understanding nausea. *Annales Academiae Medicae Silesiensis, 60,* 175182.

Stern, R. M., Koch, K. L., Leibowitz, H. W., Lindblad, I., Shupert, C., & Stewart, W. R. (1985). Tachygastria and motion sickness. *Aviat Space Environ Med, 56,* 1074–1077.

Stern, R. M., Koch, K. L., Stewart, W. R., & Lindblad, I. M. (1987a). Spectral analysis of tachygastria recorded during motion sickness. *Gastroenterology, 92,* 92–97.

Stern, R. M., Koch, K. L., Stewart, W. R., & Vasey, M. W. (1987b). Electrogastrography: Current issues in validation and methodology. *Psychophysiology, 24,* 55–64.

Stern, R. M., Ray, W. J., & Quigley, K. (2000). *Psychophysiological recording* (2nd ed.). New York: Oxford University Press.

Stern, R. M., Uijtdehaage, S. H., Muth, E. R., & Koch, K. L. (1994). Effects of phenytoin on vection-induced motion sickness and gastric myoelectric activity. *Aviat Space Environ Med, 65,* 518–521.

Stern, R. M., Vitellaro, K., Thomas, M., & Koch, K. L. (2004). Electrogastrographic biofeedback: A technique for enhancing normal gastric activity. *Neurogastroenterol Motil, 16,* 753–757.

Sternini, C. (2007). Taste receptors in the gastrointestinal tract: 4. Functional implications of bitter taste receptors in gastrointestinal chemosensing. *Am J Physiol Gastrointest Liver Physiol, 292,* G457–461.

Sternini, C., Wong, H., Pham, T., De Giorgio, R., Miller, L. J., Kuntz, S. M., Reeve, J. R., Walsh, J. H., & Raybould, H. E. (1999). Expression of cholecystokinin A receptors in neurons innervating the rat stomach and intestine. *Gastroenterology, 117,* 1136–1146.

Stewart, J. J., Wood, M. J., Wood, C. D., & Mims, M. E. (1991). Effects of ginger on motion sickness susceptibility and gastric function. *Pharmacology, 42,* 111–120.

Stockhorst, U., Enck, P., & Klosterhalfen, S. (2007). Role of classical conditioning in learning gastrointestinal symptoms. *World J Gastroenterol, 13,* 3430–3437.

Stockhorst, U., Klosterhalfen, S., & Steingrüber, H. J. (1998). Conditioned nausea and further side-effects in cancer chemotherapy: A review. *J Psychophysiol, 12*(Suppl. 1), 14–33.

Stockhorst, U., Spennes-Saleh, S., Körholz, D., Göbel, U., Schneider, M. E., Steingrüber, H.-J., & Klosterhalfen, S. (2000). Anticipatory symptoms and anticipatory immune responses in pediatric cancer patients receiving chemotherapy: Features of a classically conditioned response? *Brain Behav Immun, 14,* 198–218.

Stockhorst, U., Steingrüber, H.-J., Enck, P., & Klosterhalfen, S. (2006). Pavlovian conditioning of nausea and vomiting. *Auton Neurosci, 129,* 50–57.

Stockhorst, U., Wiener, J. A., Klosterhalfen, S., Klosterhalfen, W., Aul, C., & Steingrüber, H. J. (1998). Effects of overshadowing on conditioned nausea in cancer patients: An experimental study. *Physiol Behav, 64,* 743–753.

Stoddard, C. J., Smallwood, R., Brown, B. H., & Duthie, H. L. (1975). The immediate and delayed effects of different types of vagotomy on human gastric myoelectrical activity. *Gut, 16,* 165–170.

Stokes, T. (2006). The earth-eaters. *Nature, 444,* 543–544.

Stott, J. R. R. (1986). Mechanisms and treatment of motion illness. In C. B. Davis, G. V. Lake-Bakaar, & D. G. Grahame-Smith (Eds.), *Nausea and vomiting: Mechanisms and treatment* (pp. 110–129). Berlin: Springer-Verlag.

Stott, J. R. R. (1990). Adaptation to nauseogenic motion stimuli and its application in the treatment of airsickness. In G. H. Crampton (Ed.), *Motion and space sickness* (pp. 373–390). Boca Raton, FL: CRC Press.

Stricker, E. M., McCann, M. J., Flanagan, L. M., & Verbalis, J. G. (1988). Neurohypophyseal secretion and gastric function: Biological correlates of nausea. In H. Takagi, Y. Oomura, M. Ito, & M. Otsuka (Eds.), *Biowarning system in the brain: A Naito Foundation symposium* (pp. 295–307). Tokyo: University of Tokyo Press.

Suntharalingam, G., Perry, M. R., Ward, S., Brett, S. J., Castello-Cortes, A., Brunner, M. D., & Panoskaltsis, N. (2006). Cytokine storm in a phase 1 trial of the anti-CD28 monoclonal antibody TGN1412. *N Engl J Med, 355,* 1018–1028.

Suri, K. B., Crampton, G. H., & Daunton, N. G. (1979). Motion sickness in cats: A symptom rating scale used in laboratory and flight tests. *Aviat Space Environ Med, 50,* 614–618.

Symonds, M., & Hall, G. (1999). Overshadowing not potentiation of illness-based contextual conditioning by a novel taste. *Animal Learning and Behaviour, 27,* 379–390.

Symonds, M., & Hall, G. (2000). Contextual conditioning with an illness US is attenuated by the anti-emetic Ondansetron. *Psychobiology, 28,* 360–366.

Szurszewski, J. H. (1975). Mechanisms of action of pentagastrin and acetylcholine on the longitudinal muscle of the canine antrum. *J Physiol, 252,* 335–361.

Tack, J., Talley, N. J., Camilleri, M., Holtmann, G., Hu, P., Malagelada, J.-R., & Stanghellini, V. (2006). Functional gastrointestinal disorders. In D. A. Drossman (Ed.), *Rome III: The functional gastrointestinal disorders* (pp. 419–486). Lawrence, KS: Allen Press.

Takeda, N., Hasegawa, S., Morita, M., & Matsunaga, T. (1993a). Pica in rats is analogous to emesis: An animal model in emesis research. *Pharmacol Biochem Behav, 45,* 817–821.

Takeda, N., Hasegawa, S., Morita, M., Horii, A., Uno, A., Yamatodani, A., & Matsunaga, T. (1995a). Neuropharmacological mechanisms of emesis: 1. Effects of antiemetic drugs on motion- and apomorphine-induced pica in rats. *Methods Find Exp Clin Pharmacol, 17,* 589–590.

Takeda, N., Hasegawa, S., Morita, M., Horii, A., Uno, A., Yamatodani, A., & Matsunaga, T. (1995b). Neuropharmacological mechanisms of emesis: 2. Effects of antiemetic drugs on cisplatin-induced pica in rats. *Methods Find Exp Clin Pharmacol, 17,* 647–652.

Takeda, N., Morita, M., Hasegawa, S., Horii, A., Kubo, T., & Matsunaga, T. (1993b). Neuropharmacology of motion sickness and emesis. A review. *Acta Otolaryngol Suppl, 501,* 10–15.

Takeda, N., Morita, M., Kubo, T., Yamatodani, A., Watanabe, T., Wada, H., & Matsunaga, T. (1986). Histaminergic mechanism of motion sickness: Neurochemical and neuropharmacological studies in rats. *Acta Otolaryngol, 101,* 416–421.

Talley, N. J. (2003). Diabetic gastropathy and prokinetics. *Am J Gastroenterol, 98,* 264–271.

Talley, N. J., Camilleri, M., Burton, D., Thomforde, G., Koch, K., Rucker, M. J., Peterson, J., Zinsmeister, A. R., & Earnest, D. L. (2006). Double-blind placebo-controlled study to evaluate the effects of tegaserod on gastric motor, sensory, and myoelectrical function in healthy volunteers. *Aliment Pharmacol Ther, 24,* 859–867.

Talley, N. J., Phillips, S. F., Haddad, A., Miller, L. J., Twomey, C., Zinsmeister, A. R., & Ciociola, A. (1989). Effect of selective 5HT3 antagonist (GR 38032F) on small intestinal transit and release of gastrointestinal peptides. *Dig Dis Sci, 34,* 1511–1515.

Talley, N. J., Young, J., Bytzer, P., Hammer, J., Leemon, M., Jones, M., & Horowitz, M. (2001). Impact of gastrointestinal symptoms in diabetes mellitus on health-related quality of life. *Am J Gastroenterol, 96,* 71–76.

Tanihata, S., Igarashi, H., Suzuki, M., & Uchiyama, T. (2000). Cisplatin-induced early and delayed emesis in the pigeon. *Br J Pharmacol, 130,* 132–138.

Tatewaki, M., Strickland, C., Fukuda, H., Tsuchida, D., Hoshino, E., Pappas, T. N., & Takahashi, T. (2005). Effects of acupuncture on vasopressin-induced emesis in conscious dogs. *Am J Physiol Regul Integr Comp Physiol, 288,* R401–408.

Tattersall, F. D., Rycroft, W., Cumberbatch, M., Mason, G., Tye, S., Williamson, D. J., Hale, J. J., Mills, S. G., Finke, P. E., MacCoss, M., Sadowski, S., Ber, E., Cascieri, M., Hill, R. G., MacIntyre, D. E., & Hargreaves, R. J. (2000). The novel NK_1 receptor antagonist MK-0869 (L-754,030) and its water soluble phosphoryl prodrug, L-758,298, inhibit acute and delayed cisplatin-induced emesis in ferrets. *Neuropharmacology, 39,* 652–663.

Tattersall, F. D., Rycroft, W., Francis, B., Pearce, D., Merchant, K., MacLeod, A. M., Ladduwahetty, T., Keown, L., Swain, C., Baker, R., Cascieri, M., Ber, E., Metzger, J., MacIntyre, D. E., Hill, R. G. and Hargreaves, R. J. (1996). Tachykinin NK_1 receptor antagonists act centrally to inhibit emesis induced by the chemotherapeutic agent cisplatin in ferrets. *Neuropharmacology, 35,* 1121–1129.

Tattersall, F. D., Rycroft, W., Marmont, N., Cascieri, M., Hill, R. G., & Hargreaves, R. J. (1995). Enantiospecific inhibition of emesis induced by nicotine in the house musk shrew (Suncus murinus) by the neurokinin 1 (NK_1) receptor antagonist CP-99,994. *Neuropharmacology, 34,* 1697–1699.

Taylor, I. L., Byrne, W. J., Christie, D. L., Ament, M. E., & Walsh, J. H. (1982). Effect of individual L-amino acids on gastric acid secretion and serum gastrin and pancreatic polypeptide release in humans. *Gastroenterology, 83,* 272–278.

Taylor, N. B., Hunter, J., & Johnson, W. H. (1957). Antidiuresis as a measurement of laboratory induced motion sickness. *Can J Biochem Physiol, 35,* 1017–1027.

Taylor R. (1996). Successful management of hyperemesis gravidarum using steroid therapy. *Quart J Med, 89,* 103–107.

Temkin, O. (1956). *Soranus' gynecology.* Baltimore: The Johns Hopkins University Press.

Teng, N. (2000). Oncology. In R. H. Blum, W. L. Heinrichs, & A. Herxheimer (Eds.), *Nausea and vomiting* (pp. 437–451). London: Whurr.

Terry-Nathan, V. R., Gietzen, D. W., & Rogers, Q. R. (1995). Serotonin3 antagonists block aversion to saccharin in an amino acid-imbalanced diet. *Am J Physiol Regul Integr Comp Physiol, 268,* R1203–1208.

Thomas, C. (2000). The economic impact of nausea and vomiting. In R. H. Blum, W. L. Heinrichs, & A. Herxheimer (Eds.), *Nausea and vomiting* (pp. 190–206). London: Whurr.

Thomas, M., Woodhead, G., Masood, N., & Howard, R. (2007). Motion sickness as a predictor of postoperative vomiting in children aged 1–15. *Paediat Anaesth, 17,* 61–63.

Thomford, N. R., & Sirinek, K. R. (1975). Intravenous vasopressin in patients with portal hypertension: Advantages of continuous infusion. *J Surg Res, 18,* 113–117.

Thompson, D. G., & Malagelada, J. R. (1982). Vomiting and the small intestine. *Dig Dis Sci, 27,* 1121–1125.

Thompson, P. I., Bingham, S., Andrews, P. L. R., Patel, N., Joel, S. P., & Slevin, M. L. (1992). Morphine 6-glucuronide: A metabolite of morphine with greater emetic potency than morphine in the ferret. *Br J Pharmacol, 106,* 3–8.

Thompson, R. G., Gottlieb, A., Organ, K., Koda, J., Kisicki, J., & Kolterman, O. G. (1997). Pramlintide: A human amylin analogue reduced postprandial plasma glucose, insulin, and C-peptide concentrations in patients with type 2 diabetes. *Diabet Med, 14,* 547–555.

Thornton, W. E., Moore, T. P., Pool, S. L., & Vanderploeg, J. (1987). Clinical characterization and etiology of space motion sickness. *Aviat Space Environ Med, 58,* 1–8.

Tiersch, T. R., & Griffith, J. S. (1988). Apomorphine-induced vomiting in rainbow trout (Salmo gairdneri). *Comp Biochem Physiol A Comp Physiol, 91,* 721–725.

Tierson, F. D., Olsen, C. L., & Hook, E. B. (1986). Nausea and vomiting of pregnancy and association with pregnancy outcome. *Am J Obstet Gynecol, 155,* 1017–1022.

Tinbergen, N. (1963). On aims and methods of ethology. *Zeitschrift für Thierpsychologie, 20,* 410–433.

Tonato, M. (1994). Antiemetics in cancer chemotherapy: Historical perspective and current state of the art. *Support Care Cancer, 2,* 150–160.

Tonato, M., Roila, F., & Del Favero, A. (1993). Nausea in anti-cancer therapy: Measurement and mechanisms. In P. L. R. Andrews & G. J. Sanger (Eds.), *Emesis in anti-cancer therapy: Mechanism and treatment* (pp. 61–70). London: Chapman and Hall Medical.

Toorop, R. J., Scheltinga, M. R., Huige, M. C., & Luirink, M. R. (2007). Excessive vomiting abolished by carotid denervation. *Auton Neurosci, 133,* 175–177.

Torii, Y., Saito, H., & Matsuki, N. (1991). 5-Hydroxytryptamine is emetogenic in the house musk shrew, Suncus murinus. *Naunyn Schmiedebergs Arch Pharmacol, 344,* 564–567.

Torii, Y., Shikita, M., Saito, H., & Matsuki, N. (1993). X-irradiation-induced emesis in Suncus murinus. *J Radiat Res (Tokyo), 34,* 164–170.

Tougas, G., Eaker, E. Y., Abell, T. L., Abrahamsson, H., Boivin, M., Chen, J., Hocking, M. P., Quigley, E. M., Koch, K. L., Tokayer, A. Z., Stanghellini, V., Chen, Y., Huizinga, J. D., Rydén, J., Bourgeois, I., & McCallum, R. W. (2000). Assessment of gastric emptying using a low fat meal: Establishment of international control values. *Am J Gastroenterol, 95,* 1456–1462.

Travagli, R. A., Hermann, G. E., Browning, K. N., & Rogers, R. C. (2006). Brainstem circuits regulating gastric function. *Ann Rev Physiol, 68,* 279–305.

Travers, J. B., & Norgren, R. (1986). Electromyographic analysis of the ingestion and rejection of sapid stimuli in the rat. *Behav Neurosci, 100,* 544–555.

Travers, S. P., & Travers, J. B. (2005). Reflex topography in the nucleus tractus solitarius. *Chem Senses, 30*(Suppl. 1), i180–i181.

Treisman, M. (1977). Motion sickness: An evolutionary hypothesis. *Science, 197,* 493–495.

Tremblay, P. B., Kaiser, R., Sezer, O., Rosler, N., Schlenz, C., Possinger, K., Roots, I., & Brockmoller, J. (2003). Variations in the 5-hydroxytryptamine type 3B receptor gene as predicters of the efficacy of antiemetic treatment in cancer patients. *J Clin Oncol, 21,* 2147–2155.

Tribollet, E., Barberis, C., Dreifuss, J. J., & Jard, S. (1988). Autoradiographic localization of vasopressin and oxytocin binding sites in rat kidney. *Kidney Int, 33,* 959–965.

Tsuchiya, M., Fujiwara, Y., Kanai, Y., Mizutani, M., Shimada, K., Suga, O., Ueda, S., Watson, J.W. and Nagahisa, A. (2002). Anti-emetic activity of the novel nonpeptide tachykinin NK_1 receptor antagonist ezlopitant (CJ-11,974) against acute and delayed cisplatin-induced emesis in the ferret. *Pharmacology, 66,* 144–152.

Tucci, S., Rada, P., & Hernandez, L. (1998). Role of glutamate in the amygdala and lateral hypothalamus in conditioned taste aversion. *Brain Res, 813,* 44–49.

Tung, C. F., Chang, C. S., Chen, G. H., Kao, C. H., & Wang, S. J. (1997). Comprehensive gastric emptying study for type-II diabetes mellitus dyspeptic patients. *Scand J Gastroenterol, 32,* 884–887.

Tuor, U. I., Kondysar, M. H., & Harding, R. K. (1988). Emesis, radiation exposure, and local cerebral blood flow in the ferret. *Radiat Res, 114,* 537–549.

Turgut, S., Ozalp, G., Dikmen, S., Savli, S., Tuncel, G., & Kaioggullari, N. (2007). Acupressure for postoperative nausea and vomiting in gynaecological patients receiving patient-controlled analgesia. *Eur J Anaesthesiol, 24,* 87–91.

Turner, M., & Griffin, M. J. (1999). Motion sickness in public road transport: Passenger behavior and susceptibility. *Ergonomics, 42,* 444–461.

Tye, V. L., Mulhern, R. K., Barclay, D. R., Smith, B. F., & Bieberich, A. A. (1997). Variables associated with anticipatory nausea and vomiting in pediatric cancer patients receiving ondansetron antiemetic therapy. *J Pediat Psychol, 22,* 45–58.

Tyler, D. B. (1946). The influence of placebo, body position, and medication on motion sickness. *Amer J Physiol, 146,* 458–466.

Uchino, M., Kuwahara, M., Ebukuro, S., & Tsubone, H. (2006). Modulation of emetic response by carotid baro- and chemoreceptor activations. *Auton Neurosci, 128,* 25–36.

Ueno, N., Inui, A., Asakawa, A., Takao, F., Tani, S., Komatsu, Y., Itoh, Z., & Kasuga, M. (2000). Erythromycin improves glycemic control in patients with Type II diabetes mellitus. *Diabetologia, 43,* 411–415.

Ueno, S., Matsuki, N., & Saito, H. (1987). Suncus murinus: A new experimental model in emesis research. *Life Sci, 41,* 513–518.

Ueno, S., Matsuki, N., & Saito, H. (1988). Suncus murinus as a new experimental model for motion sickness. *Life Sci, 43,* 413–420.

Uijtdehaage, S. H. J., Stern, R. M., & Koch, K. L. (1992). Effects of eating on vection-induced motion sickness, cardiac vagal tone, and gastric myoelectrical activity. *Psychophysiology, 29,* 193–201.

Uijtdehaage, S. H. J., Stern, R. M., & Koch, K. L. (1993). Effects of scopolamine on autonomic profiles underlying motion sickness susceptibility. *Aviat Space Environ Med, 64,* 1–8.

Unno, T., Hashimoto, M., Arai, S., & Kurosawa, M. (2002). Reduction of food intake following X-ray irradiation of rats: Involvement of visceral afferent nerves. *Auton Neurosci, 96,* 119–125.

Van Belle, S., Lichinitser, M. R., Navari, R. M., Garin, A. M., Decramer, M. L., Riviere, A., Thant, M., Brestan, E., Bui, B., Eldridge, K., De Smet, M., Michiels, N., Reinhardt, R.R., Carides, A.D., Evans, J.K. and Gertz, B.J. (2002). Prevention of cisplatin-induced acute and delayed emesis by the selective neurokinin-1 antagonists, L-758,298 and MK-869. *Cancer, 94,* 3032–3041.

van der Kooy, D., Koda, L. Y., McGinty, J. F., Gerfen, C. R., & Bloom, F. E. (1984). The organization of projections from the cortex, amygdala, and hypothalamus to the nucleus of the solitary tract in rat. *J Comp Neurol, 224,* 1–24.

van der Kooy, D., Swerdlow, N. R., & Koob, G. F. (1983). Paradoxical reinforcing properties of apomorphine: Effects of nucleus accumbens and area postrema lesions. *Brain Res, 259,* 111–118.

van der Voort, I. R., Becker, J. C., Dietl, K. H., Konturek, J. W., Domschke, W., & Pohle, T. (2005). Gastric electrical stimulation results in improved metabolic control in diabetic patients suffering from gastroparesis. *Exp Clin Endocrinol Diabetes, 113,* 38–42.

Van Lawick-Goodall, H., & Van Lawick-Goodall, J. (1970). *Innocent killers.* London: Collins.

Van Oudenhove, L., Coen, S. J., & Aziz, Q. (2007). Functional brain imaging of gastro-intestinal sensation in health and disease. *World J Gastroenterol, 13,* 3438–3445.

Van Sickle, M. D., Oland, L. D., Ho, W., Hillard, C. J., Mackie, K., Davison, J. S., & Sharkey, K. A. (2001). Cannabinoids inhibit emesis through CB1 receptors in the brainstem of the ferret. *Gastroenterology, 121,* 767–774.

Van Sickle, M. D., Oland, L. D., Mackie, K., Davison, J. S., & Sharkey, K. A. (2003). Delta9-tetrahydrocannabinol selectively acts on CB1 receptors in specific regions of dorsal vagal complex to inhibit emesis in ferrets. *Am J Physiol Gastrointest Liver Physiol, 285,* G566–576.

Van Thiel, D. H., Gavaler, J. S., Joshi, S. N., Sara, R. K., & Stremple, J. (1977). Heartburn of pregnancy. *Gastroenterology, 72,* 666–668.

Van Thiel, D. H., Gavaler, J. S., & Stremple, K. K. (1976). Lower esophageal pressure in women using sequential oral contraceptives. *Gastroenterology, 71,* 232–234.

Vandenbergh, J., Dupont, P., Fischler, B., Bormans, G., Persoons, P., Janssens, J., & Tack, J. (2005). Regional brain activation during proximal stomach distention in humans: A positron emission tomography study. *Gastroenterology, 128,* 564–573.

Vavilova, N. M., & Kassil, V. G. (1984). Conditioned reflex taste aversion during dog ontogeny. *Zh Vyssh Nerv Deiat Im I P Pavlova, 34,* 662–668.

Vera, G., Chiarlone, A., Martin, M. I., & Abalo, R. (2006). Altered feeding behaviour induced by long-term cisplatin in rats. *Auton Neurosci, 126,* 81–92.

Verbalis, J. G., McCann, M. J., McHale, C. M., & Stricker, E. M. (1986a). Oxytocin secretion in response to cholecystokinin and food: Differentiation of nausea from satiety. *Science, 232,* 1417–1419.

Verbalis, J. G., McHale, C. M., Gardiner, T. W., & Stricker, E. M. (1986b). Oxytocin and vasopressin secretion in response to stimuli producing learned taste aversions in rats. *Behav Neurosci, 100,* 466–475.

Verbalis, J. G., Richardson, D. W., & Stricker, E. M. (1987). Vasopressin release in response to nausea-producing agents and cholecystokinin in monkeys. *Am J Physiol Regul Integr Comp Physiol, 252,* R749–753.

Vig, M. M. (1990). Nicotine poisoning in a dog. *Vet Hum Toxicol, 32,* 573–575.

Villablanca, J. R., Harris, C. M., Burgess, J. W., & de Andres, I. (1984). Reassessing morphine effects in cats: 1. Specific behavioral responses in intact and unilaterally brain-lesioned animals. *Pharmacol Biochem Behav, 21,* 913–921.

Walsh, J. W., Hasler, W. L., Nugent, C. E., & Owyang, C. (1996). Progesterone and estrogen are potential mediators of gastric slow wave dysrhythmias in nausea of pregnancy. *Am J Physiol Gastrointest Liver Physio, 270,* G506–514.

Walton, J., Beeson, P. B., & Bodley Scott, R. (Eds.). (1986). *The Oxford companion to medicine* (Vol. 2). Oxford: Oxford University Press.

Wang, S. C., & Glaviano, V. V. (1954). Locus of emetic action of morphine and hydergine in dogs. *J Pharmacol Exp Ther, 111,* 329–334.

Warwick-Evans, L. A., Masters, I. J., & Redstone, S. B. (1991). A double-blind placebo controlled evaluation of acupressure in the treatment of motion sickness. *Aviat Space Environ Med, 62,* 776–778.

Watcha, M. F., & Smith, I. (1994). Cost-effectiveness analysis of anti-emetic therapy for ambulatory surgery. *J Clin Anesthesiol, 6,* 370–377.

Watcha, M. F., & White, P. F. (1992). Postoperative nausea and vomiting: Its etiology, treatment, and prevention. *Anesthesiology, 77,* 162–184.

Watson, M., McCarron, J., & Law, M. (1992). Anticipatory nausea and emesis, and psychological morbidity: Assessment of prevalence among out-patients on mild to moderate chemotherapy regimens. *Brit J Cancer, 66,* 862–866.

Watson, P. J., Hawkins, C., McKinney, J., Beatey, S., Bartles, R. R., & Rhea, K. (1987). Inhibited drinking and pica in rats following 2-deoxy-D-glucose. *Physiol Behav, 39,* 745–752.

Wegener, M., Borsch, G., Schaffstein, J., Luerweg, C., & Leverkus, F. (1990). Gastrointestinal transit in patients with insulin-treated diabetes mellitus. *Digestive Dis, 8,* 23–26.

Weigel, M. M., Reyes, M., Caiza, M. E., Tello, N., Castro, N. P., Cespedes, S., Duchicela, S., & Betancourt, M. (2006). Is the nausea and vomiting of early pregnancy really feto-protective? *J Perinat Med, 34,* 115–122.

Weigel, M. M., & Weigel, R. M. (1989). Nausea and vomiting of early pregnancy and pregnancy outcome: An epidemiological study. *Br J Obstet Gynaecol, 96,* 1304–1311.

Weigel, R. M., & Weigel, M. M. (1989). Nausea and vomiting of early pregnancy and pregnancy outcome: A meta-analytical review. *Br J Obstet Gynecol, 96,* 1312–1318.

Weinstein, S. E., & Stern, R. M. (1997). Comparison of Marezine and Dramamine in preventing symptoms of motion sickness. *Aviat Space Environ Med, 68,* 890–894.

Welzl, H., D'Adamo, P., & Lipp, H. P. (2001). Conditioned taste aversion as a learning and memory paradigm. *Behav Brain Res, 125,* 205–213.

Werntoft, E., & Dykes, A. K. (2001). Effect of acupressure on nausea and vomiting during pregnancy: A randomized, placebo-controlled pilot study. *J Reprod Med, 46,* 835–839.

Westman, H. R. (1999). Post-operative complications and unanticipated hospital admissions. *Semin Pediatr Surg, 8,* 23–29.

Weytjens, C., Keymeulen, B., Van Haleweyn, C., Somers, G., & Bossuyt, A. (1998). Rapid gastric emptying of a liquid meal in long-term Type 2 diabetes mellitus. *Diabet Med, 15,* 1022–1027.

White, P. F. (2004). Prevention of postoperative nausea and vomiting: A multimodal solution to a persistent problem. *N Engl J Med, 350,* 2511–2512.

White, P. F., & Shafer, A. (1988). Nausea and vomiting: Causes and prophylaxis. *Seminar in anesthesia, 6,* 300–308.

White, P. F., & Watcha, M. E. (1999). Postoperative nausea and vomiting: Prophylaxis versus treatment. *Anesth Analg, 89,* 1337–1339.

Whitehead, S. A., Andrews, P. L. R., & Chamberlain, G. V. P. (1992). Characterisation of nausea and vomiting in early pregnancy: A survey of 1000 women. *J Obstet Gynaecol, 12,* 364–369.

Whitehead, S. A., Holden, W. A., & Andrews, P. L. R. (1992). Pregnancy sickness. In A. L. Bianchi, L. Grelot, A. D. Miller, & G. L. King (Eds.), *Mechanisms and control of emesis* (pp. 297–306). Eastleigh, UK: John Libbey Publishing.

WHO (2009). Diabetes fact sheet. Retrieved May 15, 2009, from http://www.who.int/mediacentre/factsheets/fs312/en/index.html

Wickham, R. (1999). Nausea and vomiting. In C. H. Yarbo, M. H. Frogge, & M. Goodman (Eds.), *Cancer symptom management* (2nd ed., pp. 228–263). Boston: Jones and Bartlett.

Wilhelm, S. M., Dehoorne-Smith, M. L., & Kale-Pradhan, P. B. (2007). Prevention of postoperative nausea and vomiting. *Ann Pharmacother, 41,* 68–78.

Wilkens, E. P., & Yates, B. J. (2005). Pretreatment with ondansetron blunts plasma vasopressin increases associated with morphine administration in ferrets. *Anesth Analg, 101,* 1029–1033.

Willems, J. L., & Lefebvre, R. A. (1986). Peripheral nervous pathways involved in nausea and vomiting. In C. J. Davis, G. V. Lake-Bakaar, & D. G. Grahame-Smith (Eds.), *Nausea and vomiting: Mechanisms and treatment* (pp. 56–64). Berlin: Springer-Verlag.

Willett, C. J., Rutherford, J. G., Gwyn, D. G., & Leslie, R. A. (1987). Projections between the hypothalamus and the dorsal vagal complex in the cat: An HRP and autoradiographic study. *Brain Res Bull, 18,* 63–71.

Williamson, M. J., Higgins, S. C., & Stern, R. M. (2003). Factors that predict number of sessions to adapt to a rotating drum, retention, and transfer to carsickness [Abstract]. *Neurogastroenterol Motil, 15,* 348.

Williamson, M. J., Levine, M. E., & Stern, R. M. (2005). The effects of meals of varying nutritional composition on subjective and physiological markers of nausea in response to optokinetic motion. *Digestion, 72,* 254–260.

Willms, B., Werner, J., Holst, J. J., Orskov, C., Creutzfeldt, W., & Nauck, M. A. (1996). Gastric emptying, glucose responses, and insulin secretion after a liquid test meal: Effects of exogenous glucagon-like peptide-1 (GLP-1)-(7-36) amide in type 2 (noninsulin-dependent) diabetic patients. *J Clin Endocrinol Metab, 81,* 327–332.

Wilm, S., & Helmert, U. (2006). The prevalence of fullness, heartburn, and nausea among persons with or without diabetes mellitus. *Z Gastroenterol, 44,* 373–377.

Wilpizeski, C. R., Lowry, L. D., El Raheb, M., Eyyunni, U., Contrucci, R. B., & Goldman, W. S. (1985). Experimental motion sickness induced in squirrel monkeys by continuous off-axis horizontal rotation. *Am J Otolaryngol, 6,* 1–22.

Wilpizeski, C. R., Lowry, L. D., Green, S. J., Smith, B. D., Jr., & Melnick, H. (1987). Subjective concomitants of motion sickness: Quantifying rotation-induced illness in squirrel monkeys. *Otolaryngol Head Neck Surg, 97,* 433–440.

Winbery, S. L., & Blaho, K. E. (2001). Dyspepsia in pregnancy. *Obstet Gynecol Clin N Am, 28,* 333–350.

Wiseman-Orr, M. L., Nolan, A. M., Reid, J., & Scott, E. M. (2004). Development of a questionnaire to measure the effects of chronic pain on health-related quality of life in dogs. *Am J Vet Res, 65,* 1077–84.

Wiseman-Orr, M. L., Scott, E. M., Reid, J., & Nolan, A. M. (2006). Validation of a structured questionnaire as an instrument to measure chronic pain in dogs on the basis of effects on health-related quality of life. *Am J Vet Res, 67,* 1826–1836.

Wolf, S. (1943). The relation of gastric function to nausea in man. *J Clin Invest, 22,* 877–882.

Wolf, S. (1949). Studies on nausea: Effects of ipecac and other emetics on the human stomach and duodenum. *Gastroenterology, 12,* 212–218.

Wolf, S. (1965). *The stomach.* New York: Oxford University Press.

Wolf, S., & Wolff, H. G. (1948). *Human gastric function.* New York: Oxford University Press.

Wood, C. D. (1990). Pharmacological countermeasures against motion sickness. In G. H. Crampton (Ed.), *Motion and space sickness* (pp. 343–352). Boca Raton, FL: CRC Press.

Wood, J. R., Camilleri, M., Low, P. A., & Malagelada, J. R. (1985). Brainstem tumor presenting as an upper gut motility disorder. *Gastroenterology, 89,* 1411–1414.

Woods, S. C., Figlewicz, D. P., Madden, L., Porte, D., Jr., Sipols, A. J., & Seeley, R. J. (1998). NPY and food intake: Discrepancies in the model. *Regul Pept, 75–76,* 403–408.

Wooten, R. L., & Meriwether, T. W., 3rd (1961). Diabetic gastric atony: A clinical study. *JAMA, 176,* 1082–1087.

Wotjak, C. T., Kubota, M., Liebsch, G., Montkowski, A., Holsboer, F., Neumann, I., & Landgraf, R. (1996). Release of vasopressin within the rat paraventricular nucleus in response to emotional stress: A novel mechanism of regulating adrenocorticotropic hormone secretion? *J Neurosci, 16,* 7725–7732.

Wu, C-Y., Tseng, J-J., Chou, M-M, Lin, S-K., Poon, S-K., & Chen, G-H. (2000). Correlation between *Helicobacter pylori* infection and gastrointestinal symptoms in pregnancy. *Advan Ther, 17,* 152–158.

Wu, M., Harding, R. K., Hugenholtz, H., & Kucharczyk, J. (1985). Emetic effects of centrally administered angiotensin II, arginine vasopressin, and neurotensin in the dog. *Peptides, 6*(Suppl. 1), 173–175.

Wu, Q., Zhao, Z., & Shen, P. (2005). Regulation of aversion to noxious food by Drosophila neuropeptide Y- and insulin-like systems. *Nat Neurosci, 8,* 1350–1355.

Xing, J., Qian, L., & Chen, J. (2006). Experimental gastric dysrhythmias and its correlation with in vivo gastric muscle contractions. *World J Gastroenterol, 12,* 3994–3998.

Xu, L. H., Koch, K. L., Summy-Long, J., Stern, R. M., Seaton, J. F., Harrison, T. S., Demers, L. M., & Bingaman, S. (1993). Hypothalamic and gastric myoelectrical responses during vection-induced nausea in healthy Chinese subjects. *Am J Physiol, 265,* E578–584.

Xu, X., Brining, D. L., & Chen, J. D. (2005). Effects of vasopressin and long pulse-low frequency gastric electrical stimulation on gastric emptying, gastric and intestinal myoelectrical activity and symptoms in dogs. *Neurogastroenterol Motil, 17,* 236–244.

Xu, X., Pasricha, P. J., & Chen, J. D. (2007). Feasibility of gastric electrical stimulation by use of endoscopically placed electrodes. *Gastrointest Endosc, 66,* 981–986.

Yamamoto, K., Asano, K., Matsukawa, N., Imaizumi, M., & Yamatodani, A. (2010). Time-course analysis of pica in rats using an automatic feeding monitoring system. *J Pharmacol Toxicol Meth,* in press.

Yamamoto, K., Matsunaga, S., Matsui, M., Takeda, N., & Yamatodani, A. (2002). Pica in mice as a new model for the study of emesis. *Methods Find Exp Clin Pharmacol, 24,* 135–138.

Yamamoto, K., Nakai, M., Nohara, K., & Yamatodani, A. (2007). The anti-cancer drug-induced pica in rats is related to their clinical emetogenic potential. *Eur J Pharmacol, 554,* 34–39.

Yamamoto, K., Ngan, M. P., Takeda, N., Yamatodani, A., & Rudd, J. A. (2004). Differential activity of drugs to induce emesis and pica behavior in Suncus murinus (house musk shrew) and rats. *Physiol Behav, 83,* 151–156.

Yamamoto, K., Nohara, K., Furuya, T., & Yamatodani, A. (2005). Ondansetron, dexamethasone, and an NK_1 antagonist block radiation sickness in mice. *Pharmacol Biochem Behav, 82,* 24–29.

Yamamoto, K., Takeda, N., & Yamatodani, A. (2002). Establishment of an animal model for radiation-induced vomiting in rats using pica. *J Radiat Res (Tokyo), 43,* 135–141.

Yamamoto, T., Suzuki, Y., Kojima, K., Sato, T., Tanemura, M., Kaji, M., Yamakawa, Y., Yokoi, M., & Suzumori K. (2001). Pneumomediastinum secondary to hyperemesis gravidarum during early pregnancy. *Acta Obstet Gynecol Scand, 80,* 1143–1145.

Yates, B. J., Grelot, L., Kerman, I. A., Balaban, C. D., Jakus, J., & Miller, A. D. (1994). Organization of vestibular inputs to nucleus tractus solitarius and adjacent structures in cat brain stem. *Am J Physiol Regul Integr Comp Physiol, 267,* R974–983.

Yates, B. J., Miller, A. D., & Lucot, J. B. (1998). Physiological basis and pharmacology of motion sickness: An update. *Brain Res Bull, 47,* 395–406.

Yen Pik Sang, F. D., Billar, J. P., Golding, J. F., & Gresty, M. A. (2003). Behavioral methods of alleviating motion sickness: Effectiveness of controlled breathing and a music audiotape. *J Travel Med, 10,* 108–111.

Yen Pik Sang, F., Billar, J., Gresty, M. A., & Golding, J. F. (2005). Effects of a novel motion desensitization training regime and controlled breathing on habituation to motion sickness. *Perceptual and Motor Skills, 1001,* 244–256.

Yen Pik Sang, F. D., Golding, J. F., & Gresty, M. A. (2003). Suppression of sickness by controlled breathing during mildly nauseogenic motion. *Aviat Space Eviron Med, 74,* 998–1002.

Yeshrun, Y., Lapid, H., Doudai, Y., & Sobel, N. (2009). The privileged brain representation of first olfactory associations. *Curr Biol, 19,* 1869–1874.

Yoo, H. J., Ahn, S. H., Kim, S. B., Kim, W. K., & Han, O. S. (2005). Efficacy of progressive muscle relaxation training and guided imagery in reducing chemotherapy side effects in patients with breast cancer and in improving quality of life. *Support Care Cancer, 13,* 826–833.

Yoshida, M. M., Schuffler, M. D., & Sumi, S. M. (1988). There are no morphologic abnormalities of the gastric wall or abdominal vagus in patients with diabetic gastroparesis. *Gastroenterology, 94,* 907–914.

Yoshikawa, T., Yoshida, N., & Oka, M. (2001). Central antiemetic effects of AS-8112, a dopamine D2, D3, and 5-HT(3) receptor antagonist, in ferrets. *Eur J Pharmacol, 431,* 361–364.

You, C. H., & Chey, W. Y. (1984). Study of electromechanical activity of the stomach in humans and in dogs with particular attention to tachygastria. *Gastroenterology, 86,* 1460–1468.

You, C. H., Chey, W. Y., Lee, K. Y., Menguy, R., & Bortoff, A. (1981). Gastric and small intestinal myoelectrical dysrhythmia associated with chronic intractable nausea and vomiting. *Ann Intern Med, 95,* 449–451.

Yu, X., Yang, J., Hou, X., Zhang, K., Qian, W., & Chen, J. D. Z. (2009). Cisplatin-induced gastric dysrhythmia and emesis in dogs and possible role of gastric electrical stimulation. *Dig Dis Sci, 54,* 922–927.

Yung, C. (1984). A review of clinical trials of lithium in medicine. *Pharmacol Biochem Behav, 21,* 51–55.

Zabara, J., Chaffee, R. B., Jr., & Tansy, M. F. (1972). Neuroinhibition in the regulation of emesis. *Space Life Sci, 3,* 282–292.

Zachariae, R., Paulsen, K., Mehlsen, M., Jensen, A. B., Johansson, A., & von der Maase, H. (2007). Anticipatory nausea: The role of individual differences related to sensory perception and autonomic reactivity. *Ann Behav Med, 33,* 69–79.

Zaman, S., Woods, A. J., Watson, J. W., Reynolds, D. J., & Andrews, P. L. R. (2000). The effect of the NK1 receptor antagonist CP-99,994 on emesis and c-fos protein induction by loperamide in the ferret. *Neuropharmacology, 39,* 316–323.

Zelano, C., Montag, J., Johnson, B., Khan, R., & Sobel, N. (2007). Dissociated representations of irritation and valence in human primary olfactory cortex. *J Neurophysiol, 97,* 1969–1976.

Zerbe, R. I. (1985). Genetic factors in normal and abnormal regulation of vasopressin secretion. In R. W. Schrier (Ed.), *Vasopressin* (pp. 213–220). New York: Raven Press.

Zhang, Y., Lu, H., & Bargmann, C. I. (2005). Pathogenic bacteria induce aversive olfactory learning in Caenorhabditis elegans. *Nature, 438,* 179–184.

Zhao, J., Frokjaer, J. B., Drewes, A. M., & Ejskjaer, N. (2006). Upper gastrointestinal sensory-motor dysfunction in diabetes mellitus. *World J Gastroenterol, 12,* 2846–2857.

Zhu, H., Sallam, H., Chen, D. D., & Chen, J. D. (2007). Therapeutic potential of synchronized electrical stimulation for gastroparesis: enhanced motility in dogs. *Am J Physiol, 293,* R1875–1881.

Zhu, J. X., Zhu, X. Y., Owyang, C., & Li, Y. (2001). Intestinal serotonin acts as a para-crine substance to mediate vagal signal transmission evoked by luminal factors in the rat. *J Physiol, 530,* 431–442.

Zhu, Y. R., Cowles, V. E., Herranz, E. S., Schulte, W. J., & Condon, R. E. (1992). Arginine vasopressin inhibits phasic contractions and stimulates giant contractions in monkey colon. *Gasteroenterology, 102,* 868–874.

Ziavra, N. V., Yen Pik Sang, F. D., Golding, J. F., Bronstein, A. M., & Gresty, M. A. (2003). Effect of breathing supplemental oxygen on motion sickness in healthy adults. *Mayo Clin Proc, 78,* 574–578.

Zick, S. M., Ruffin, M. T., Lee, J., Normolle, D. P., Siden, R., Alrawi, S., & Brenner, D. E. (2009). Phase II trial of encapsulated ginger as a treatment for chemotherapy-induced nausea and vomiting. *Support Care Cancer, 17,* 563–572.

Ziegler, D., Schadewaldt, P., Pour Mirza, A., Piolot, R., Schommartz, B., Reinhardt, M., Vosberg, H., Brösicke, H., & Gries, F. A. (1996). [13C]octanoic acid breath test for non-invasive assessment of gastric emptying in diabetic patients: Validation and relationship to gastric symptoms and cardiovascular autonomic function. *Diabetologia, 39,* 823–830.

Author Index

Note: Page references followed by "*f*" and "*t*" denote figures and tables, respectively.

Subject Index

Note: Page numbers followed by "*f*" and "*t*" denote figures and tables, respectively.